ISBN 978-0-7624-4589-9
Library of Congress Control Number: 2011944643

E-book ISBN 978-0-7624-4590-5

9   8   7   6   5   4   3
Digit on the right indicates the number of this printing

Cover and interior design by Susan Van Horn
Edited by Jennifer Kasius
Typography: Avenir, Mrs. Eaves, and Filosofia

Running Press Book Publishers
2300 Chestnut Street
Philadelphia, PA 19103-4371

Visit us on the web!
www.runningpresscooks.com

EAT MORE
of what you
LOVE

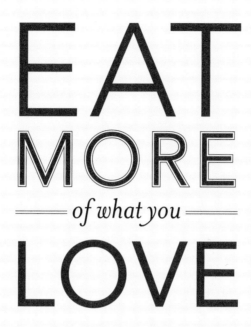

MARLENE KOCH

Photographs by
STEVE LEGATO

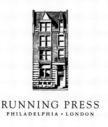

Running Press
PHILADELPHIA · LONDON

I dedicate this book to Stephen and James

You give me more to love every day . . .

table of contents

MORE FROM MARLENE

Introduction

What if I told you that you could enjoy all the foods you love without having to worry about excess sugar, fat, or calories, or that you could eat all the foods you love and still lose weight while keeping your blood sugar in check, or, perhaps best of all, that you could feed your family the great-tasting dishes they love, more healthfully? Well, with this book, you can!

I passionately believe that no one wants to give up the foods they love, and what's more, I believe with equal passion that they shouldn't have to. Instead, as a nutritionist and bona fide food lover, I believe—actually, I *know*—that good health and great taste can go delectably hand-in-hand. In fact, there are over 300 delicious reasons I know this—and they're all found in *Eat What You Love: More Than 300 Incredible Recipes Low in Sugar, Fat, and Calories.* I created *Eat What You Love* and the 300 guilt-free recipes in it so everyone could enjoy the foods they love, no matter what their diet.

I could not be more honored by the incredible response to it, from readers (thank you!)—and from my very own family, who, like many Americans, are challenged by some of today's most pressing health concerns, such as diabetes and weight control. It delights me to hear readers say they never knew healthy could be so tasty, but I must say that it's the success stories of better health that truly inspire me to continue to do what I do. Countless readers have shared the wonderful news that *Eat What You Love* helped them lose weight, control their blood sugar, lower their blood pressure, and feed their families more healthfully. Many of those same readers (and my fabulous Facebook fans) also requested more of my healthy recipes. You're holding in your hands my response. *Eat More of What You Love* lets you eat even *more* of what you love!

In this book you will find 200 brand-new recipes for even more of the foods we love to eat. Whether what you love is ooey, gooey, creamy, cheesy, or fried, you will find it here—with less sugar and fat, fewer calories, and simply more yum. So many of my readers (and maybe you're one?) have shared what they would like more of—and I listened. Here at your fingertips are more Southern recipes like Chicken Chicken Fried Steak with Cream Gravy, more super-quick and easy recipes and lots more classic comfort foods, more fabulous restaurant makeovers, such as PF Chang-Style Mongolian Beef, and even more family favorites like Pizza Pasta Pie. You'll also find more burger recipes and another oft-requested favorite: pizza! For slow-cooker enthusiasts, I am really excited to share that I have, for the first time, included an entire chapter of easy, tasty, slow-cooker recipes for no-fuss dinners that are ready when you are. As an avid baker (and lover of all things sweet), I *always* make sure that there are plenty of recipes for dessert lovers in my books and this one is no exception. My Amazing Pecan Pie Cups (with less than a teaspoon of sugar in each!) are, well, truly amazing; my Unbelievable Whoopie Pies contain a fraction of the usual fat; and, yes, I've included an *entire chapter* of cupcakes!

In addition to the scrumptious recipes, you'll also find more beautiful photos, more healthy-eating cooking tips, more fun and informative "Dare to Compares," and more options on sweeteners. *(Whew!)* You'll also discover an entire section devoted just to menus (including bonus menus from my first *Eat What You Love* cookbook), and I've included tips for eating gluten-free (with several great gluten-free desserts).

Eat More of What You Love stands alone as a wonderful collection of over 200 delicious recipes, but it's also a perfect companion to the original *Eat What You Love*. I didn't repeat a single recipe (with the exception of my always requested Unbelievable Chocolate Cake) and I have broadened the range of recipes (for example, in *Eat What You Love* I offered several frittata recipes, so here I added several breakfast bakes) to provide lots of tasty options for mixing and matching recipes between both books. Whether this is your first *Eat What You Love* cookbook or you are coming back for *more*, I guarantee this cookbook can help you and your family look and feel your very best—all while eating what you love!

My best to you and yours,

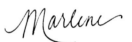

MORE HEALTHY EATING TIPS

THE HARDEST FOODS TO GIVE UP ARE THOSE WE LOVE THE BEST. These are the foods we eat most often, and all too often the ones we eat most of! Unfortunately, these foods aren't usually the ones that are the best for us. While wholesome foods are delicious, it's foods high in sugar and fat that send powerful "happy" signals to our brains and *give-me-more* signals to our mouths. If you're like me, just reading words like "creamy," "cheesy," "crunchy," "salty," and "sweet" is enough to make your mouth water (and to set off your cravings). It's no wonder that depriving ourselves of our favorite foods rarely, if ever, works. That's why I am thrilled to report that I have found an easier path to better health, and instead of sacrificing the foods you love, you can actually eat more of them! In this book you will find over 200 easy recipes and healthy cooking tips guaranteed to help you reduce the sugar, fat and calories (*and* keep carbs and sodium in check) in the delicious foods you love. Eating the scrumptious, creamy, cheesy, crunchy, sweet results will not only make your body healthier, it will make your tastebuds very, very happy!

As a professional cook, my top priority is to make everything taste great, but as a nutritionist (who passionately believes *everyone* should be able to enjoy the delectable, crave-worthy foods they love), it's my responsibility to do so with good health in mind. To help you get started on the road to healthy eating, here are some healthy tips:

1. CALORIES COUNT!

Calories count—they always have and they always will. A calorie is simply a measure of the amount of energy that a food provides. The wonderful thing about calories is that they provide the fuel for everything we do (including breathing). The bad thing about calories is that when we eat too many of them we gain weight (and it's *really* easy to eat too many calories). I am sure you have heard it before, but it's worth repeating: the very best thing you can do for your health is to balance the calories you eat with the calories you burn. In other words, maintain a healthy weight. For most people this means budgeting between 1,800 and 2,400 calories a day. (To calculate your own daily budget, go to www.marlenekoch.com and click on the Personal Calorie Calculator.) Alternatively, if you want to lose weight, you have to burn more calories than you eat.

> The very best thing you can do for your health is to balance the calories you eat with the calories you burn.

Now here's a weight loss secret: it doesn't matter which diet you follow (low-fat, low-carb, or high-protein), or if you count grams of carbs, fat, or "points"—your body *only* counts calories! That's why the recipes in this book have been crafted to give you more bang for your calorie buck. No calorie counting is required. Simply cook and enjoy the delicious foods you love while effortlessly reducing or keeping your calories in check. In fact, you don't need to look any further than the "Dare to Compare" feature found with many of the recipes to see just how enormous the calorie savings are when you are eating "more of what you love." All the foods you love are here, all with the same great taste. The only thing missing is extra calories!

2. THE BIG FAT TRUTH (ABOUT FAT!)

The truth is that the subject of dietary fat is widely debated even among health professionals. But here are some solid facts. First, we all need some fat in our diets. Fat not only provides flavor, aroma and creamy or crispy textures to food (some of my favorite fat attributes!), it also makes skin supple, hair shiny, and helps the body absorb essential vitamins like A, D, E and K. Second—and most important when it comes to your health—unlike calories, all fats are not created equal. While some fats, like transfats (mostly found in commercial crackers, baked goods, and some margarines) and saturated fats (found in butter, meat, and full-fat cheeses) can raise your risk for heart disease, healthy fats, like monounsaturated, polyunsaturated, and omega-3 polyunsaturated fats (found primarily in nuts, seeds, avocados, liquid oils, and fish) can actually reduce your risk for heart disease and a host of other ailments. Hence, healthy eating guidelines recommend that most of the fats you eat are "healthy" fats, that less than 10%

> The bottom line is that choosing healthier fats and eating less of them will whittle your waist and improve your health.

of your daily calories come from saturated fats, and that trans-fats be strictly limited.

Third—and extremely important when it comes to your weight—is the fact that all fat, good and bad, is very dense in calories (fat has more than *twice* the calories per gram of either carbohydrates or protein). Since eating extra calories translates to extra weight, *all* fats should be eaten in moderation.

The bottom line is that choosing healthier fats and eating less of them will whittle your waist and improve your health. Living proof can be found in members of the National Weight Control Registry (an organization comprised of those who have lost a substantial amount of weight and kept it off). A recent poll revealed that virtually all members of the organization follow a low-fat diet. The great news is that with my recipes you can do the same

thing (and your tastebuds will never know it!). Moreover, good-for-you fats, such as those found in nuts, canola oil, olive oil, and salmon, are given star billing in this book, while less healthy fats, such as those found in meat, cheese, and chocolate, are creatively curbed to keep you and yours satisfied *and* healthy. The biggest, best part of all is that I have used my culinary tricks to slash the fat in the rich-tasting foods we love most, from creamy shakes and dips, to crispy appetizers and entrees and luscious, rich-tasting desserts—all while maintaining the original fabulous flavors we also love (and that's the truth!).

3. THE WHOLE STORY ABOUT CARBS

Do you love carbs? Well, most people do (myself included), and that's okay, because carbohydrates, or carbs, are the body's preferred energy source. Just as gas fuels a car, carbohydrates are the fuel for all the wonderful things you do, like exercising or playing with your kids, grandkids, or pets. The problem is that too many of us get our carbs from baskets full of bread, big bowls of mashed potatoes, heaping platters of plain pasta and stupendous slabs of sugar-laden cake—and yes, indulging in carbs like this (along with the fat that usually accompanies them) can get us into trouble. But there's some good news here: We all need *some* carbs in our diet, and like fats, all carbs are not created equal. Refined carbohydrates like sugar and unfortified white bread raise blood sugar quickly and offer little nutrition beyond calories, but the more complex carbs such as whole grains, whole fruit, beans, and vegetables are gentler on blood sugar and packed with valuable nutrients. With this fact in mind, every recipe in this book was created to be what I call carb-conscious. Whenever possible, I use more nutritious slow-burning complex carbs such as white whole-wheat flour, wholesome oats, fiber-rich beans, and fresh and frozen fruits, along with a varied assortment of non-starchy veggies. You'll also find fewer refined carbs like sugar, white rice, or breads that offer no fiber.

I also dug deeper into my bag of culinary tricks to keep the *total* amount of carbs in check for every recipe so that even those on carbohydrate-controlled diets—

> Whole grains, whole fruit, beans, and vegetables are gentler on blood sugar and packed with valuable nutrients.

such as those for diabetes or weight loss—can enjoy the foods they love. (For more information on carbohydrate-controlled diets see page 20.) P.S. You are also in for some carb-loving surprises: If one of your crave-worthy carbs is potatoes, page 212 will give you all the healthy reasons potatoes get my vote!

4. THE NOT-SO-SWEET SCOOP ON SUGAR

One might think that because I have written four reduced-sugar cookbooks that I, like many sugar naysayers, am completely against sugar, but I'm not. I actually love sugar, not only for its sweet taste, but for the wonderful properties it imparts in cooking and baking. I also believe that small amounts of sugar can be incorporated into all diets. So why is my scoop not so sweet? All carbohydrates are composed of sugar molecules and all carbs eventually break down to glucose. While starches (fruits, vegetables, bread, and pasta) are composed of many sugar molecules, sugars (such as honey, molasses, white and brown sugars, and fructose) are made up of just one or two sugar molecules. Because of sugar's simple structure, the body breaks it down more quickly than starches—and it enters our bloodstream more rapidly. On the positive side, this makes sugar a quick source of energy; regrettably, though (especially for those of us who love sugar), research shows that supplying our bodies with too much sugar also has a lot of bitter consequences. Unlike more complex starches that offer vitamins and minerals, sugar is simply full of empty calories, ones that can lead to weight gain, and in turn increase the risk of type 2 diabetes. Moreover, sugar has been shown to weaken the immune system and increase the risk of heart disease and several types of cancer.

While the average American consumes 20 teaspoons of sugar a day, the newest guidelines set forth by the American Heart Association (which also apply to those who have diabetes) recommend that women consume no more than 6 teaspoons and men no more than 9 teaspoons of *added* sugars per day. The message is that for your health—and your waistline—minimizing added sugars is one of the sweetest things you can do! But this doesn't mean you have to forgo the delicious sweet foods and treats you love. I am so proud of the sweet collection of reduced-sugar recipes in this book (for example, my Unbelievable Whoppie Pies

---

For your health—and your waistline—minimizing added sugars is one of the sweetest things you can do!

---

have just one teaspoon of sugar in each, including the filling!). I am also excited to tell you about the guide on page 54 which gives you more sweetening options for my recipes than ever before. While sucralose no-calorie sweeteners like Splenda are still my favorite sugar swappers, I've also listed no-calorie sweetener packets in many of the recipes. Either Splenda or natural stevia-based Truvia packets can be used in these recipes (in beverage and non-baked recipes you can use any no-calorie sweetener packet that you enjoy). In case you simply prefer real sugar, I've provided tips for that as well. With more sumptuously sweet recipes than ever, I guarantee that no matter what sweetener you use there won't be a single sweet tooth left unsatisfied.

5. GET FIT WITH FIBER

It always makes me happy to report that there is something we can and should eat more of instead of less. Fiber is one of those things. And while eating it is not quite as exciting as, say, eating chocolate cake, it is really good for you. Fiber is actually a type of carbohydrate, but unlike other carbohydrates, it cannot be digested. This means that fiber also has no calories and does not raise blood sugar. Mother Nature packages fiber in two forms—non-soluble and soluble. Non-soluble fiber is what most people know as roughage. It's the type of fiber found in seeds and fruit and vegetable skins that keeps our digestive system running smoothly. Soluble fiber, though, offers a much larger range of health benefits. The latest research shows that adding soluble fiber to your diet can reduce the risk of everything from breast and colon cancer to heart disease and obesity. A higher fiber diet can speed up weight loss, slow the rise of blood sugar, and keep you feeling full.

> A higher fiber diet can speed up weight loss, slow the rise of blood sugar, and keep you feeling full.

Eating 20 to 35 grams of fiber a day will help you reap the most health benefits. To support you in this effort I've incorporated great-tasting, higher-fiber ingredients throughout the book. White whole-wheat flour, instant brown rice, beans, light breads, and high-fiber tortillas are a few of the easy-to-find fiber-rich superstar ingredients you will find. If you haven't yet tried any of these products, never fear: only those recipes that passed my own family's white-flour-loving tastebuds made the cut.

6. GET LEAN WITH PROTEIN

From counseling weight loss and diabetes clients to feeding my own family, I know just how satisfying it is to eat protein-rich food. So it comes as no surprise that emerging studies continue to support what I have known for some time: beefing up the (lean) protein in your diet is a powerful tool in the battle of the bulge. Here's why:

1) protein requires more calories to digest and turn into fuel than either carbohydrates or fat; 2) protein helps you feel full faster and stay full longer; and 3) protein reduces appetite. Protein has also been shown to minimize the loss of lean muscle when dieting (and muscle burns the most calories!) Last, and most important, to get lean by eating protein, the protein you eat needs to be lean.

While most people tend to eat the majority of their daily protein at dinner, research dictates that you get the greatest appetite-curbing effect if you eat protein-rich foods at every meal, especially breakfast. In this book, I've included plenty of delicious, satisfying protein-rich recipes to help create a lean healthy you. For breakfast you'll find plenty of egg-ceptional dishes to get your day rolling; for lunch, lots of great entrée salads and sandwiches (including three new juicy

> Beefing up the (lean) protein in your diet is a powerful tool in the battle of the bulge.

burger recipes) to keep you energized and alert all afternoon; and for dinner, an array of generously portioned, protein-packed entrees, from crispy chicken and tender beef to flavorful pork and creamy seafood. Who said anything about dieting?

7. SHAKE OFF THE SODIUM

As a cooking instructor to chefs, I can tell you that chefs commonly criticize home cooks for not adding enough salt. Perhaps that explains why it is not uncommon to find restaurant meals (or even a single dish) that can include *thousands* of milligrams of sodium. Because on average higher sodium intake is correlated with higher blood pressure, leading to a higher risk for heart disease, the most recent Dietary Guidelines for Americans recommend that we consume no more than 2,300

> The easiest way to keep sodium in check is to cook at home.

milligrams of sodium, or the equivalent of one teaspoon of added salt a day (with even less for select populations and those who already have high blood pressure). With current consumption closer to 4,000 milligrams per day per person, most of us could benefit from shaking off a little salt.

As someone who loves to cook, I am happy to share that the easiest way to keep sodium in check is to cook at home. While some ingredients, such as canned vegetables, have added sodium, the highest levels of sodium are often found in fully prepared foods and meals. When you cook with fresh ingredients and from recipes that keep sodium in check (like those in this book), shaking off some of the sodium is easy. The tricks I use to reduce sodium include packing my recipes with loads of flavor, using reduced-sodium products, such as reduced-sodium broth, and healthier preparation techniques, like draining and rinsing canned goods before adding them to the recipe. Rest assured that even the recipes in this book with slightly higher sodium levels are still far lower than their traditional sky-high salty counterparts. If you desire a lower sodium level, please feel free to adjust the recipe, and read page 116 for more information on sodium and shopping for the lowest sodium ingredients.

MORE ABOUT DIABETES

MY VERY FIRST COOKBOOK WAS BORN AS A RESULT OF A COOKING school request that I teach a class featuring sugar-free desserts. Ironically, the class never took place, but I was struck by the challenge of creating truly wonderful-tasting treats with less sugar that *everyone*, including those with diabetes, could enjoy with less worry. Two of my family members have diabetes, so I know firsthand how difficult it can be to think your favorite foods are forbidden. For them, and everyone like them, I have made it my mission to take the word "diet" right out of **diabet**es. After *Eat What You Love* was published, one kind reader wrote to me to say, "I have had diabetes for 40 years and food has never tasted this good." Many others have shared how my recipes have helped them control their blood sugar, lose weight, and even reduce their need for diabetes medications. Best of all, they said doing so was not difficult, but delicious! Receiving such news truly thrills me as much as being able to tell you that every tempting recipe in this book is perfect for those with diabetes, and all the people who love them! In these pages you will find pasta, pizza, potatoes, and of course plenty of mouth-watering desserts; they're here for *all* to enjoy—and they're all worry-free.

DIABETES—THE BASICS

To understand diabetes, it is important to understand two things that normally circulate in your blood—glucose and insulin. When you have diabetes, your body can't properly use or store the glucose (or sugar) in your blood that is produced from the carbohydrates (both starch and sugar) you eat. In type 1 diabetes this happens because the body completely stops producing insulin, a hormone that helps move glucose out of your blood and into your cells for energy. (Insulin acts as a key that opens your otherwise "locked" cells, enabling glucose to enter them.) In type 2 diabetes, the body either does not produce enough insulin or the cells simply ignore or *resist* the insulin that you produce (creating what is called "insulin resistance"). When you do not produce enough insulin, or it cannot do its job properly, glucose accumulates in the blood to levels that can have severe consequences.

If you or someone you love has diabetes, you are not alone. An estimated 26 million people in the United States have diabetes and that number is rising rapidly. What you may not realize is that before most people develop type 2 diabetes they have "prediabetes," a condition in which blood sugar is higher than normal but not quite high enough to warrant diabetes medications. A staggering 79 million, or *one in three Americans, have prediabetes*, and most don't know it.* (The majority of people with prediabetes will go on to develop type 2 diabetes within 10 years.)

> The single factor that contributes the greatest risk (for type 2 diabetes) is not whether diabetes runs in your genes but the size of the jeans you wear!

Although there are many factors that contribute to type 2 diabetes, including genetics, ethnicity, and age, the single factor that contributes the greatest risk is not whether diabetes runs in your genes, but the size of the jeans you wear! When it comes to decreasing your risk for type 2 diabetes, maintaining a healthy weight trumps all. The great news is that as many as 8 out of 10 cases of type 2 diabetes can be prevented by weight loss, regular physical activity, and a diet high in fiber and low in saturated fat and trans-fats. If you already have prediabetes, it is often the case that you can actually reverse it. It has been clinically proven that the combination of modest weight loss (losing as little as 5 to 7 percent of your body weight) and moderate exercise (30 minutes of walking five days a week) can delay or even prevent the onset of type 2 diabetes in persons with prediabetes. And last, if you have type 2 diabetes, there is no better time for you to take control of your health.

I am excited to share that *Eat More of What You Love* can help you do just that.

Every delectable recipe in this book has been carefully designed with diabetes in mind—*and* with a clear focus on the fact that eating is one of life's greatest pleasures. In fact, it's my pleasure to share with you that you *can* eat all the foods you love while keeping your carbs, blood sugar, and weight in check. For more specific information on meal planning and on how each recipe and its accompanying nutrition information can help, keep reading.

* The American Diabetes Association recommends that all persons who are overweight and 45 years of age or older be tested for prediabetes. It is also recommended that you have a blood test screening for diabetes by a qualified health care provider if you are younger than 45 and overweight, or have a family history of diabetes or high blood pressure, are African-American, Hispanic or Native-American, or have had gestational diabetes.

MORE MEAL PLANNING

LET ME START BY SAYING THAT MEAL PLANNING IS NOT REQUIRED in order to enjoy the delicious food or reap the health benefits from this cookbook. You are more than welcome to simply enjoy the incredible recipes knowing that each comes with a better-for-you "bonus." Many of the readers of my original *Eat What You Love* cookbook shared with me that they simply cooked from the book, and to their pleasant surprise, their clothes got looser and their energy higher—without ever counting a single calorie, carb, food exchange, or "point." But for many others, however, as the old saying goes, "when you fail to plan, you plan to fail." This old adage is backed up by studies which show that when it comes to achieving health goals, whether it's losing weight, keeping blood sugar in check (which is vital for those with diabetes), or simply eating more healthfully, a little planning can go a long way. That being said, a "meal plan" is a simple tool that can help you decide what, when, and how much you eat. This section gives you information on several types of meal plans geared toward helping you achieve your healthiest best. In this section you will also find Nutrition Tidbits (or more detailed information) about the nutritional analysis that's provided with each recipe.

THE PLATE METHOD

In *Eat What You Love*, I shared my enthusiasm for the "plate method" as an effortless, yet effective, meal planning tool. It seems the USDA likes this method too, as they recently replaced the food pyramid (as a visual representation of the dietary guidelines) with what they call "MyPlate"—an image of a plate depicting the amount and types of foods that make for the healthiest eating.

The MyPlate guidelines suggest filling half your plate with non-starchy vegetables and unsweetened fruit and the other half with a combination of starch and protein. What I love about the plate method is its simplicity. My plate (aka "Marlene's Plate") differs just slightly from the government's version in that I recommend a slightly higher portion of protein, less starch, and even more vegetables to encourage better satiety, weight control, and blood sugar management.

To create meals that are moderate in both carbs and calories, use a 9-inch dinner plate (no larger) as your guide. Fill half the plate with non-starchy vegetables and salad and then fill one-quarter of the plate with one of my starchy sides (about one serving of any recipe from the *Sides That Make the Meal* chapter) or bread. The remaining quarter should be comprised of any lean meat or seafood entrées (like those in this book). If you're dining on pasta, dish up one serving and fill the rest of the plate with salad and non-starchy veggies. To complete your meal, add one 8-ounce glass of skim or low-fat milk or yogurt and a single serving of whole fruit. (If you need to keep tighter control of your carbs, you can save either your dairy or fruit servings for snacks.)

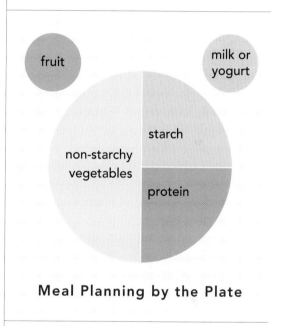

Meal Planning by the Plate

MEAL PLANNING WITH CALORIES

A sure-fire way to keep weight in check is to balance the number of calories you eat each day with what you expend. While the idea of counting calories is tedious or burdensome for some people, for others it is a way of life. According to a recent survey by the International Food Information Council Foundation, 27% of Americans routinely monitor the calories they eat—but only 9% (or 1 out of 10), are able to accurately estimate the number of calories they should consume each day.

The number of calories you require depends on many factors, including your sex, age, height, current weight, and activity level. Setting a daily calorie "budget" also takes into account your goals (whether you are trying to lose, maintain, or gain weight, and how quickly). I believe that everyone, whether or not they choose to diligently track their daily caloric intake, should know the number of calories they require. Without knowing how many calories you require, it's as if you are going on a shopping spree each day—only without knowing how much you are allowed to spend! To assist you in determining your personal calorie budget, you will find a Personal Calorie Calculator that can help you determine a daily budget at www.marlenekoch.com.

I've designed every recipe in this book to be a calorie-counting bargain. I've carefully monitored the calories in the ingredients to build recipes that are founded on good nutrition *and* great taste (while slashing the extra calories that commonly come from unnecessary fat and excess sugar). The end result is designer calorie taste with a bargain calorie price! To give you a *general estimate* (and to put my recipes' calorie counts and "Dare to Compares" in perspective): *a moderately active woman usually requires between 1,800 and 2,200 calories per day, and a man, 2,200 to 2,700 calories, for weight maintenance.*

CARBOHYDRATE COUNTING

A healthy diet for anyone—and that includes people with diabetes—is one that includes wholesome, good-for-you foods such as carbohydrate-rich fruits and vegetables, whole grains, and low-fat dairy. That said, of all the nutrients you eat, carbohydrates have the greatest impact on blood glucose. Thus, controlling the amount of carbohydrates you eat is vital for controlling blood sugar, (especially if you have diabetes).

Carbohydrate counting is a meal-planning tracking system that helps you monitor the carbohydrates you eat. Like calories, the amount of carbohydrates you individually need varies based on several factors, including gender, weight, and activity. To keep blood sugar in check and on an even keel (and your energy level optimum), it's best to spread the carbohydrates you eat evenly throughout the day. *A carb-counting budget for diabetes or weight loss averages 45 grams of carbohydrates per meal for most women and 60 grams for most men. In addition, snacks should range between 15 and 22 grams of carbohydrate.* (For a personalized carbohydrate budget, go to www.marlenekoch.com and click on my Carbohydrate Budget Calculator.)

At the end of each recipe, you'll find the total amount of carbohydrates and "Carbohydrate Choices." Many diabetes educators use "carbohydrate choices" to budget carbs for each meal and snacks. Carbohydrate choices are simply a calculation of the total number of carbs in a food divided by 15 (see *Carbohydrate Choices Chart* below). Thus, each carbohydrate choice = 15 grams of carbohydrate. Most women average 3 carb choices per meal and men 4 carb choices per meal. Snacks average 1 to 1½ carb choices.

One last note: While counting carbs is relatively easy, keeping within a carbohydrate budget can be challenging. The recipes in this book are fantastic for keeping blood sugar in check and stretching any carbohydrate budget. If you need more information on carbohydrate counting or a personalized menu plan, a registered dietitian or certified diabetes educator can help you.

USING FOOD EXCHANGES

The exchange system, a popular method of meal planning for those with diabetes, groups similar foods together, such as starches or fruit, to form "exchange lists." The foods within each list contain a similar amount of calories, carbohydrates, protein, and fat, and affect blood sugar similarly. This means that one food in the group can be "exchanged" or traded for another. For example, the value of a starch exchange is 80 calories, 15 grams of carbohydrate and 1 to 2 grams of fat. The equal value in the starch group is a single slice of bread, one-half cup of cooked oatmeal, or a quarter of a large bagel. So when you follow a meal plan based on the exchange system you can "exchange" a slice of toast for a half cup of cooked oatmeal or a quarter of a bagel. By varying the number of servings among the various groups, the exchange system ensures that all your nutrient needs are met and that the trifecta of carbs, fat, and calories is kept in check. The number of servings you are allowed to choose from each group at each meal or snack is based on your individual needs and can be determined by a qualified health provider such as a registered dietitian or certified diabetes educator.

Carbohydrates	Carbohydrate Choices
0–5	0
6–10	½
11–20	1
21–25	1½
26–35	2
36–40	2½
41–50	3
51–55	3½
56–65	4

I have included exchanges for every recipe for those of you who use the exchange system. The food exchanges and values are those set forth by the American Diabetes and American Dietetic Associations. The individual food groups include:

- STARCH (breads, pasta, rice, beans, potatoes and corn)

- VEGETABLE (all non-starchy vegetables)

- FRUIT (all fruits and fruit juices)

- MILK (nonfat and low-fat yogurt)

- MEAT (lean and medium fat meats, cheese, and eggs)

- FAT (oil, butter, margarine, nuts, and other added fats)

- CARBOHYDRATE (sugar and desserts)

NUTRITION TIDBITS

A complete nutritional analysis complements every recipe so you will be able to make smart and healthy choices based on your personal needs. The information was calculated using ESHA Nutrition Food Processor software in conjunction with manufacturers' food labels.

- FOOD EXCHANGES follow the guidelines set forth by the American Diabetes and American Dietetic Associations.

Values have been rounded to the nearest one-half for ease of use. (For more information see Food Exchanges on page 21.)

- CARBOHYDRATE CHOICES have been calculated in accordance with the American Diabetes Association. See Carbohydrate Counting and the Choices Conversion Chart on page 21 for more information.

- WEIGHT WATCHERS and WINNING POINTS are registered trademarks of Weight Watchers International, Inc. For all my weight-watching friends I have made a comparison using the new "Plus" points. Comparisons are rounded to the nearest whole number.

I take pride in offering realistic portion sizes that satisfy. There is nothing more annoying than getting excited about the nutrition numbers only to find they relate to a mere bite. I also try to be very realistic when it comes to how recipes are measured and/or normally served. For example, for a recipe that includes four chicken breasts and states that it "Makes Four Servings," each person gets one chicken breast and an equal portion of sauce. Because sauces can reduce down in the cooking process, the exact amount of a pan sauce may not always be consistent (and there is almost always one person who takes more than his or her share!). Measurements by the cup or spoonful are also provided where it is realistic that a food will be measured in this way. Casseroles and such that don't lend themselves to such neat measures are often apportioned into more realistic serving sizes like "one-fourth or one-sixth of the dish."

As the mother of two athletic boys, I am also well aware that appetites and caloric needs vary. So, like me, you may need to adjust the portions to your own or your family's needs and desires; just remember to adjust the nutritional information accordingly. Here are a few other useful tidbits about the recipes:

GARNISHES that are normally eaten (e.g., sprinkled green onions or powdered sugar) are always included in the nutritional analysis.

OPTIONAL INGREDIENTS are not included in the nutritional analysis.

ITEMS THAT ARE ADDED TO TASTE are also not included. If a choice is given, the first item listed was used for the nutritional analysis.

Above all, eating is one of life's greatest pleasures. I have created this book so that everyone can eat what they love—and love doing it. So feel free to peek at the numbers (they are sure to make you smile!), but the main thing is to simply enjoy!

Eat What You Love

INCREDIBLE INGREDIENTS
(from A to Z)

EVERY RECIPE IN THIS BOOK HAS BEEN CREATED WITH THE INCREDIBLE combination of delicious, healthy, and easy in mind—but having all three come together in perfect harmony is not always easy. I often spend hours at the market (and even more time in the kitchen) comparing similar ingredient choices before selecting those for a recipe. Most of those I use are everyday basic pantry staples like dry pasta, canned tomato products and beans, all-purpose flour, and spices. Others are those common to a healthy kitchen, such as reduced-sodium chicken broth, light soy sauce, low-fat dairy products, fresh vegetables, and lean meats. In this section you will find more information and tips on select ingredients, including substitutions, to make your shopping easier and to help you get the same incredible results that I do. Use this information as a guide, but please, feel free to adjust ingredients, especially spices, to impart the flavors you love best. Do note, however, that baking is a more exact science. As such, for baked goods (with the exception of add-ins such as nuts), it's important to follow the recipes as written for the best results.

AGAVE NECTAR

Agave nectar, or syrup, is a mild-tasting sweet syrup made from the agave plant. Like honey, agave is high in fructose, sweeter than sugar (1.3 times as sweet), and has more calories. When buying agave for its lower glycemic index (the rate at which it raises blood sugar), be sure to look for the word "raw" on the label. (Note: As it is still a concentrated sugar, agave nectar should be used in moderation.) For information on substituting agave in more of my recipes see page 54.

BREADS

I am happy to say that in the bread aisle there are more "light" choices than ever for those who are calorie and/or carb-conscious. All "100-calorie" products can be substituted for one another. When choosing other bread products, be sure to read the label carefully to note the calorie differences. "Light" breads not only have fewer calories and carbs (about 45 and 9 per piece, respectively), they contain more fiber (a double bonus when it comes to keeping blood sugar in check).

BUTTERMILK

Buttermilk adds great flavor to recipes and tenderizes baked goods. To make your own, place 1 tablespoon of vinegar or lemon juice in a measuring cup, add enough low-fat milk to make 1 cup, and let it sit for 5 minutes before using. Alternately, mix ½ cup nonfat or low-fat plain yogurt with ½ cup low-fat milk.

COCOA POWDERS

Dutch processing reduces cocoa's natural acidity and bitterness, mellowing the cocoa and imparting a richer, darker color. I particularly like Hershey's Special Dark Cocoa powder (found right next to the regular Hershey's cocoa powder), but any unsweetened cocoa powder may be used in the recipes unless otherwise noted.

COOKING AND BAKING SPRAYS

The difference between cooking and baking sprays is that baking sprays add flour to the oil, making them a convenient way to "grease and flour" a pan (especially in hard to coat spots). Be sure to select a flavorless vegetable-oil or canola-oil-based spray and remember to keep the "trigger finger" light—two to three seconds is all it should take. (A dusting of flour can be used with a cooking spray if you don't have baking spray on hand.)

COTTAGE CHEESE

Cottage cheese is an exceptional ingredient when it comes to cutting calories and fat and adding hunger-curbing protein to recipes—especially when it's creamed. The simple trick to creaming it, whether alone or with other ingredients, is to blend it (with an immersion blender or in a food processor) until no curds are left. Low-fat or 2% cottage cheese is my choice for the best outcome.

CREAM CHEESE

I always come back to Philly—for cream cheese, that is. Philadelphia brand cream cheeses are my top taste pick and are worth every penny, especially for reduced fat and nonfat cream cheeses. Neufchatel cheese can be used in place of light tub-style cream cheese in any of the recipes. Nonfat cream cheese has fewer calories, but does not have the taste or texture to stand on its own. Substituting additional nonfat cream cheese will affect the taste and texture of the product and is not recommended.

DAIRY PRODUCTS
(Milk and cheese)

Because taste comes first, as a rule of thumb I choose reduced- or low-fat dairy products over nonfat products. If you have nonfat brands you prefer, you may use them, but the texture may change. Unsweetened soy and almond milk can be used as alternatives for low-fat milk in most recipes (note: they will not work in recipes that call for sugar-free pudding mix), as can Lactaid brand dairy products. When it comes to low-fat cheeses I often use Sargento Brand. (See page 189 for more information about cheese.)

EGGS AND EGG SUBSTITUTES

To keep the total fat, cholesterol, and calories in check, and still maintain the taste and texture of whole eggs, I use a higher ratio of egg whites to yolk (or only egg whites when appropriate). I generally prefer this over using egg substitutes, especially for baking. There are some recipes such as smoothies and egg casseroles in which egg substitutes work well. If you choose to make additional substitutions, it is helpful to keep the following in mind: 1 large egg = 2 large egg whites = 1/4 cup liquid egg substitute

FLAVORINGS

Good-quality spices and flavorings make a big flavor difference in all recipes and even more so in reduced-sugar and/or reduced-fat recipes. Vanilla extract is best when "real"; alternate flavorings like lemon and coconut can be found next to the vanilla; and dried spices should still be fragrant when you open the jars.

FLOURS

Some tips about flours: all-purpose flour is the gold standard for traditional baking as it has the perfect amount of protein and offers a mild taste and light texture and can be used anywhere flour is called for. Cake flour has less protein and is used specifically to create a lighter, more tender crumb. To "make" 1 cup of cake flour, place

2 tablespoons of cornstarch in a one-cup measure and fill it with all-purpose flour. For good health with great taste, white whole-wheat flour is my choice. Although it tastes like and bakes up similarly to white flour, it has the wholesome fiber of whole wheat. The most common brand is King Arthur. White whole-wheat flour can be replaced with all-purpose flour or with a 50/50 blend of white and whole wheat, or whole wheat pastry flours.

LEAN GROUND BEEF AND GROUND TURKEY

Lean ground beef and turkey make it possible to put many of our favorite foods back on a healthy table. For the recipes in this book, I used 93% lean ground beef and turkey. I often combine beef and turkey to create a flavorful leaner ground meat, but all of one or the other can be used in any of the recipes. (See page 259 for more information on ground meat and how to reduce the fat content in regular ground beef.)

LIGHT WHIPPED TOPPING

The gold standard for me when it comes to light whipped topping is Lite Cool Whip sold in a tub in the freezer section of most markets. Light whipped topping has only a fraction of the fat of real whipped cream and adds a great deal of flavor and creaminess to recipes. Be sure to thaw before using. (Note: My preference is light, not nonfat whipped topping. The additional calorie savings are not worth the difference in taste and texture.)

MARGARINE OR BUTTER

In the margarine versus butter battle, I specify margarine first as it has far less saturated fat. My current favorite is Smart Balance. We had good results in all recipes even with the tub (the Original Buttery Spread). You may also substitute any brand of stick margarine you prefer, but I recommend you choose one with little or no trans-fat. In general, soft and tub margarines with less than 65% fat by weight do not work as their water content is too high. For flavor, butter can't be beat, but because it contains eight grams of saturated fat in each tablespoon, I only use butter when a small amount can make big taste difference (or it is a must-have as in the Sugar-Free Lemon Shortbread). You are welcome to indulge and use butter wherever you choose.

MAYONNAISE

With 100 calories per tablespoon, regular mayo is a "gotta-go" ingredient if you want to reduce the fat in your favorite mayo-based foods. I carefully crafted the recipes for great taste and less fat by using light mayonnaise. Low-fat mayonnaise will not give you the same delicious results. (Tip: After testing mixtures of mayonnaise (at every fat level) with yogurt, and every other common mayonnaise replacement, the winner for best taste and texture as a replacement for full fat mayo was a 50/50 blend of light mayonnaise and low-fat or non-fat plain yogurt.

NONFAT HALF-AND-HALF

Nonfat or fat-free half-and-half has the creamy richness of regular half-and-half but without the fat. The only quality substitute for nonfat half-and-half is real half-and-half (which of course adds fat and calories). Nonfat milk is not a fitting substitute.

OATS

You can use old-fashioned oats, rolled oats, and the quick-cooking variety interchangeably. I personally prefer the larger-cut, old-fashioned or rolled variety, especially for toppings. Instant oatmeal cannot be substituted for old-fashioned or quick-cooking oats.

OILS

All liquid oils contain the same amount of fat, so it's the flavor (or lack of) that primarily determines the type I select. For flavorless oil, I prefer canola, which is high in monounsaturated fat—but any flavorless vegetable oil can be substituted. For a bit more flavor, I like olive oil. The reality is that most of the time regular or virgin olive oil is all you need. When I specify extra-virgin olive oil, it's because the flavor it adds is worth the extra cost. In the Asian-style recipes you will often find sesame oil. Made from sesame seeds, sesame oil has a distinct flavor and there is no substitute. Look for it in the Asian food section of your market.

ORANGE JUICE (Light)

Light orange juice, such as Trop 50 (made by Tropicana) offers the taste of regular orange juice but with only half the sugar, carbs, and calories. If you see instead a simple listing of "orange juice" as an ingredient, it means that the difference in carbs and calories between using regular and light orange juice was not significant.

PASTA

Today's pasta aisle is a far cry from yesteryear when the only choices were white or whole wheat. Today a myriad of different flours and grains are used for pastas—many of them with the same delicious and yet more nutritious results. Ronzoni Smart Taste is the newest of the bunch. I love it because it has double the fiber and more protein than regular pasta, but the same great traditional white pasta taste my family loves. I also recommend trying whole wheat or whole grain "blend" pastas which offer the benefits of whole wheat without the heavy wheat taste. Ancient Harvest

Quinoa Pasta is a tasty gluten-free alternative. Finally, a word about pasta shapes: although I specify various shapes for all the pasta dishes based on the sauce and other ingredients, feel free to vary the shape based on your own preference and what you have on hand.

PRUNE PUREE

Puréed prunes are great for low-fat baking. I find it most convenient to keep on hand a couple of containers of baby food "prunes" (specifically, Gerber Prunes and Apples sold in a two-pack). To make your own prune purée, combine 1¼ cups pitted prunes and 6 tablespoons very hot water in a food processor and blend until smooth. You can store the purée in a covered container in the refrigerator for one to two months.

SWEETENERS (No-Calorie Granulated Sweetener)

Sucralose-based no-calorie sweeteners such as Splenda brand or other generic equivalents, which are made from sugar, are still my favorite go-to sugar alternatives. You will find several types of sucralose sweeteners next to the sugar in most

markets. The easiest to measure (and what every recipe was tested with) is the "no-calorie sweetener" sold in a yellow box or a large bag. It measures 1:1 for sugar and has 96 calories and 24 grams of carbohydrate per cup. Please note: Splenda Sugar Blend for Baking is a 50/50 combination of regular granulated sugar and sucralose and while it works well, it is not specified in any of the recipes. It has half the calories of sugar (384 per cup) and half the carbs (96 grams per cup). If you want to use it instead of the no-calorie granulated sweetener, *use half as much—as it has twice the sweetening effect.* Where I specify packets you may also use Truvia (see below). Other sweeteners such as the pink and blue packets will NOT work well in baked goods. Refer to page 54 and Stevia in this section for more information.

STEVIA (Truvia)

Stevia is a sweet-tasting sugar substitute derived from the stevia plant. When it comes to most sugar substitutes, all brands that are packaged the same way are equal, but this is not the case with stevia products, which vary widely in taste and quality. Despite the "natural" claims, only the

---

* I am often asked about the safety of sucralose, so here is some additional information: leading health experts and organizations, including the Center for Science in the Public Interest (CSPI), WebMD, the Mayo Clinic and the American Diabetes and Dietetic Associations, have carefully examined all the research and confirm that sucralose is safe for everyone, including pregnant women.

highly purified rebiana (or Reb-A) form of stevia has actually been approved as a safe food additive. Truvia is a tabletop brand that meets this guideline and the only other no-calorie sweetener I recommend for baking. (When compared to sucralose-based no-calorie sweeteners, Truvia works best in recipes that require less sugar substitute, and more natural sugar. You'll notice that some recipes, like those for cupcakes, suggest "(like Splenda)," and for those recipes *only* a sucralose-based no-calorie granulated sweetener (or real sugar) should be used. (See page 54 for more information). Truvia can be used wherever I give the packet equivalent. (If you want to use bulk Truvia, check the package for conversion guidelines.)

TORTILLAS

Reduced-carbohydrate, high-fiber tortillas are widely available and are found next to the regular tortillas. In addition to the traditional flour variety you will also find many flavors to choose from. Mission Carb Balance and La Tortilla Factory Smart and Delicious Wraps are two brands to look for. (Mission Carb Balance are the perfect swap for regular white tortillas and thin pizza crusts.) When shopping, look for wraps that offer over 10 grams of fiber each. 100% corn tortillas are a great gluten-free substitute.

YOGURT

While I do not specify Greek yogurt in most recipes that call for yogurt due to its extra cost, I do highly recommend it. Greek-style yogurts are strained, which removes much of the liquid whey. The result is a creamier, thicker texture, more protein (as much as double!), and fewer carbs and less sugar when compared to traditional American-style yogurts. Plain nonfat or low-fat (2%) Greek yogurt can be used anywhere I call for yogurt. TIP: To make your own Greek-style yogurt, simply use a yogurt strainer or line a strainer with cheesecloth and place it over a bowl. Add "American-style" plain yogurt and let it drain for several hours or until extra thick.

ZESTS

I love the fresh taste of citrus zests. Orange, lemon, and lime are interchangeable in most recipes. To zest a piece of fresh fruit, just wash it and grate off the brightly colored outer layer (rind) of the whole fruit (avoid going deeper into the bitter white pith). Zest is best when finely grated. If you do not have a zester, simply use a box grater and then mince finely with a knife before adding the zest to the recipe.

Eat What You Love
MORE RECIPES

super sippers, smoothies, and shakes

Iced Tea Lemonade

"Honest" Cranberry Lemonade

Cherry Lemonade Freeze

Peachy Green Tea Blast

Orange Cream "Soda"

Strawberry Banana Orange Julius

Mango Tango Smoothie

Frosty Caramel Frappe

Strawberry Shortcake Milkshake

Jump For Java Smoothie

Berry Slim Protein Shake

Frosty Chocolate and Vanilla Malts

Thin-Mint Cookie Milkshake

Deep Dark Hot Chocolate Mix

From a *refreshing* bottle of iced cold tea, to the newest *tempting* coffee sensation, to that sweet satisfying smoothie that helps get us through the day—sweet beverages are *hard to resist*. In fact, they are so hard to resist that they are the number one source of sugar in the American diet! It goes without saying, of course, that all that sugar (and in the case of *creamy* beverages, fat) brings with it not-so-sweet caloric consequences. If that weren't enough, studies suggest that when you drink too many calories you're more likely to gain weight than if you eat too many. A quick peek at some of today's most popular *temptations* reveals exactly how weighty the nutrition consequences can be. A single bottle of iced tea can easily contain 250 calories, a medium-sized creamy coffee drink from the Golden Arches packs in 550 calories (and more unhealthy fat than a Quarter Pounder with Cheese), and that seemingly "healthy" mango *smoothie* comes with 620 not-so-healthy calories and the equivalent of 36 teaspoons of sugar (enough to make anyone's blood sugar soar)!

In this chapter you will find my *better-for-you* takes on all of these popular beverages (and a whole lot more) to help you curb the calories, but not the taste, *in your glass*. My Iced Tea Lemonade is just 25 calories a glass, my McDonald's-style Frosty Caramel Frappe clocks in at 120 calories (and under 3 grams of fat), and my Mango-Tango Smoothie is a *slim* 100 calories—with no added sugar. If you prefer a *luscious* waist-whittling shake, you are going to love my new Berry Slim Protein Shake. If natural is what you seek, my "Honest" Cranberry Lemonade fits the bill. And last, but definitely not least, you'll find more of my incredible milkshake creations and two old-fashioned *frosty* malts. *Guilt-free* temptation has finally met its glass!

Iced Tea Lemonade

THE IDEA OF COMBINING EQUAL PARTS OF ICED TEA and lemonade is said to have started with the legendary Arnold Palmer, who would drink the "50/50" mixture to refresh and invigorate himself after a round of golf. This popular mix is also sold as a half-and-half, or over at Starbucks, as a fancy-sounding "Shaken" Iced Tea Lemonade. To get the shaken effect—for a fraction of the bucks—simply fill a shaker (or any container with a lid) with ice and then add the tea mixture. Shake vigorously for 10 seconds, pour into a glass, and serve.

MAKES **1** SERVING

1 black tea bag

¾ cup very hot water

2 tablespoons fresh lemon juice

Pinch of lemon zest

3 tablespoons granulated no-calorie sweetener (or 4 packets)

¾ cup crushed ice

Lemon wedge (optional)

1. In a medium-sized mug or glass measuring cup, steep the tea bag in very hot water for 3 minutes. Remove the tea bag and add the lemon juice, zest and sweetener. Stir and cool to room temperature. (When cooled slightly, you may move the tea to the refrigerator to speed up cooling or store for later use.)

2. To serve, pour tea mixture over crushed ice in a glass. If desired, garnish with a fresh lemon wedge.

DARE TO COMPARE: Whether purchased at a coffee shop or at a store, the sugar content found in most iced tea/lemonade blends is anything but refreshing. While the smallest version at Starbucks will "only" set you back 100 calories and a day's worth of added sugar, the contents of a can or bottle often exceeds 250 calories and 16 teaspoons (or two days' worth) of added of sugar.

NUTRITION INFORMATION PER SERVING: Calories 25 | Carbohydrate 6g (Sugars 1g) | Total Fat 0g (Sat Fat 0g) | Protein 0g | Fiber 0g | Cholesterol 0mg | Sodium 0mg | Food Exchanges: Free Food | Carbohydrate Choices: 0 | Weight Watcher Plus Point Comparison: 0

"Honest" Cranberry Lemonade

LIKE THE HONEST TEA BRAND BEVERAGES, this completely natural sipper combines the great taste of real juice and just a touch of sugar to create a drink that delivers less than half the usual sugar and calories. If you're wondering how it gets its sweet taste with lots of lemon flavor— but not lots of sugar— the trick is lemon extract. With a natural lemon taste (and far less bitterness than lemon juice), versatile lemon extract can easily be found in the market with the extracts.

MAKES **1** SERVING

½ cup light cranberry juice (like Hansen's)*

1 tablespoon lemon juice

1 teaspoon lemon extract

1 teaspoon granulated sugar

½ teaspoon lemon zest

½ cup crushed ice

1. Pour cranberry juice, ⅓ cup water, lemon juice, lemon extract, sugar and zest into a tall glass. Stir well.

2. Carefully add crushed ice to glass and stir again. Enjoy!

Marlene Says: *To make this into a sparkling beverage, substitute seltzer or any brand of carbonated plain or lemon-flavored water, even sugar-free lemon lime soda, for the ⅓ cup of water.*

*   Hansen's light juices are
    100% natural, but any
    light cranberry juice blend
    can be substituted.

NUTRITION INFORMATION PER SERVING: Calories 45 | Carbohydrate 10g (Sugars 5g) | Total Fat 0g (Sat Fat 0g) | Protein 0g | Fiber 0g | Cholesterol 0mg | Sodium 0mg | Food Exchanges: ½ fruit | Carbohydrate Choices: ½ | Weight Watcher Plus Point Comparison: 1

Cherry Lemonade Freeze

LISTED AS ONE OF THE WORST BEVERAGES in America by the folks at Eat This, Not That, the Wild Cherry Lemonade Mixer from Auntie Anne's is wildly popular, and with good reason. The taste combination of tart lemon and sweet cherry is undeniably hard to resist. Unfortunately, with 28 teaspoons of sugar in a large drink, it certainly earns its "worst" title. This wonderful variation delivers the same great taste combo, but instead of gobs of sugar you'll get an entire serving of whole fruit and a third of your day's worth of Vitamin C in every irresistible glass. That makes this a beverage "best." (P.S. This is just as delicious when made with frozen strawberries.)

MAKES **2** SERVINGS

1½ cups light lemonade*

1 cup frozen dark cherries

1½ cups crushed ice

⅛ teaspoon almond extract

1. Place light lemonade and cherries in a blender. Blend to mix.

2. Add crushed ice and almond extract and blend on high until the ice is completely incorporated.

DARE TO COMPARE: A large Wild Cherry Lemonade Mixer at Auntie Anne's contains 470 calories and 28 teaspoons sugar. Even if you order the smallest size they sell, you're looking at 2 days' worth of added sugar.

* *To make light lemonade, use 1 packet light lemonade drink mix (like Crystal Light On the Go) and 1½ cups water, or add 1 cup water, ¼ cup fresh lemon juice, and 4 packets of no-calorie sweetener to the blender.*

NUTRITION INFORMATION PER SERVING (1½ cups): Calories 50 | Carbohydrate 12g (Sugars 10g) | Total Fat 0g (Sat Fat 0g) | Protein 1g | Fiber 2g | Cholesterol 0mg | Sodium 0mg | Food Exchanges: 1 Fruit | Carbohydrate Choices: 1 | Weight Watcher Plus Point Comparison: 1

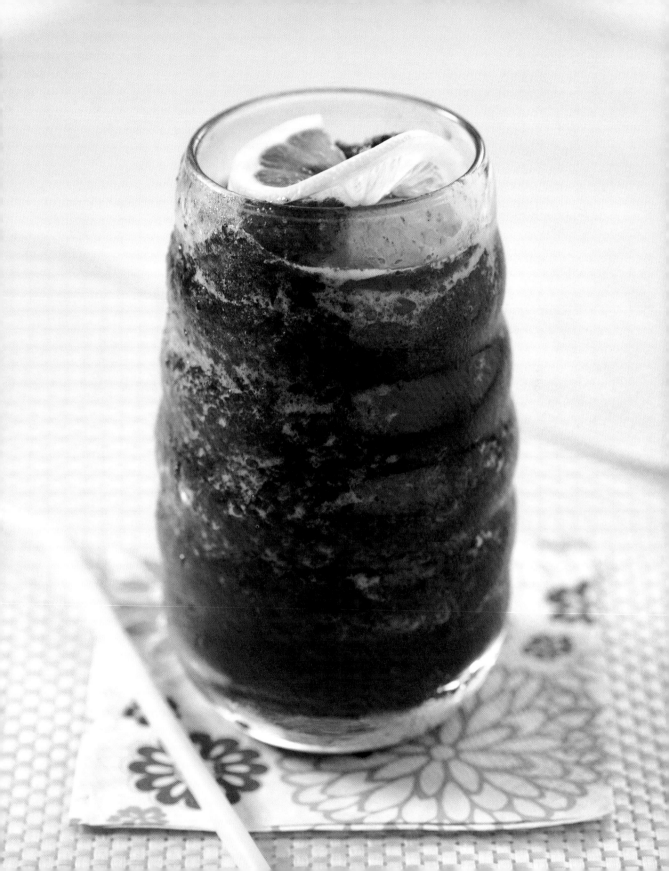

Peachy Green Tea Blast

THE SWEET TASTE OF PEACH combined with the health benefits of green tea has turned this iced-tea flavor into a bestseller. I was especially delighted when I discovered that canned peach nectar imparts the same wonderfully peachy taste as pureed fresh or frozen peaches— only without the mess or fuss! Better yet, this homemade version contains more real fruit and a fraction of the sugar of the bottled brands. This peach of a tea is perfect for entertaining.

MAKES **1** SERVING

3¼ cups water

3 green tea bags

¾ cup peach nectar
(like Kerns)

¼ cup granulated
no-calorie sweetener
(or 6 packets)*

Crushed ice

1. Pour the water into a small saucepan and bring to a low boil. Let cool 1 minute. Add tea bags and steep for 10 minutes. Remove tea bags and discard.

2. Pour tea into a pitcher. Add peach nectar and sweetener and stir. Let cool. Serve over crushed ice

* A popular version of this tea is made with agave nectar. If you would like to do the same, substitute 3 tablespoons agave nectar for the sweetener and add 45 calories and 11 grams carbohydrate to each serving.

Marlene says: *Recent studies show that green tea, in addition to its ability to fight heart disease and cancer, can also raise your metabolism to help your body burn extra calories. We can all drink to that!*

NUTRITION INFORMATION PER SERVING (1 cup): Calories 30 | Carbohydrate 8g (Sugars 6g) | Total Fat 0g (Sat Fat 0g) | Protein 0g | Fiber 0g | Cholesterol 0mg | Sodium 0mg | Food Exchanges: ½ Fruit | Carbohydrate Choices: ½ | Weight Watcher Plus Point Comparison: 1

Orange Cream "Soda"

THIS DRINK MADE MY DAY. Because most of my recipes are thoroughly researched before I ever set foot in the kitchen, I relish those that come about unexpectedly. One day as we were testing various iced tea combinations my focus turned to the glass of orange juice in my hand. Inspiration struck and thirty minutes later, after a wild firestorm of orange juice drink combinations, this simple, crazy-good, orange cream "soda" was born.

MAKES **1** SERVING

¾ cup crushed ice

½ cup light orange juice

¼ cup diet tonic water

2 teaspoons nonfat half-and-half

Sliced fresh orange (optional)

1. Place crushed ice in a 12-ounce glass.

2. Pour light orange juice and tonic water over crushed ice. Pour half-and-half on top of drink and then lightly stir. Garnish with fresh orange slice, if desired, and drink immediately.

Marlene Says: *The splash of nonfat half-and-half is what makes this drink. Milk does not give the same result. Because the amount is so small, regular half-and-half is a fine substitute.*

NUTRITION INFORMATION PER SERVING: Calories 35 | Carbohydrate 8g (Sugars 6g) | Total Fat 0g (Sat Fat 0g) | Protein 1g | Fiber 0g | Cholesterol 0mg | Sodium 10mg | Food Exchanges: ½ Fruit | Carbohydrate Choices: ½ | Weight Watcher Plus Point Comparison: 1

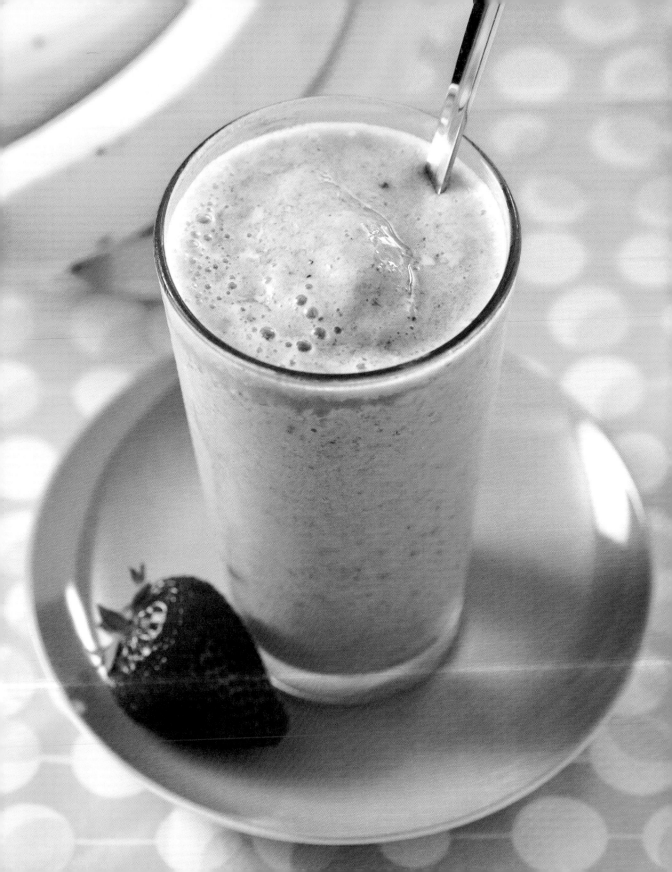

Strawberry Banana Orange Julius®

STRAWBERRIES + ORANGE JUICE + BANANA = one seriously delicious drink. This slimmed down version of the familiar fruity, frothy, and fabulous "Julius" drink supplies the protein of one egg (without the fat), and 1½ servings of real fruit in just 130 calories. It takes three of my Strawberry Banana Orange Juliuses to equal the calories of a single small Strawberry Banana Julius from an Orange Julius stand.

MAKES **1** SERVING

⅓ cup frozen strawberries

⅓ cup light orange juice

½ small banana

¼ cup liquid egg substitute

4 teaspoons granulated no-calorie sweetener (or 2 packets)

2 tablespoons low-fat milk

¼ teaspoon vanilla extract

½ cup crushed ice

1. Place all the ingredients except the ice in a blender. Blend to mix.

2. Add crushed ice and blend on high until the ice is completely incorporated.

NUTRITION INFORMATION PER SERVING: Calories 130 | Carbohydrate 25g (Sugars 15g) | Total Fat 0g (Sat Fat 0g) | Protein 8g | Fiber 3g | Cholesterol 0mg | Sodium 115mg | Food Exchanges: 1 ½ Fruit, 1 Lean Meat | Carbohydrate Choices: 1 ½ | Weight Watcher Plus Point Comparison: 3

Mango Tango Smoothie

USING FROZEN MANGO MAKES IT EASY to enjoy this fruit's wonderful taste all year long. I have purposely kept this smoothie simple, having the mango only "tango" with orange juice and a touch of milk. Pineapple extract is optional for an extra taste of the tropics, without adding any extra sugar or calories.

MAKES **1** SERVING

½ cup frozen mango

½ cup light orange juice

2 tablespoons low-fat milk

2 teaspoons granulated
no-calorie sweetener
(or 1 packet)

½ teaspoon pineapple
extract (optional)

¾ cup crushed ice

1. Place all the ingredients except the ice in a blender. Blend to mix.

2. Add crushed ice and blend on high until the ice is completely incorporated.

DARE TO COMPARE: A medium Mango Fruit Blast Smoothie at Baskin Robbins contains a startling 620 calories, more than 2 meals' worth of carbohydrates, and a whopping 144 grams of sugar (the equivalent of 36 teaspoons of sugar in a single smoothie!).

NUTRITION INFORMATION PER SERVING: Calories 100 | Carbohydrate 25g (Sugars 25g) | Total Fat 0g (Sat Fat 0g) | Protein 1g | Fiber 2g | Cholesterol 0mg | Sodium 15mg | Food Exchanges: 1 ½ Fruit | Carbohydrate Choices: 1 ½ | Weight Watcher Plus Point Comparison: 3

Frosty Caramel Frappe

IF YOU LOVE THE MCCAFE CARAMEL FRAPPE at McDonald's you're in for a treat. My taste testers and I found our take on this popular Frappe just as creamy, sweet, and addictive as the original. In fact, the only thing missing is 75% of the calories and 90% of the original sugar and fat. I'm loving it!

MAKES **1** SERVING

½ cup low-fat milk

¼ teaspoon instant coffee powder

¼ cup light, no-sugar-added butter pecan ice cream

1 tablespoon sugar-free caramel syrup (like Smuckers)

2 teaspoons granulated no-calorie sweetener (or 1 packet)

½ cup crushed ice

Light whipped cream (optional)

1. Place all the ingredients, except the ice, in a blender. Blend to mix.

2. Add crushed ice and blend on high until the ice is completely incorporated. Top with a squirt of light whipped cream, if desired.

DARE TO COMPARE: Not loving it – a medium Caramel Frappe with 550 calories, 24 grams of fat (15 of them saturated), and 71 grams of sugar, packs more saturated fat and calories than a Quarter Pounder with Cheese and more sugar than five Hot Apple Pies.

NUTRITION INFORMATION PER SERVING: Calories 120 | Carbohydrate 21g (Sugars 6g) | Total Fat 2.5g (Sat Fat 1g) | Protein 4g | Fiber 0g | Cholesterol 5mg | Sodium 110mg | Food Exchanges: 1 carbohydrate, ½ Low-Fat milk | Carbohydrate Choices: 1 ½ | Weight Watcher Plus Point Comparison: 3

Strawberry Shortcake Milkshake

THE DAY WE TESTED THIS I turned to my kitchen assistant and proudly declared it my most fabulous milkshake yet. With a layer of sweet strawberry topping nestled between two layers of French-vanilla milkshake and topped with a squirt of light whipped cream, it not only tastes fabulous but it looks absolutely fabulous too. For the best effect, be sure to use a tall clear glass and have a long spoon ready to dig for any bits of strawberry topping that don't make it up the straw. Better-for-you just got even better.

MAKES **1** SERVING

¼ cup frozen strawberries, thawed

1 teaspoon granulated no-calorie sweetener (or ½ packet)

½ cup low-fat milk

1 tablespoon French vanilla sugar-free instant pudding mix

½ cup light, no-sugar-added vanilla ice cream

½ cup crushed ice

Light whipped cream (optional)

1. In a small bowl, mash strawberries and sweetener together. Set aside.

2. Combine the milk and pudding mix in a blender. Blend to mix. Allow the pudding to set for 1 minute. Add ice cream and crushed ice to blender and blend on high until the ice is completely incorporated and the shake is thick and creamy.

3. Pour one-half of the milkshake into a tall glass; spoon strawberry mix onto shake. Carefully spoon remaining milkshake over strawberries. Top with squirt of light whipped cream, if desired (adds 20 calories).

Marlene Says: *To make a **Snickerdoodle Milkshake**, combine ⅔ cup low-fat milk and 1 tablespoon French vanilla sugar-free instant pudding mix. Add ½ cup vanilla ice cream and ½ cup crushed ice and blend per instructions above. Mix ½ teaspoon each cinnamon and sugar in a small dish and sprinkle on top of shake. Lightly stir and add a straw! (Nutrition stats the same as Strawberry Shortcake Milkshake.)*

NUTRITION INFORMATION PER SERVING: Calories 190 | Carbohydrate 32g (Sugars 14g) | Total Fat 5g (Sat Fat 3g) | Protein 7g | Fiber 5g | Cholesterol 5mg | Sodium 370mg | Food Exchanges: 1½ Carbohydrate, ½ Low-Fat Milk, ½ Fat | Carbohydrate Choices: 2 | Weight Watcher Plus Point Comparison: 5

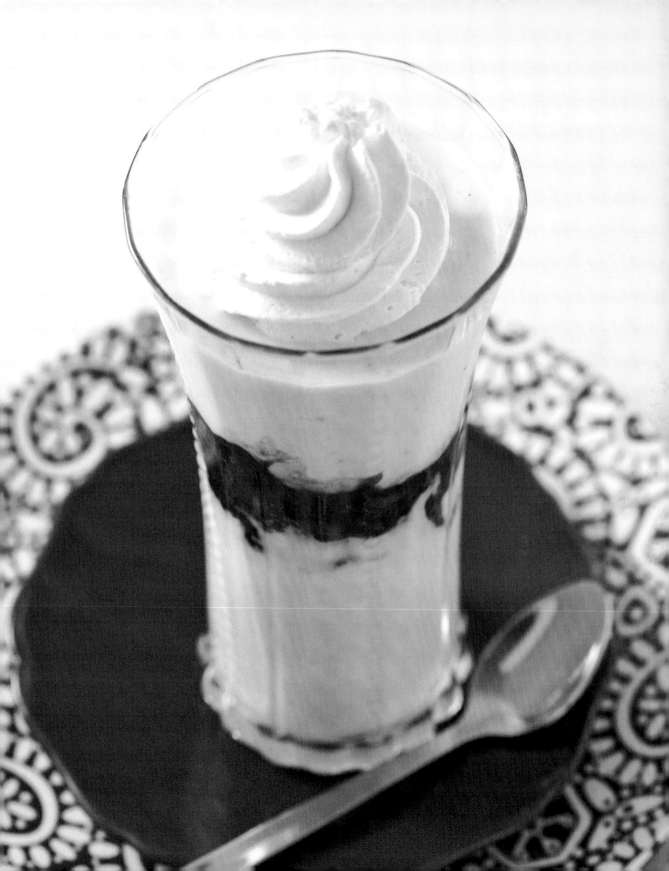

Jump for Java Smoothie

THIS GREAT GRAB-N-GO smoothie is sure to put extra bounce in your step. Cool and creamy, it's a lot more filling—and a whole lot more fun—than an ordinary cup of coffee and a piece of fruit. To pump up the protein, simply add a tablespoon of protein powder before you blend it. Vanilla protein powder pairs well, while chocolate turns it into what I call my Mocha Power Smoothie.

MAKES **1** SERVING

¾ teaspoon instant coffee

¼ cup water

½ cup low-fat milk

½ medium banana, frozen

2 tablespoons granulated no-calorie sweetener (or 3 packets)

½ cup crushed ice

Pinch of ground cinnamon

1. Place all the ingredients except the ice and cinnamon in a blender. Blend to mix.

2. Add crushed ice and blend on high until the ice is completely incorporated. Sprinkle on cinnamon and stir.

Marlene Says: *Feel free to moo-ve the low-fat milk over and replace it with either light soy milk or regular almond milk (subtracts 25 calories).*

NUTRITION INFORMATION PER SERVING: Calories 120 | Carbohydrate 22 (Sugars 17g) | Total Fat 1.5g (Sat Fat .5 g) | Protein 5 g | Fiber 2g | Cholesterol 0mg | Sodium 30mg | Food Exchanges: ½ Low-Fat Milk, ½ Fruit, ½ Carbohydrate | Carbohydrate Choices: 1 ½ | Weight Watcher Plus Point Comparison: 3

Berry Slim Protein Shake

IF YOU'VE BEEN LOOKING FOR A TASTY inexpensive body slimming shake, look no further. This creamy shake is high in hunger-satisfying protein and fiber, yet low in fat and calories. Best of all, this waist-whittling drink tastes great! Adding cottage cheese (which virtually disappears into the drink while adding a slight cheesecake flavor) or Greek yogurt helps bump up the protein, while frozen raspberries pack a fiber punch. Slightly lower in fiber, but with fewer seeds, strawberries and blueberries are also great berry options. To keep sugar and carbs in check, use a no-sugar-added protein powder with no more than 2 grams of carb per serving.

MAKES **1** SERVING

⅔ cup nonfat milk (or unsweetened soy milk)

¼ cup low-fat cottage cheese (or Greek yogurt)

½ cup frozen raspberries

1 tablespoon vanilla protein powder

2 teaspoons granulated no-calorie sweetener (or 1 packet)

⅛ teaspoon almond extract

⅔ cup crushed ice

1. Place half the milk and cottage cheese (or yogurt) in a blender. Blend well until mixture is smooth. Add the remaining ingredients, except the ice, and blend briefly.

2. Add crushed ice and blend on high until the ice is completely incorporated.

DARE TO COMPARE: This shake rocks it with twice the protein and less than one-half the sugar of the most popular canned-beverage meal replacement. Vary the berry and protein powder combinations and you have more flavor variations than you'll ever find on the grocery store shelf.

NUTRITION INFORMATION PER SERVING: Calories 170 | Carbohydrate 22g (Sugars 10g) | Total Fat 1.5g (Sat Fat 0.5g) | Protein 18g | Fiber 4g | Cholesterol 10mg | Sodium 340mg | Food Exchanges: 2 ½ Very Lean Meat, ½ Nonfat Milk, ½ Fruit | Carbohydrate Choices: 1 ½ | Weight Watcher Plus Point Comparison: 4

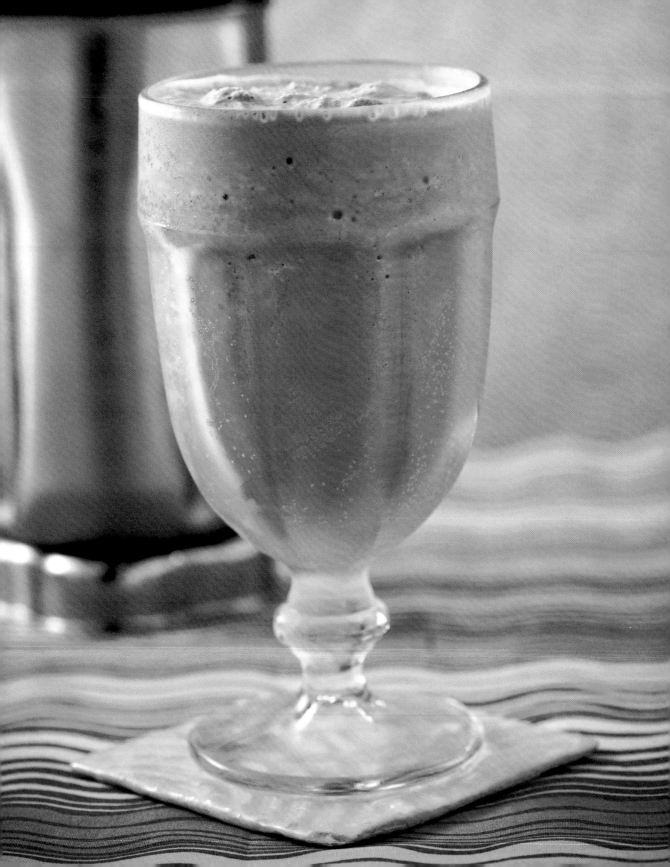

Frosty Chocolate and Vanilla Malts

FOR MANY PEOPLE (my husband included), no milkshake satisfies quite like a malted milkshake. As someone who's concerned about his health (and his waistline), my husband is not usually tempted, but if there's a malt on the menu, his willpower absolutely disappears. Needless to say, he was thrilled when he got a taste of this frosty malted milkshake. It's pure satisfaction.

MAKES **1** SERVING

⅔ cup low-fat milk

1½ tablespoons malted milk powder (like Carnation brand)

½ cups light, no-sugar-added chocolate or vanilla ice cream

½ cup crushed ice

1. Combine milk and malted milk powder in a blender. Blend to mix.

2. Add ice cream and crushed ice and blend on high until the ice is completely incorporated and the shake is thick and creamy.

Marlene Says: *Malted milk powder is a combination of flour, barley (which gives it its signature earthy flavor), and powdered milk. Malted milk powder not only flavors milkshakes, it makes them thicker.*

NUTRITION INFORMATION PER SERVING: Calories 200 | Carbohydrate 30g (Sugars 17g) | Total Fat 7g (Sat Fat 3.5g) | Protein 9g | Fiber 4g | Cholesterol 5mg | Sodium 130mg | Food Exchanges: 2 Carbohydrate, ½ Low-Fat Milk | Carbohydrate Choices: 2 | Weight Watcher Plus Point Comparison: 6

Thin-Mint Cookie Milkshake

IN MY HOUSE the thought of Girl Scouts means one thing – cookies –Thin Mint cookies, to be exact. Apparently, our family is not alone. The minty sensations account for 25% of all the Girl Scout cookies sold each year. If you are also a Thin-Mint fan, this is the perfect shake for you. You can also use this recipe to concoct the St. Patty's Day favorite, a Shamrock shake, by simply switching to vanilla ice cream.

MAKES **1** SERVING

⅔ cup low-fat milk

1 tablespoon vanilla sugar-free instant pudding mix

½ cup light, no-sugar-added cookies and cream ice cream

2 drops green food coloring

scant ¼ teaspoon mint extract

⅔ cup crushed ice

1. Combine the milk and pudding mix in a blender. Blend to mix. Allow pudding to set for 1 minute.

2. Add ice cream, green food coloring, mint extract, and crushed ice to blender and blend on high until the ice is completely incorporated and shake is thick and creamy.

DARE TO COMPARE: Not-so-thin-mint. The *smallest* Crème de Menthe™ milkshake you can order at Cold Stone Creamery serves up a mind-boggling 1,160 calories, 67 grams of fat (including two full days' worth of saturated fat), and 109 grams (or the equivalent of 28 teaspoons) of sugar!

NUTRITION INFORMATION PER SERVING: Calories 200 | Carbohydrate 31g (Sugars 11g) | Total Fat 7g (Sat Fat 3g) | Protein 8g | Fiber 4g | Cholesterol 5mg | Sodium 425 mg | Food Exchanges: 1 ½ Carbohydrate, ½ Low-Fat Milk, ½ Fat | Carbohydrate Choices: 2 | Weight Watcher Plus Point Comparison: 5

Deep Dark Hot Chocolate Mix

LOW-CALORIE HOT CHOCOLATE MIX is great to have on hand when chocolate cravings hit. This homemade dark hot chocolate mix is equivalent to an entire box of dark hot cocoa packets. The secret to its "deep, dark" color and flavor is Dutch-processed cocoa. I use Hershey's brand Special Dark Cocoa, but any unsweetened cocoa will do. Your result may not be quite as dark, but will still be plenty delicious. Stored in a tightly sealed container, the mix will stay fresh for several months.

MAKES **8** SERVINGS

⅔ cup non-fat dry milk

⅓ cup powdered non-dairy creamer

⅓ cup cocoa powder (preferably Dutch-process)

½ cup granulated no-calorie sweetener (or 12 packets)

1 tablespoon cornstarch

1. In a small container with a lid, combine all ingredients and shake well.

2. To make one serving of hot chocolate, measure 3 tablespoons of the mix into a mug. Add 6 ounces very hot or boiling water and whisk or stir well.

OR TRY THIS: *For **Peppermint Hot Chocolate** add 1/16th teaspoon (4 drops) mint extract or 2 crushed sugar-free peppermints to prepared hot chocolate. For an "Almond Joy," add 2 to 3 drops each of coconut and almond extract. This mix can also be used to create the Frozen Hot Chocolate Frosty on page 68 in my book* Eat What You Love.

NUTRITION INFORMATION PER SERVING (1 cup): Calories 55 | Carbohydrate 9g (Sugars 3g) | Total Fat 1.5g (Sat Fat 1.5g) | Protein 2g | Fiber 1g | Cholesterol 0mg | Sodium 40mg | Food Exchanges: ½ Carbohydrate | Carbohydrate Choices: ½ | Weight Watcher Plus Point Comparison: 2

fresh baked breads, muffins, and coffee cakes

Triple Lemon Blueberry Muffins

Cream Cheese Filled Pumpkin Muffins

Any Day Sunshine Muffins

Whole Grain Oatmeal Muffins

Favorite Focaccia Muffins

Cheddar Bay-Style Biscuits

Bran-ana Nut Mini-Loaves

Marvelous Marble Poundcake

Razzle-Dazzle Lemon Loaf

Chocolate Zucchini Bread

Berry Best Old-Fashioned Coffee Cake

Chocolate Chip Quick Cake

I've never been overly *tempted* by breakfast pastries or donuts, but put a *tasty* muffin or a slice of coffeecake or quick bread in front of me, and my resolve quickly fades. The problem is that as much as *I love* the taste of *quick breads*, I hate the sky-high calories, sugar, and fat that most commercial muffins, biscuits, and coffeecakes are packed full of. Once a well-kept secret, the astronomical numbers are clear for all to see now that restaurants and coffee shops must display the caloric content of the food they serve. A single *pumpkin muffin* contains a staggering 490 calories, and a rather modest-looking slice of lemon loaf is equally *rich*. The sugar content is not on display, but if you're watching sugar or counting carbs, I guarantee you that those numbers are just as staggering, with as much as a day's worth of added sugar in a single piece of coffeecake or crumb-topped muffin.

That's why I am especially excited to share the recipes in this chapter with you. The chapter starts with *scrumptious* Triple Lemon Blueberry Muffins and ends with Chocolate Chip Quick Cake, one of the quickest coffeecake recipes you will ever make. In between are more *easy-to-make* quick breads for every meal and every occasion, including my Cream Cheese Filled Pumpkin Muffins (whose 170 equally *satisfying* calories I am happy to show), *savory* rosemary-scented Favorite Focaccia Muffins, Raspberry Swirl Lemon Loaf, and one of my holiday favorites—deep, dark, *delicious* Chocolate Zucchini Bread.

NOTE: *Muffins and slices of quick bread freeze quite well. Simply slice and tightly wrap leftovers (if you are lucky enough to have any) in plastic wrap, and freeze. Unwrap and warm these individual servings in the microwave to bring back their fresh-baked goodness.*

SUGAR

Cooking, and especially baking, sweet foods with less sugar can be challenging as sugar not only adds sweetness to recipes, but also has the unique ability to add texture, structure, volume, and even color. In contrast, while low- and no-calorie substitutes are super at sweetening, they do not have sugar's other qualities. Moreover, with so many different sugar substitutes on the market, it can be hard to know which one to choose. To help you, here's what I have found:

SUCRALOSE (aka Splenda®). All of my sweet recipes were tested with granulated and/or packets of no-calorie sucralose-based sweeteners. I have yet to find another sweetener that's safer, easier to find, more economical, and delivers better tasting results for all cooking and baking applications. Generic no-calorie sucralose products perform identically to Splenda brand. If you prefer to use Splenda Sugar Blend for Baking, reduce the amount of sweetener in the recipe by half. It tastes and works great, but does add some calories and carbs.

STEVIA (Truvia® brand). There are many types and brands of all-natural stevia-based sweeteners and they differ greatly in safety, strength, and taste. Truvia is the only brand that passed my recipe taste tests, and Truvia packets, or its bulk equivalent, can be used wherever I specify no-calorie sweetener packets.* Truvia works great in drinks, sauces and cold or unbaked desserts. For baking, Truvia works best when combined with some real sugar. (Note: The end result may be slightly drier than recipes made with sucralose or sugar).

AGAVE NECTAR, or syrup, is a honey-like syrup derived from the agave plant. Agave is sweeter than sugar *and* has more carbs and calories (15 carbs and 60 calories per tablespoon versus 12 carbs and 48 calories for sugar). Agave syrup may raise blood sugar less than other sugars, but should be used in moderation. In baking, agave requires recipes developed specifically for a liquid sweetener. For use in beverages, dressings and sauces, use one-third less agave than the specified amount of sweetener.

Many readers simply prefer to use real sugar when making my recipes. Even with real sugar my reduced-fat recipes are healthier than their counterparts. When using granulated sugar in baked good recipes omit ¼ teaspoon of baking soda per cup of flour and expect to increase baking time by as much as 7 to 10 minutes for cakes, 5 minutes for muffins, and 3 to 5 minutes for cookies. Check all baked goods according to the recipe's test for doneness.

TIP: *When opting for sugar over a no-calorie sweetener you can reduce the sugar by up to one-fourth in most recipes with the only effect being slightly reduced sweetness.*

---

* *Use only the number of specified packets (or a conversion rate of 1 packet equaling 2 teaspoons granulated no-calorie sweetener). Do not open the packets and try to measure the contents.*

Triple Lemon Blueberry Muffins

MAKING TRULY BETTER-FOR-YOU MUFFINS (ones that are low in sugar and fat) is often a challenge. Reducing the fat can make them dry, while reducing the sugar can alter height, browning, and texture. Bursting with the taste of fresh lemon, plump with blueberries, and crowned with a touch of sugar, these muffins are better-for-you baking at its triple best.

MAKES **12** SERVINGS

1 (6-ounce) container light lemon yogurt

½ cup low-fat milk

3 tablespoons margarine or butter, melted

1 large egg

1 teaspoon vanilla extract

1 teaspoon lemon zest

½ teaspoon lemon extract

2 cups all-purpose flour

½ cup granulated no-calorie sweetener (or 12 packets)

2 tablespoons and 2 teaspoons granulated sugar, divided

1 tablespoon baking powder

½ teaspoon baking soda

1 cup fresh blueberries

1. Preheat oven to 375°F. Lightly spray 12 muffin cups with nonstick cooking spray (or line with paper or foil liners).

2. In a medium bowl, whisk together the first seven ingredients (yogurt through lemon extract). Set aside.

3. In a large bowl, stir together the next five ingredients (flour through baking soda using 2 tablespoons of sugar). Add blueberries and stir lightly to coat with flour. Make a well in the center and add the yogurt mixture. Using a large spoon, stir until dry ingredients are just moistened.

4. Spoon the batter evenly into the prepared muffin tins, filling each cup two-thirds full. Evenly sprinkle the 2 remaining teaspoons of sugar over the muffins.

5. Bake for 17 to 20 minutes or until center springs back when lightly touched. Cool for 5 minutes before removing to a wire rack.

Marlene Says: *These are at their "berry" best when made with fresh berries and eaten while warm. If using frozen blueberries, do not thaw them. To freeze, wrap cooled muffins tightly in plastic wrap. To serve, thaw, unwrap and microwave 30 to 45 seconds to warm.*

NUTRITION INFORMATION PER SERVING (1 muffin): Calories 130 | Carbohydrate 23g (Sugars 4g) | Total Fat 3g (Sat Fat 1g) | Protein 4g | Fiber 1g | Cholesterol 20mg | Sodium 150mg | Food Exchanges: 1½ Starch | Carbohydrate Choices: 1½ | Weight Watcher Plus Point Comparison: 4

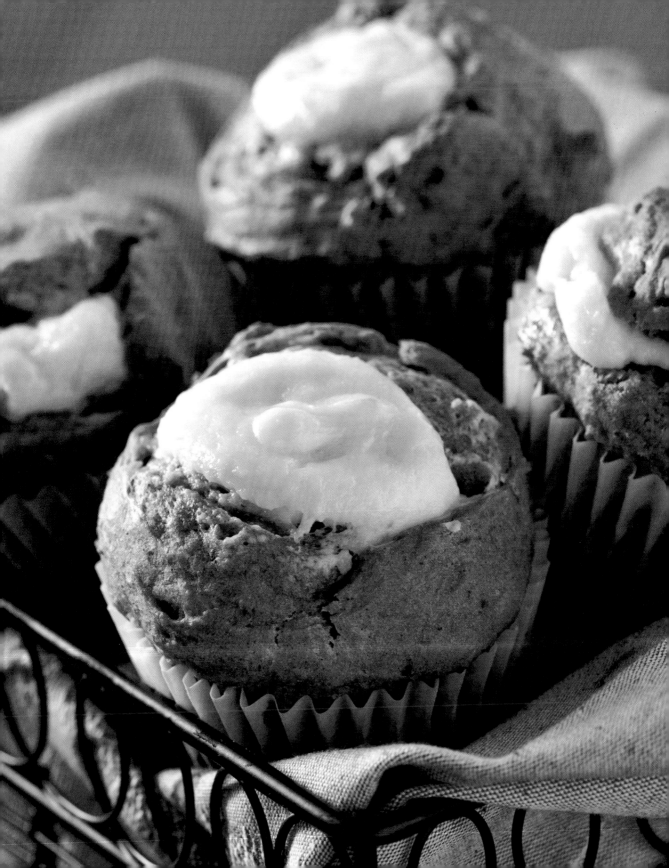

Cream Cheese Filled Pumpkin Muffins

EACH FALL STARBUCKS rolls out their beloved pumpkin muffins. I must admit, the moist, spicy muffins filled with sweet cream cheese are everything you could ask for in a pumpkin muffin—and more. Unfortunately, the "more" also means more sugar, more fat, and more calories! This marvelous makeover also offers everything you could ask for—only with 70% fewer calories and a mere fraction of the added sugar and fat. Enjoy.

¼ cup plus 2 tablespoons light tub-style cream cheese

2 teaspoons powdered sugar

4 teaspoons plus ¾ cup granulated no-calorie sweetener (like Splenda), divided

1¾ cups all-purpose flour

1½ teaspoons baking powder

½ teaspoon baking soda

2 teaspoons cinnamon

1 teaspoon ginger

¼ teaspoon cloves

1 large egg

2 large egg whites

¾ cup canned pumpkin

⅓ cup unsweetened applesauce

3 tablespoons canola oil

2 tablespoons molasses

1. Preheat the oven to 375°F. Line 12 muffin cups with paper or foil cupcake liners.

2. In a small bowl thoroughly blend the cream cheese, powdered sugar and 4 teaspoons sweetener. Set aside. In a medium bowl whisk next six ingredients (flour through cloves).

3. In another medium bowl, with an electric mixer, beat the ¾ cup sweetener, egg, and egg whites for 3 to 4 minutes, or until doubled in volume. Turn mixer to low and blend in the pumpkin, applesauce, oil and molasses. Using a large spoon, stir in the flour mixture just until the dry ingredients are incorporated.

4. Spoon 3 tablespoons of batter into each muffin cup. Make an indent in each muffin by pressing the end of a wet teaspoon into the batter. Press a heaping teaspoon of the cream cheese mixture into the indent. Top each muffin with another tablespoon of batter, spreading it to cover most of the cream cheese.

5. Bake for 18 to 20 minutes or until the center springs back when lightly touched. Cool for 5 minutes before moving muffins to wire rack for complete cooling.

DARE TO COMPARE: Treat or trick? A single pumpkin muffin at Starbucks has 490 calories, 24 grams of fat, 10 teaspoons of sugar, and a meal's worth of carbohydrates.

NUTRITION INFORMATION PER SERVING (1 muffin): Calories 140 | Carbohydrate 21g (Sugars 4g) | Total Fat 4.5g (Sat Fat 1.5g) | Protein 4g | Fiber 1g | Cholesterol 20mg | Sodium 150mg | Food Exchanges: 1½ Starch, ½ Fat | Carbohydrate Choices: 1½ | Weight Watcher Plus Point Comparison: 4

Any Day Sunshine Muffins

THESE QUICK ALL-NATURAL MUFFINS made sweet with low-sugar orange marmalade are guaranteed to add an extra bit of sunshine to any breakfast table. For variety, feel free to substitute apricot, raspberry, or strawberry low-sugar jam for the orange marmalade.

MAKES **12** SERVINGS

2 large eggs

4 tablespoons margarine or butter, melted

½ cup low-fat milk

¾ cup low-sugar orange marmalade (like Smuckers)

1 tablespoon orange zest

1¾ cups all-purpose flour

3 tablespoons granulated sugar

2 teaspoons baking powder

½ teaspoon baking soda

12 teaspoons low-sugar orange marmalade

1. Preheat the oven to 375°F. Lightly spray 12 muffin cups with non-stick baking spray (or line with paper or foil liners).

2. In a medium bowl, whisk together first 5 ingredients (eggs through zest). Set aside.

3. In a large bowl, combine the flour, sugar, baking soda, and baking powder and stir. Make a well in the center and add the marmalade mixture. Using a large spoon, stir just until the dry ingredients are moistened.

4. Spoon the batter evenly into prepared muffin tins, filling each cup two-thirds full.

5. Bake for 15 minutes or until the center springs back when lightly touched. Cool for 5 minutes before removing to a wire rack. Serve each muffin with 1 teaspoon jam.

Marlene Says: *Smuckers uses only the sweetness of natural fruit to produce its flavor-packed low-sugar jam. It tastes as sweet as the regular variety but with half the sugar and calories.*

NUTRITION INFORMATION PER SERVING (1 muffin): Calories 155 | Carbohydrate 25g (Sugars 11g) | Total Fat 4g (Sat Fat 1g) | Protein 4g | Fiber 1g | Cholesterol 35mg | Sodium 140mg | Food Exchanges: 1½ Starch, ½ Fat | Carbohydrate Choices: 2 | Weight Watcher Plus Point Comparison: 4

Whole Grain Oatmeal Muffins

OLD-FASHIONED OATMEAL and white whole-wheat flour lend the goodness of whole grain to these wholesome muffins. While many whole grain muffins are heavy or taste overly wheaty, that's not the case here. The addition of brown sugar and cinnamon makes them extra tasty, while cutting in the shortening keeps them nice and light.

MAKES **12** SERVINGS

1 cup low-fat milk

1 large egg

1 large egg white

1 teaspoon vanilla extract

1 cup old-fashioned rolled oats

⅔ cup white whole-wheat flour

⅔ cup all-purpose flour

½ cup granulated no-calorie sweetener (or 12 packets)

2 tablespoons brown sugar

1 tablespoon baking powder

¼ teaspoon baking soda

2 teaspoons ground cinnamon

¼ cup shortening

1. Preheat the oven to 375°F. Lightly spray 12 muffin cups with non-stick baking spray (or line with paper or foil liners).

2. In a medium bowl, whisk together the first four ingredients (milk through vanilla). Set aside.

3. In a large bowl, combine the next 8 ingredients (oats through cinnamon). Using your fingertips, a pastry blender, or a fork, cut the shortening into the flour mixture until the shortening is incorporated. Make a well in the center and add the milk mixture. Using a large spoon, stir until the dry ingredients are just moistened.

4. Spoon the batter evenly into prepared muffin tins, filling each cup two-thirds full.

5. Bake for 12 to 15 minutes or until the center springs back when lightly touched. Cool for 5 minutes before removing to a wire rack.

Marlene Says: *While "measures like sugar" sucralose-based sweeteners are still my preference for baking, when you see "or packets" after the no-calorie sweetener measurement, you can choose from either Splenda or Truvia (stevia-based) packets (or their generic equivalents).*

NUTRITION INFORMATION PER SERVING (1 muffin): Calories 140 | Carbohydrate 18g (Sugars 3g) | Total Fat 5.5 g (Sat Fat 1.5g) | Protein 4g | Fiber 3g | Cholesterol 20mg | Sodium 105mg | Food Exchanges: 1 Starch, 1 Fat | Carbohydrate Choices: 1 | Weight Watcher Plus Point Comparison: 3

Favorite Focaccia Muffins

WHEN MY BOYS WERE YOUNG one of their favorite places to eat was an Italian restaurant where the bread baskets were filled with warm Focaccia bread. Scented with fresh rosemary and dusted with Parmesan cheese, the bread made the meal. The first time he ate one of my focaccia muffins, my son James said they reminded him of that beloved restaurant. Needless to say, these have since become a family favorite.

MAKES **12** SERVINGS

¾ cup chopped onion

1 large egg

1½ cups low-fat buttermilk

3 tablespoons olive oil

2 cups all-purpose flour

1 tablespoon granulated sugar

1 tablespoon baking powder

1 teaspoon finely chopped fresh rosemary

½ cup and 1 tablespoon grated Parmesan cheese

½ teaspoon baking soda

½ teaspoon garlic powder

1. Preheat the oven to 400°F. Lightly spray 12 muffin cups with non-stick baking spray.

2. Place onions in microwave-safe bowl. Spray onions lightly with cooking spray and microwave on high for 2 minutes or until soft and translucent. In a medium bowl, whisk together the egg, buttermilk, and olive oil. Add the cooked onions and set aside.

3. In a large bowl, combine the remaining ingredients (flour through garlic powder using ½ cup of the Parmesan cheese). Create a well in the center and add the egg mixture. Using a large spoon, stir until the dry ingredients are just incorporated.

4. Spoon the batter evenly into prepared muffin tins, filling each cup two-thirds full.

5. Sprinkle each muffin with ¼ teaspoon of the remaining Parmesan cheese. Bake for 18 to 20 minutes or until lightly browned. Cool for 5 minutes before removing from tins. Serve warm.

Marlene Says: *These savory muffins add a great twist to the usual bread basket. Try them with 15-Minute Roasted Red Pepper Soup (page 123); Fast Fix Ratatouille (page 182) or Good and Easy Garlic Chicken (page 238).*

NUTRITION INFORMATION PER SERVING (1 muffin): Calories 150 | Carbohydrate 20g (Sugars 4g) | Total Fat 6g (Sat Fat 1.5g) | Protein 6g | Fiber 1g | Cholesterol 20mg | Sodium 240mg | Food Exchanges: 1 Starch, 1 Fat | Carbohydrate Choices: 1 | Weight Watcher Plus Point Comparison: 4

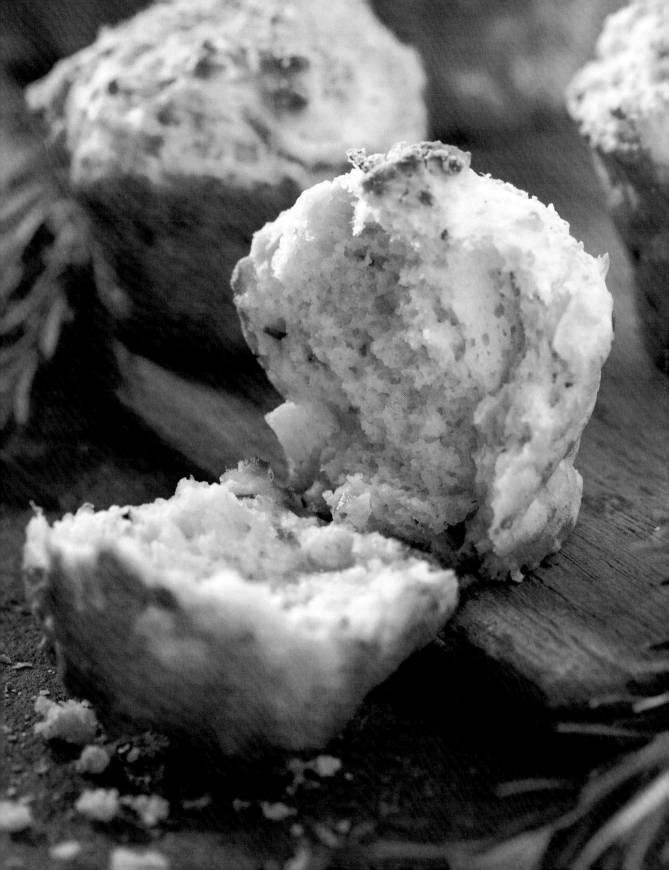

Cheddar Bay-Style Biscuits

WHEN IT COMES TO A POPULAR BISCUIT, the Cheddar Bay Biscuit served at Red Lobster, with its signature brush of butter and garlic, takes the prize. My version uses a healthy baking mix, sharper cheddar, and Old Bay seasoning to create a drop-style biscuit with more deliciously savory flavor and less fat. But of course, just like those at Red Lobster, these also come with a prize-winning brush of butter and garlic on top.

2 cups reduced-fat baking mix (like Bisquick Heart Smart)

½ teaspoon Old Bay seasoning

⅔ cup shredded reduced-fat sharp cheddar cheese

¾ cup low-fat buttermilk

2 tablespoons butter, melted

½ teaspoon garlic powder

1. Preheat the oven to 425°F. Lightly spray a large non-stick cookie sheet with non-stick cooking spray.

2. In a large bowl, mix together the baking mix and Old Bay seasoning. Add the cheddar and stir with a large spoon or spatula until just combined. Add the buttermilk and mix until just combined.

3. Remove mixture from bowl and mix slightly with hands, if needed, to finish combining. Divide dough into 12 equal drop biscuits (about ¼ cup of dough each) and place onto a prepared cookie sheet 2 inches apart. Bake for 13 to 15 minutes or until golden brown.

4. Remove from oven. In a small bowl, combine butter and garlic powder. Brush tops of biscuits with butter. Serve warm.

NUTRITION INFORMATION PER SERVING (1 biscuit): Calories 110 | Carbohydrate 15g (Sugars 2g) | Total Fat 3.5g (Sat Fat 1g) | Protein 4g | Fiber 0g | Cholesterol 0mg | Sodium 330mg | Food Exchanges: 1 Starch | Carbohydrate Choices: 1 | Weight Watcher Plus Point Comparison: 3

Bran-ana Nut Mini-Loaves

WONDERFULLY MOIST, THIS FIBER-RICH BANANA BREAD is loaded with the great taste of fresh bananas. My favorite way to bake this batter is to create two mini-loaves so I can use one and freeze the other. If you prefer to make one large loaf, bake the batter in a 9 x 5-inch loaf pan at 350°F for 50 to 60 minutes.

MAKES **12** SERVINGS

1 cup mashed banana
(about 2 medium bananas)

1 cup unsweetened
shredded bran cereal

¼ cup low-fat buttermilk

1 large egg

2 tablespoons canola oil

1 tablespoon molasses

1 teaspoon vanilla extract

½ cup white whole-wheat
flour

½ cup all-purpose flour

¼ cup granulated
no-calorie sweetener (or
6 packets)

2 teaspoons baking powder

1 teaspoon baking soda

⅓ cup chopped pecans

1. Preheat the oven to 375°F. Spray two small loaf pans with non-stick baking spray (or preheat oven to 350°F for one large loaf).

2. In a medium bowl, stir together the first 7 ingredients (banana through vanilla extract). Set aside for at least 5 minutes to soften bran.

3. In a large bowl, combine both flours, no-calorie sweetener, baking soda, baking powder, and pecans. Stir. Make a well in the center and add the banana mixture. Using a large spoon, stir just until the dry ingredients are incorporated.

4. Spoon batter into prepared loaf pans.

5. Bake for 30 minutes or until center springs back when lightly touched.

6. Remove from oven and let cool in pans for 10 minutes. Remove loaves from pans and allow to cool completely before cutting.

DARE TO COMPARE: Just because something is made with fruit doesn't mean it's better for you. One piece of Starbucks' Banana Nut Loaf packs 490 calories and more sugar and carbs than their Double Iced Cinnamon Roll.

NUTRITION INFORMATION PER SERVING (1 slice): Calories 120 | Carbohydrate 19g (Sugars 12g) | Total Fat 4.5 g (Sat Fat 1g) | Protein 3.5g | Fiber 4g | Cholesterol 0mg | Sodium 210mg | Food Exchanges: 1 Starch, 1 Fat | Carbohydrate Choices: 1 | Weight Watcher Plus Point Comparison: 3

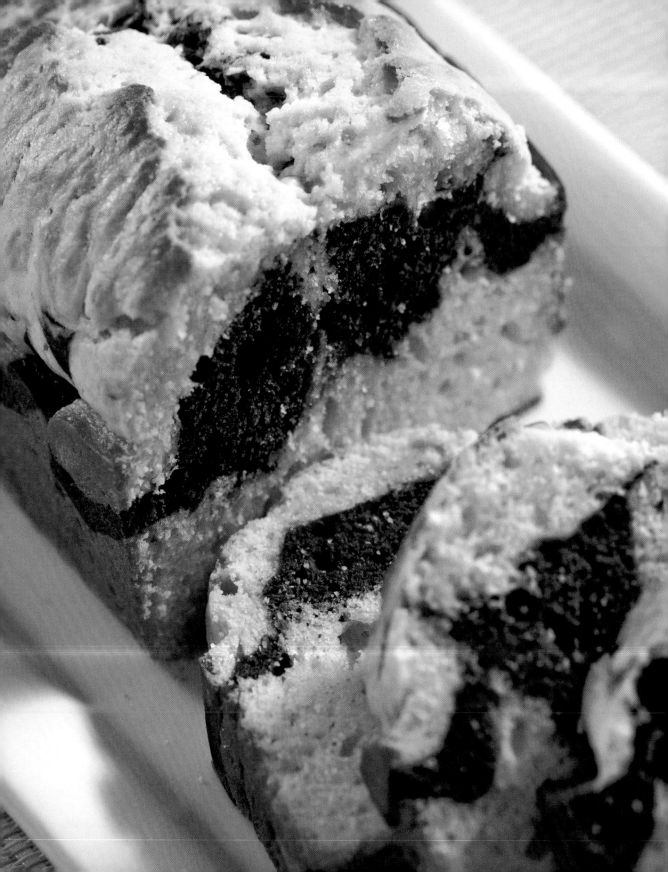

Marvelous Marble Poundcake

A GORGEOUS DARK CHOCOLATE SWIRL entwined with moist vanilla poundcake makes this marvelous loaf a real showstopper whether you eat it for breakfast—or for dessert! And while it may look complicated, it's really quite easy to make. This recipe makes a large loaf, so be sure to use a 9 x 5-inch (rather than 8 x 4-inch) loaf pan.

MAKES **12** SERVINGS

6 tablespoons margarine or butter

⅔ cup granulated sugar

⅔ cup granulated no-calorie sweetener (like Splenda)

2 large eggs

2 large egg whites

1½ teaspoons vanilla extract

2 ¼ cups cake flour

¾ teaspoon baking soda

⅛ teaspoon salt

¾ cup light sour cream

3 tablespoons cocoa powder (preferably Dutch-process)

2 tablespoons low-fat milk

1. Preheat oven to 325°F. Lightly spray a 9 x 5-inch loaf pan with non-stick baking spray.

2. In a large bowl, with an electric mixer, beat the margarine and sugar until very light and creamy (about 4 minutes). Add the sweetener and beat to incorporate. Add eggs and then egg whites, one by one, beating each time until creamy. Beat in vanilla extract.

3. Sift together flour, baking soda, and salt. By hand, stir one-half of the flour mixture into the creamed mixture. Stir in half of sour cream and repeat, stirring each time until ingredient is just incorporated.

4. Remove 1 cup of the batter and place in a small bowl. Sift the cocoa into the batter, add the milk, and lightly mix. Pour about two-thirds of the remaining batter into the prepared pan. Spoon dollops of the chocolate batter on top. Spoon remaining one-third of the plain batter between chocolate dollops. With a knife, swirl the batter gently to create a marbled effect.

5. Bake for 55 to 65 minutes or until a toothpick inserted into the center comes out clean. Cool in pan, on a wire rack, for 10 minutes before removing from pan.

Marlene Says: *Cake flour has a lower gluten content and produces a fine tender crumb. In a pinch you can substitute 1⅔ cups all-purpose flour plus ¼ cup cornstarch for the cake flour.*

NUTRITION INFORMATION PER SERVING (1 slice): Calories 190 | Carbohydrate 29g (Sugars 13g) | Total Fat 7g (Sat Fat 2.5g) | Protein 4g | Fiber 1g | Cholesterol 40mg | Sodium 180mg | Food Exchanges: 2 Starch, 1 Fat | Carbohydrate Choices: 2 | Weight Watcher Plus Point Comparison: 5

Razzle-Dazzle Lemon Loaf

LIKE MY MARVELOUS MARBLE POUNDCAKE, this is another coffeehouse favorite. I start with the same fabulous poundcake base as I do for my marble loaf but instead infuse it with the great taste of lemon and a dazzle of sweet raspberry puree. Rich, moist, and decadent, this is truly a treat any time of day.

MAKES **12** SERVINGS

2 tablespoons sugar-free raspberry jam

¾ cup frozen unsweetened raspberries, thawed

⅔ cup plus 1 tablespoon granulated no-calorie sweetener (like Splenda)

6 tablespoons margarine or butter, softened

⅔ cup granulated sugar

2 large eggs

2 large egg whites

1½ teaspoons vanilla extract

1½ teaspoon lemon zest

2¼ cups cake flour

¾ teaspoon baking soda

⅛ teaspoon salt

¾ cup light sour cream

2 teaspoons powdered sugar

1. Preheat oven to 325°F. Lightly spray a 9 x 5-inch loaf pan with non-stick baking spray. In a small bowl, combine jam, raspberries and 1 tablespoon of sweetener.

2. In a large bowl, with an electric mixer, beat margarine and sugar until light and creamy (about 4 minutes). Add sweetener and beat to incorporate. Add eggs and then egg whites, one by one, beating each time until creamy. Beat in vanilla extract and lemon zest.

3. Sift together flour, baking soda, and salt. By hand, stir half of flour mixture into creamed mixture. Stir in half of sour cream and then repeat the process, gently mixing each time until flour and sour cream is just incorporated.

4. Place half of the batter in prepared pan. Spoon raspberry mixture on top of the batter and spread to within ¼ inch of the edges. Carefully top with remaining batter and spread smoothly.

5. Bake for 55 to 65 minutes or until a toothpick inserted into the center comes out clean. Cool in pan, on a wire rack, for 10 minutes before removing from pan. Cool completely before dusting with powdered sugar.

DARE TO COMPARE: Starbucks incredibly popular Iced Lemon Pound cake serves up 490 calories, 23 grams of fat and 65 grams of carbohydrate per slice. This recipe saves you a trip to the coffee shop and 290 calories!

NUTRITION INFORMATION PER SERVING (1 slice): Calories 200 | Carbohydrate 30g (Sugars 13g) | Total Fat 7g (Sat Fat 2.5g) | Protein 4g | Fiber 1g | Cholesterol 40mg | Sodium 180mg | Food Exchanges: 2 Starch | Carbohydrate Choices: 2 | Weight Watcher Plus Point Comparison: 5

Chocolate Zucchini Bread

*I wish I could eat this every day—it's **that** good. The orange-chocolate combination is utterly delicious and the zucchini, while it imparts no taste, keeps the bread marvelously moist. The fact that this bread has only one-third the sugar and half the fat of most zucchini bread recipes is, of course, an added bonus. A healthy bread that tastes totally decadent—what's not to love?*

MAKES **12** SERVINGS

¼ cup canola oil

¼ cup brown sugar

⅔ cup granulated no-calorie sweetener (like Splenda)

1 large egg

1 large egg white

½ cup unsweetened applesauce

1 teaspoon vanilla extract

1½ cups grated zucchini

1½ cups all-purpose flour

2 teaspoons orange zest

½ cup cocoa powder (preferably Dutch-process)

1 teaspoon baking powder

¾ teaspoon baking soda

1. Preheat oven to 350°F. Spray a 9 x 5-inch loaf pan with non-stick baking spray.

2. In a medium bowl, whisk together the oil, brown sugar, sweetener, eggs, applesauce and vanilla. With a large spoon, stir in the grated zucchini and mix until well combined.

3. In a medium bowl, combine remaining ingredients. Create a well in the center and add the zucchini mixture. Stir until the dry ingredients are just moistened. Spoon mixture into prepared pan and smooth.

4. Bake for 50 to 55 minutes or until a toothpick inserted into the center comes out clean. Cool in pan on a wire rack for 10 to 15 minutes and then remove from pan.

Marlene Says: *This batter is fabulous for gift loaves. To make smaller loaves, fill loaf pans two-thirds full with batter and cook for 30 to 35 minutes, depending on size of pans.*

NUTRITION INFORMATION PER SERVING (1 slice): Calories 120 | Carbohydrate 19g (Sugars 6g) | Total Fat 3.5g (Sat Fat 1g) | Protein 3g | Fiber 1g | Cholesterol 20mg | Sodium 140mg | Food Exchanges: 1 Starch | Carbohydrate Choices: 1 | Weight Watcher Plus Point Comparison: 3

Berry Best Old Fashioned Coffee Cake

CROWNED WITH BROWN SUGAR, CINNAMON, AND WALNUTS, and baked in an angel food pan, this is a beauty of a coffee cake. A peek inside reveals a moist cake studded with plenty of fresh berries. Blueberries hold their shape best (and they don't dye the cake), but I leave the final choice up to you. The traditional recipe for this cake called for 38 tablespoons of sugar. An 85% reduction in sugar (and 50% in fat) makes this cake one of my best.

MAKES **12** SERVING

2 cups all-purpose flour

½ teaspoon baking soda

2 teaspoons baking powder

⅓ cup cold butter or margarine

2 cups fresh berries

2 large eggs

2 large egg whites

1½ cups granulated no-calorie sweetener (like Splenda), divided

5 tablespoons brown sugar, divided

1½ teaspoons vanilla extract

1 cup light sour cream or low-fat plain Greek yogurt

⅓ cup finely chopped walnuts

1 teaspoon cinnamon

2 teaspoons powdered sugar

1. Preheat the oven to 350°F. Lightly coat a 10-inch tube (or angel food) pan with nonstick baking spray.

2. To make the cake batter, whisk together the flour, baking soda, and baking powder large bowl. Add the butter and cut it in until it is thoroughly incorporated. Add the berries, mix gently, and set aside.

3. In a medium bowl, with an electric mixer, beat the eggs, egg whites, 1¼ cups sweetener, and 3 tablespoons brown sugar together until the eggs double in volume and the mixture is light and foamy. Stir in the vanilla and sour cream. Make a well in the center and add the flour mixture. Use a large spoon to mix until just moistened and spoon batter into the prepared pan.

4. In a small bowl combine walnuts, ¼ cup sweetener, 2 tablespoons brown sugar and 1 teaspoon cinnamon. Sprinkle over the top of the cake and bake for 45 minutes or until a toothpick inserted into the center comes out clean. Cool on a wire rack and dust with powdered sugar.

NUTRITION INFORMATION PER SERVING (1 piece): Calories 210 | Carbohydrate 28g (Sugars 7g) | Total Fat 8g (Sat Fat 3g) | Protein 5g | Fiber 1g | Cholesterol 25mg | Sodium 140 mg | Food Exchanges: 2 Starch, 1 Fat | Carbohydrate Choices: 2 | Weight Watcher Plus Point Comparison: 5

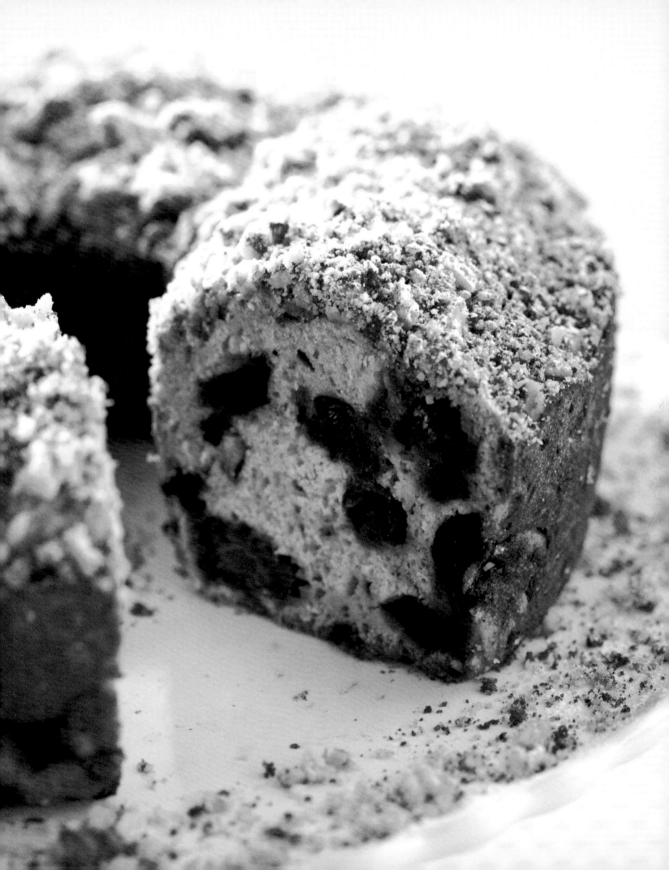

Chocolate Chip Quick Cake

HOMEMADE DOESN'T GET MUCH QUICKER THAN THIS. One bowl, a few stirs of the spoon, and 20 minutes later you have a healthy homemade coffeecake on the table. The coconut extract really adds to the great taste. Look for it in the baker's aisle with the other extracts and keep it on hand for recipes, such as my Coconut, Coconut Shrimp (page 107).

MAKES **12** SERVINGS

1¾ cup reduced-fat baking mix (like Heart Smart Bisquick)

⅓ cup granulated no-calorie sweetener (or 8 packets)

⅓ cup mini chocolate chips

⅔ cup low-fat milk

1 large egg, lightly beaten

1 tablespoon canola oil

½ teaspoon vanilla extract

¼ teaspoon coconut extract

¼ cup sliced almonds or pecans (optional)

1. Preheat oven to 350°F. Spray an 8-inch square baking pan with non-stick baking spray.

2. In a large bowl, combine baking mix, sweetener, and chocolate chips. Stir in milk, egg, oil, vanilla extract, and coconut extract. Stir just until smooth.

3. Pour into prepared baking pan. Sprinkle with sliced almonds, if desired. Bake for 12 to 15 minutes, or until the center springs back when lightly touched. Cool for 5 minutes before removing to a wire rack.

Marlene Says: *My family really enjoys this topped with the almonds or chopped pecans. The nuts add 20 calories per serving.*

NUTRITION INFORMATION PER SERVING (1 piece): Calories 110 | Carbohydrate 17g (Sugars 4g) | Total Fat 4g (Sat Fat 1.5g) | Protein 2g | Fiber 0g | Cholesterol 20mg | Sodium 220mg | Food Exchanges: 1 Starch | Carbohydrate Choices: 1 | Weight Watcher Plus Point Comparison: 3

breakfast and brunch

Grab 'n Go Oat Bars

Big Bowl Carrot Cake Oatmeal

The Elvis Oat Bowl

Denver-Style Egg White Melt

Amazing 2-Minute Egg Muggs

Chuck's Everyday Egg Scramble

Creamy Scrambled Eggs in Crispy Potato Skins

Easy Morning Egg "McMuffin®" Strata

Chile Relleño Casserole

Quick 'n Easy Quiche

Eggs Benedict

Chicken Hash

Crispy Waffles with Creamy Maple Syrup

Wholesome Silver Dollar Hots

Strawberry Cheesecake Pancake Stacks

Berry Good Breakfast Sundaes

A great day starts with a *great breakfast*! Unfortunately, less than one-third of us heed the message. Research continues to support the many benefits of eating a nutritious breakfast—including new evidence that *breakfast is a powerful weapon* in the battle of the bulge. A recent study at Harvard concluded that breakfast skippers are four times more likely to gain weight than their breakfast-loving counterparts. Add that to the evidence that shows that breakfast food is good mood and brain food and it's easy to see why people who eat breakfast tend to be *smarter, thinner, and happier*. Researchers have also zeroed in on the importance of eating protein at breakfast. They've found that protein not only provides a feeling of fullness, it helps sustain energy by keeping blood sugar on an even keel. Speaking of breakfast protein, the good old egg—one of nature's *richest* sources of *protein*—has been found to be *better for you than ever*. Recent analysis shows that eggs have 14% *less* cholesterol and 64% *more* Vitamin D than once thought.

Here you will find more than a dozen *delicious* ways to enjoy protein-rich eggs, *plus* *wholesome* oats, fluffy pancakes, crispy waffles, and a "berry good" breakfast sundae! Hurried mornings require something extra fast and that's what you'll get with nutritious Grab 'n Go Oat Bars, Amazing 2-Minute Egg Muggs, or a Denver-Style Egg White Melt. When time is not quite as tight, *proven family favorites* like the Easy Morning Egg McMuffin Strata, Crispy Waffles with Creamy Maple Syrup, or *melt-in-your-mouth* Wholesome Silver Dollar Hots will keep the family happy (and healthy). For special occasions, or special guests, a great way to start the day is with easy elegant Eggs Benedict, or with what may be the *ultimate* decadent breakfast—Strawberry Cheesecake Pancake Stacks!

Grab 'n Go Oat Bars

MAKING YOUR OWN BREAKFAST BARS has never been easier. In less than 20 minutes you'll have a dozen wholesome grab 'n go bars that you can eat for a delicious, nutritious breakfast or in-between meal snack—all at a fraction of the cost of those you buy. Cooled and sliced bars will stay fresh for up to five days in the fridge in a sealed container or, when individually wrapped, for up to two weeks (or more) in the freezer. Quick-thaw the frozen bars by popping one in the microwave for 30 seconds on high. Mmm . . .

MAKES **12** SERVING

2 cups quick oats

1 cup white whole-wheat flour

¾ cup granulated no-calorie sweetener (like Splenda)

3 tablespoons brown sugar

1 teaspoon ground cinnamon

¾ teaspoon baking soda

½ teaspoon baking powder

¼ cup dried cranberries, chopped finely

¼ cup chopped walnuts

¼ cup prune puree (or 3.5-ounce package baby food prunes)

3 tablespoons canola oil

3 egg whites

1 tablespoon molasses

1½ teaspoons vanilla extract

1. Preheat oven to 350°F. Lightly spray a 9 x 9-inch baking pan with non-stick cooking spray.

2. In a very large bowl, mix together the first 9 ingredients (oats through walnuts). Set aside. In a medium bowl, whisk together remaining 5 ingredients (prunes through vanilla). Pour prune mixture over dry ingredients. Mix with spoon until all ingredients are combined. Batter will be sticky.

3. Spread batter into baking pan and bake for 12 minutes. Do not overbake. Set baking pan on rack to cool. Cut into 12 bars.

DARE TO COMPARE: With 75% less sugar than an Oatmeal-to-Go bar, these whole grain anytime snack bars are full of healthy goodness. Feel free to get creative and mix and match various baby food purees along with different types of nuts and dried fruit.

NUTRITION INFORMATION PER SERVING (1 bar): Calories 130 | Carbohydrate 18g (Sugars 5g) | Total Fat 5g (Sat Fat 0g) | Protein 5g | Fiber 3g | Cholesterol 0mg | Sodium 90mg | Food Exchanges: 1 Starch | Carbohydrate Choices: 1 | Weight Watcher Plus Point Comparison: 3

Big Bowl Carrot Cake Oatmeal

YES, "CARROT CAKE" FOR BREAKFAST! No, you're not dreaming. I must admit that when I first came across the idea of adding shredded carrot to oatmeal I too found it a bit strange. I quickly realized, however, that since many carrot cake recipes contain oats, carrot could be a tasty addition to oatmeal— especially if you were to include all the great flavors that go into a carrot cake! With double the daily recommended value of Vitamin A, a healthy dose of fiber, and a sweet, creamy, nutty topping, this bowl of oatmeal takes the cake.

MAKES **1** SERVING

1 medium carrot finely grated (about ⅓ cup)

Pinch salt

½ cup old-fashioned oats

2 teaspoons brown sugar, divided

½ teaspoon ground cinnamon

⅛ teaspoon ground ginger

⅛ teaspoon nutmeg

4 teaspoons granulated no-calorie sweetener (or 2 packets)

½ teaspoon vanilla extract

1 tablespoon chopped pecans

2 teaspoons nonfat half-and-half

1. In a small saucepan, combine the grated carrot, 1½ cups water and salt and bring to a boil. Reduce heat and simmer for 2 minutes. Add oats and simmer for 5 additional minutes. Stir in 1 teaspoon of brown sugar and spices and simmer for 2 more minutes.

2. Remove from heat and add sweetener and vanilla extract. Let sit for 1 to 2 minutes to thicken.

3. Top with chopped pecans, half-and-half, and remaining teaspoon of brown sugar.

Marlene Says: *The trifecta of adding additional water, fiber-rich carrot, and rich pecans produces a "big" bowl of oatmeal that's sure to satisfy.*

NUTRITION INFORMATION PER SERVING: Calories 255 | Carbohydrate 38g (Sugars 7g) | Total Fat 7g (Sat Fat 1g) | Protein 8g | Fiber 6g | Cholesterol 0mg | Sodium 260mg | Food Exchanges: 2 Starch, 1 Fat | Carbohydrate Choices: 2 | Weight Watcher Plus Point Comparison: 6

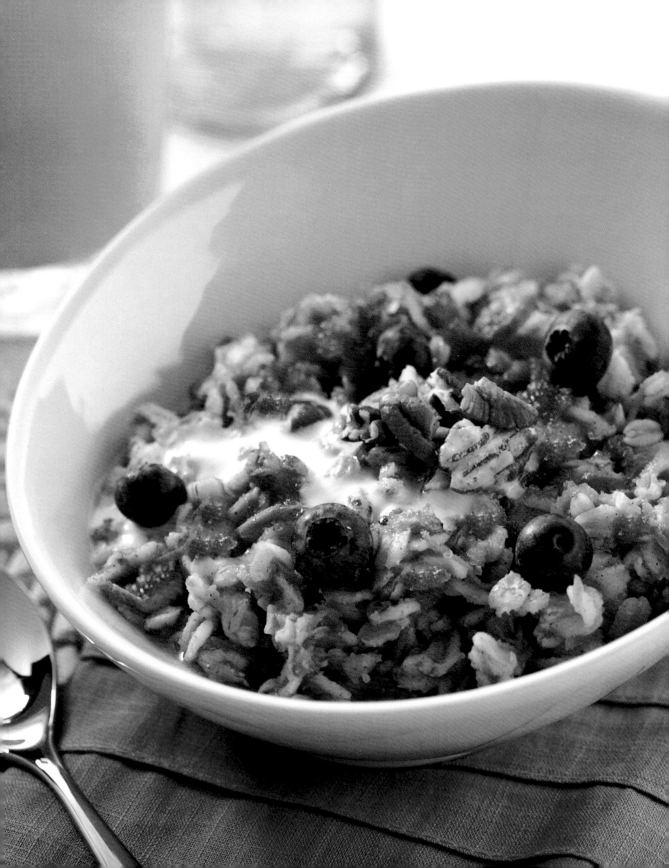

The Elvis Oat Bowl

*DARE I SUGGEST that if Elvis had started his day with this delicious belly-filling oatmeal he might have been more fit? While the King of Rock & Roll was no health nut, he **was** onto something with his love of the flavorful combination of peanut butter and bananas. If he had only added oats he would have found himself with a dynamic trio of ingredients that not only provide a satisfying breakfast, but keep blood sugar stable and waistlines trim.*

MAKES **1** SERVING

⅓ cup old-fashioned oats

1 cup water

Pinch salt

1 tablespoon peanut butter (I like mine smooth)

3 tablespoons sugar-free maple syrup

One-half small banana, thinly sliced (about ¼ cup)

½ tablespoon chopped peanuts, optional

1. In a small saucepan, add oats to water and bring to a boil. Reduce heat and simmer for 6 to 7 minutes or until most of the water is absorbed. Stir in peanut butter and 2 tablespoons of the syrup.

2. Spoon into a bowl and arrange banana slices across the top. Drizzle on the remaining syrup and sprinkle with chopped peanuts for extra flavor and crunch, if desired.

Marlene Says: *For the creamiest oatmeal, always combine uncooked oats with cold water and then bring to a boil, rather than stirring the oats into boiling water.*

NUTRITION INFORMATION PER SERVING: Calories 250 | Carbohydrate 34g (Sugars 9g) | Total Fat 9g (Sat Fat 2) | Protein 9g | Fiber 5g | Cholesterol 0g | Sodium 260mg | Food Exchanges 1 ½ Starch, ½ Fruit, 1 High Fat Meat | Carbohydrate Choices 1 ½ | Weight Watcher Plus Point Comparison: 7

Denver-Style Egg White Melt

WHILE BREAKFAST SANDWICHES have recently soared in popularity, this skinny open-faced egg melt is one that I have enjoyed on my own for years. With only 170 calories and 2 grams of fat, it's a stellar choice for anyone watching their carbs or calories. The sautéed onions and peppers really perk up the flavor of plain egg whites; for extra sizzle try adding diced jalapeño.

MAKES **1** SERVING

2 slices lean deli-style ham, thinly sliced (about ½ ounce)

3 tablespoons finely diced onion

2 tablespoons finely diced green pepper

2 large egg whites, beaten

3 tablespoons shredded reduced-fat cheddar cheese

1 slice sourdough bread

Salt and pepper to taste

1. Spray a medium-sized skillet with non-stick cooking spray and place over medium heat. Add the ham, cook for 30 seconds on each side or until lightly browned, remove and set aside.

2. Lightly spray the pan with cooking spray again. Add the onions and cook for 3 minutes or until lightly browned. Add green pepper and cook for another 2 minutes or until peppers are soft.

3. Pour the beaten egg whites into the pan. While cooking, use a spatula to push egg mixture into a shape that will fit the size of the bread. When the underside is slightly browned, flip the eggs and cook the other side until lightly browned.

4. Top the egg white patty with shredded cheese, add 1 teaspoon of water to the pan, and cover for 30 seconds to melt the cheese. Toast the bread and place the ham on top. Remove the eggs from the pan and slide onto the ham and bread. Add salt and pepper to taste.

Marlene Says: *Feel free to add an extra piece of bread to "sandwich" this melt. Either add another piece of sourdough (a great "white" choice due to its lower glycemic index) for 70 calories, or switch to 2 slices of toasted light bread for only 20 calories more and the added bonus of 4 grams of fiber!*

NUTRITION INFORMATION PER SERVING: Calories 170 | Carbohydrate 18g (Sugars 3g) | Total Fat 2g (Sat Fat 1g) | Protein 18g | Fiber 1g | Cholesterol 10mg | Sodium 580mg | Food Exchanges: 1 Starch, 2 Lean Meat | Carbohydrate Choices: 1 | Weight Watcher Plus Point Comparison: 4

Amazing Two-Minute Egg Muggs

IF YOU'VE NEVER COOKED AN EGG IN A MUG, get ready to be amazed. These beauties puff up like mini soufflés and in just two minutes, breakfast is served—without an egg-y pan to wash! What's also amazing are the endless variations you can create with Egg Muggs (I've included two of my favorites). After testing egg substitutes, I prefer the superior flavor and texture of fresh eggs for this dish, but you can use an egg substitute if you wish.

MAKES **1** SERVING

1 large egg

1 large egg white

2 teaspoons low-fat milk or water

Pinch of salt and pepper

1. Spray a large, microwave-safe mug with non-stick cooking spray. Add eggs, milk, and salt and pepper to the mug and whisk with a fork until light and frothy.

2. Microwave on high for 1 minute. Remove mug and lightly stir eggs. Microwave for another 45 seconds or until eggs are set (eggs will puff up way beyond edge of cup during cooking and then settle down).

All-American Mugg: After microwaving egg mixture for 1 minute, add 2 tablespoons of chopped lean ham (about 2 thin slices) and 1 tablespoon shredded reduced-fat cheddar cheese. Finish cooking as in Step 2 (adds 45 calories, 5 grams protein, 2 grams fat). Season with salt and pepper.

South of the Border Mugg: Substitute salsa for milk or water. After microwaving egg mixture for 1 minute, add 1 tablespoon grated reduced-fat Mexican blend cheese. Finish cooking as in Step 2. Top with 2 teaspoons light sour cream (adds 35 calories, 3 grams protein, 2 grams fat).

NUTRITION INFORMATION PER SERVING (1 plain egg mug): Calories 100 | Carbohydrate 1g (Sugars 1g) | Total Fat 5g (Sat Fat 1.5g) | Protein 10g | Fiber 0 | Cholesterol 215mg | Sodium 125mg | Food Exchanges: 1 Medium Fat Meat, 1 Lean Meat | Carbohydrate Choices: 0 | Weight Watcher Plus Point Comparison: 2

Chuck's Everyday Egg Scramble

TASTIER THAN PLAIN SCRAMBLED EGGS and faster to fix than omelets or frittatas, egg scrambles strike the perfect balance between easy and healthy. My husband, Chuck, who whips up a healthy egg scramble most mornings, has become an expert at mixing and matching veggie drawer leftovers with fresh eggs and a bit of cheese, but this particular combo is one of his favorites. Flipping the warm pan over the omelet to melt the cheese is a quick-fix technique he is particularly proud to own.

MAKES **1** SERVING

3 tablespoons chopped onion

⅓ cup diced zucchini

¼ cup diced green or sweet peppers

3 tablespoons corn niblets (fresh, frozen, or canned)

Pinch of garlic salt

Black pepper to taste (Chuck says, use plenty)

1 large egg

2 large egg whites

2 teaspoons grated Parmesan cheese

1. Spray a non-stick skillet with cooking spray and place over medium high heat. Add the onion to the pan and cook for 1 to 2 minutes or until slightly softened. Add zucchini, peppers, corn and spices and sauté for 3 to 4 minutes or until vegetables soften.

2. Whisk the egg and egg whites together in a small bowl. Pour eggs over vegetables and let sit for one minute. Using a spatula, push cooked egg mixture toward the center while letting uncooked egg flow to the edges. When most of egg is cooked, flip and cook on other side for 30 seconds to 1 minute, or just until done.

3. Slide scramble onto a plate, sprinkle with cheese (or grate cheese directly onto eggs), and immediately turn the warm skillet over to cover the scramble. Let sit 1 minute. (This is a good time to pop some bread in the toaster, if you desire). Uncover and eat!

Marlene Says: *Go ahead; clean out the veggie drawer with this one. Any non-starchy veggies—such as mushrooms, yellow squash, spinach, asparagus or broccoli—can be swapped for the onions, peppers, and zucchini, while beans can replace the corn. (Corn may sound odd with eggs, but it adds a lovely unexpected sweetness. One bite and you'll be hooked.)*

NUTRITION INFORMATION PER SERVING: Calories 180 | Carbohydrate 15g (Sugars 5g) | Total Fat 6g (Sat Fat 2.5g) | Protein 17g | Fiber 3g | Cholesterol 185mg | Sodium 360mg | Food Exchanges: 2 Low Fat Meat, 1 Vegetable, ½ Starch, 1 Fat | Carbohydrate Choices: 1 | Weight Watcher Plus Point Comparison: 4

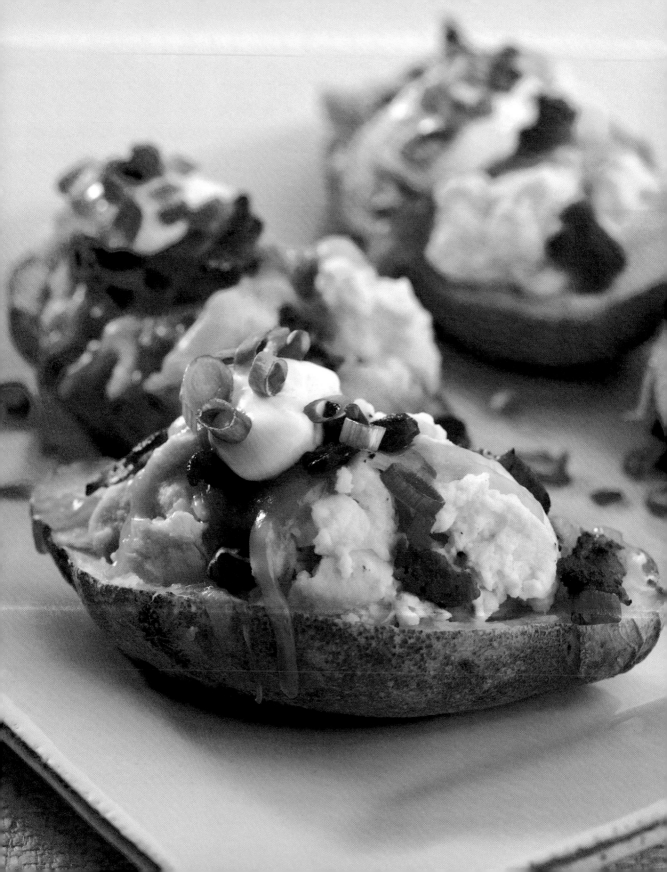

Creamy Scrambled Eggs in Crispy Potato Skins

HERE'S A DISH THAT'S SURE TO IMPRESS. My kitchen assistant Roberta was very skeptical at first about stuffing potatoes with scrambled eggs, but the end result blew away every reservation. Creamy scrambled eggs are tucked into a scooped out crispy potato skins and then topped with the usual toppings—bacon, cheese, sour cream, and green onions. I promise you, potatoes and eggs have never complemented each other better.

MAKES **4** SERVINGS

2 (12-ounce) baking potatoes, washed

4 large eggs, beaten

4 large egg whites, beaten

3 tablespoons, plus 4 teaspoons light sour cream

⅛ teaspoon each salt and black pepper

2 tablespoons chopped green onions

¼ cup shredded reduced-fat cheddar cheese

4 teaspoons real bacon bits

4 teaspoons finely chopped green onion tops

1. To prepare the potato skins, pierce potatoes with a fork and place in the microwave. Cook on high for 10 minutes. While potatoes are cooking, preheat oven to 425°F. Remove potatoes from microwave and cut lengthwise. Scoop out the potato pulp, leaving ¼ inch of potato in the skin. Place skins onto a baking sheet and lightly spray with cooking oil. Bake for 10 to 12 minutes or until skin is crispy. (Discard potato pulp or reserve for another use.)

2. While potato skins are baking, whisk together the eggs, egg whites, and 3 tablespoons of sour cream. Spray a medium-size skillet with non-stick cooking spray and place over medium low heat. Add eggs to pan and cook, stirring gently, for 2 to 3 minutes or until curds start to form. Add green onion and continue to cook for additional minute or two or until eggs are just set (eggs should be creamy, not dry).

3. Pile eggs into crispy potato skins. Top each with 1 tablespoon of cheddar cheese, 1 teaspoon light sour cream, 1 teaspoon of real bacon bits, and additional finely chopped green onion for garnish. Serve hot.

NUTRITION INFORMATION PER SERVING: Calories 230 | Carbohydrate 24g (Sugars 3g) | Total Fat 7g (Sat Fat 3g) | Protein 15g | Fiber 2g | Cholesterol 220mg | Sodium 250mg | Food Exchanges: 2 Medium Fat Meat, 1½ Starch | Carbohydrate Choices: 1 ½ | Weight Watcher Plus Point Comparison: 6

Easy Morning Egg "McMuffin®" Strata

INSPIRED BY THE CLASSIC EGG MCMUFFIN, this easy morning bake is as family friendly as it gets. Fuss-free and made with easy-to-keep-on-hand ingredients, you can make it the night before or simply assemble it in the morning, and set it aside to soak as you sip your coffee. The oven does the rest of the work. My Mickey D-loving boys enjoy it as is, but feel free to add sautéed mushrooms or a touch of hot sauce if you please.

MAKES **4** TO **6** SERVINGS

4 light English muffins (like Thomas's 100-Calorie English Muffins)

6 slices (about 3 ounces) Canadian bacon, roughly chopped

¼ cup chopped green onion

¾ cup shredded reduced-fat cheddar cheese

4 large eggs

4 large egg whites (or ½ cup liquid egg substitute)

1¾ cups low-fat milk

¾ teaspoon dry mustard

¼ teaspoon salt

⅛ teaspoon black pepper

1. Preheat oven to 350°F. Spray a 9-inch square baking dish with non-stick cooking spray.

2. Split the muffins and then tear them into medium-sized pieces. Evenly distribute muffin pieces into baking dish and top with Canadian bacon pieces. Sprinkle with green onion and shredded cheese.

3. Whisk together eggs and remaining ingredients in a medium bowl. Pour egg and milk mixture over muffin pieces. Cover and refrigerate for at least 30 minutes (can be done up to 8 hours in advance).

4. Uncover and bake for 35 to 40 minutes or until a knife inserted in the center comes out clean. Let stand 5 to 10 minutes before serving.

Marlene Says: *One hundred calorie "light" English muffins not only have fewer calories than their traditional counterparts, but significantly more fiber (up to 8 grams of fiber per muffin!). Note: This dish makes four ample servings; if you choose the six-portion yield, then it contains 210 calories, 17 carb grams, 8 fat grams, and 6 Weight Watcher Plus Comparison Points.*

NUTRITION INFORMATION PER SERVING (¼ of recipe): Calories 315 | Carbohydrate 26g (Sugars 1g) | Total Fat 12g (Sat Fat 4g) | Protein 25g | Fiber 6g | Cholesterol 230mg | Sodium 680mg | Food Exchanges: 3 Medium Fat Meat, 1 Starch, ½ Low-Fat Milk | Carbohydrate Choices: 1 ½ Weight Watcher Plus Point Comparison: 8

Chile Relleño Casserole

THIS BREAKFAST CASSEROLE has been a favorite at our family gatherings for years. Perfect for brunches, Mexican buffets, and meatless meals, it's an easy dish to fix for a crowd. I have taken the liberty of lightening my mother's recipe by reducing the amount of cheese and using low-fat milk, and with no disrespect to Mom, I think this version tastes more like a true chile relleño. Top with salsa, fresh cilantro and enchilada sauce, if desired.

MAKES **4** SERVINGS

4 large eggs, separated

1½ cups low-fat milk

½ cup all-purpose flour

¼ teaspoon salt

2 (4-ounce) cans peeled whole green chilies, drained

4 ounces (about ½ cup) reduced-fat shredded Mexican Blend cheese

1. Preheat the oven to 350°F. Spray an 11 x 7-inch (2-quart) baking pan with cooking spray.

2. In a medium bowl, whisk together the egg yolks and milk. Stir in flour and salt until smooth. Set aside. In a large bowl, with an electric mixer, beat the egg whites on high speed until soft peaks form. Gently fold the egg yolk mixture into the egg whites until no trace of whites remains.

3. Spread a very thin layer of egg mixture on the bottom of baking pan. Lay chilies on top of egg mixture, covering entire casserole. Sprinkle cheese over the chilies. Spoon the remaining egg mixture evenly over the cheese layer and spread to smooth.

4. Bake uncovered for 30 minutes or until the top is golden brown or a toothpick inserted into the center comes out clean.

Marlene Says: *I'm all for simplicity. While beating the egg whites separately is an extra step, it's worth it with this recipe as it gives this casserole the light and airy texture that is a hallmark of traditional hand-battered chile relleños.*

NUTRITION INFORMATION PER SERVING: Calories 240 | Carbohydrate 21g (Sugars 5g) | Total Fat 10g (Sat Fat 3.5g) | Protein 16g | Fiber 2g | Cholesterol 220mg | Sodium 620 mg | Food Exchanges: 2 Medium Fat Meat, 1 Starch, 1 Vegetable, 1 Fat | Carbohydrate Choices: 1 ½ | Weight Watcher Plus Point Comparison: 6

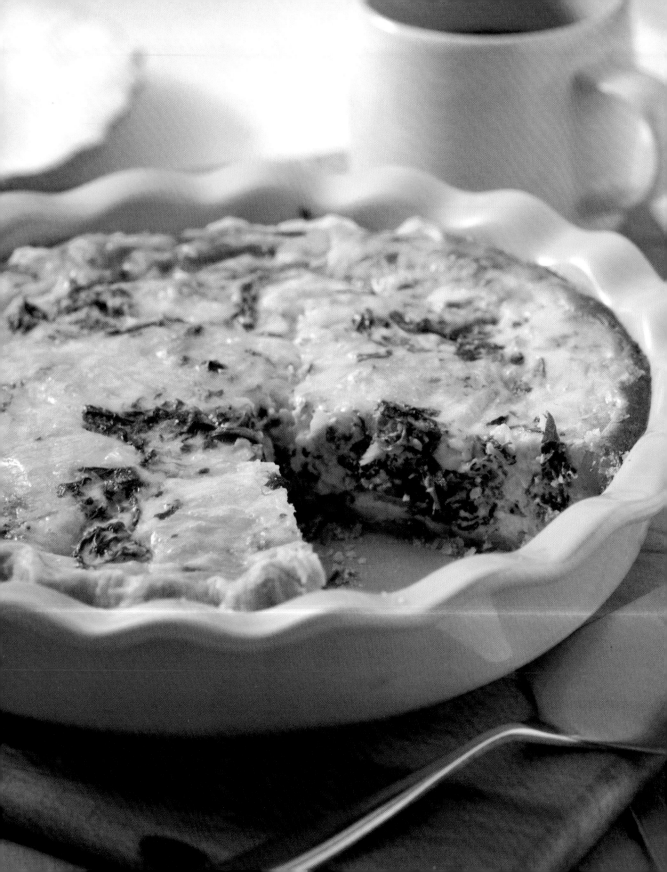

Quick 'n Easy Quiche

*QUICHE HAS BEEN ONE OF THE MOST REQUESTED RECIPES from my readers—probably because the traditional version packs more than 500 calories and 30 grams of fat in one slice! Up to the challenge, I tested many versions until I hit upon an unlikely ingredient that made this recipe work: mayonnaise. Just a touch of light mayo provides the extra creamy and dense texture quiche lovers enjoy with less fat than half-and-half or cream. And because I wanted you to have it **all**, this version features both quiche Lorraine and Florentine flavors together in perfect balance.*

MAKES **8** SERVINGS

1 (8-inch) frozen pie crust

⅓ cup minced onion

4 large eggs

4 large egg whites (or ½ cup liquid egg substitute)

⅓ cup reduced-fat mayonnaise

1 cup low-fat milk

¼ teaspoon garlic powder

¼ teaspoon liquid smoke

1 (10-ounce) package frozen spinach, thawed and squeezed dry

1 cup shredded reduced-fat Swiss cheese

1. Preheat the oven to 425°F. Using a fork, pierce pie crust all over its surface. Bake pie crust for 5 minutes. Remove from oven. Reduce oven temperature to 350°F.

2. Place onion in a small microwave-safe bowl and microwave on high for 1 minute. Set aside.

3. In a large bowl, whisk together 2 whole eggs and mayonnaise until thoroughly blended. Whisk in remaining eggs, egg whites, milk, and spices. Stir in spinach and cheese and mix until thoroughly combined. Pour into pie crust and bake for 45 minutes or until the center feels firm to the touch.

Marlene Says: *To create Quick 'n Easy Crustless Quiche Cups, ladle ½ cup of quiche mix into eight 6-ounce baking ramekins that have been lightly sprayed with non-stick cooking spray and placed on a baking sheet. Bake at 350°F for 40 to 45 minutes. (Each cup has 120 calories, 7 grams of fat, 5 grams carbohydrate, and 3 Weight Watcher Comparison Points.)*

NUTRITION INFORMATION PER SERVING: Calories 220 | Carbohydrate 13g (Sugars 3g) | Total Fat 13g (Sat Fat 4.5g) | Protein 11g | Fiber 1g | Cholesterol 135mg | Sodium 320mg | Food Exchanges: 1½ Medium Fat Meat, 1 Starch, 2 Fat | Carbohydrate Choices: 1 | Weight Watcher Plus Point Comparison: 6

Eggs Benedict

NOTHING SAYS SPLURGE LIKE A PLATE OF EGGS BENEDICT crowned with rich, silky hollandaise sauce. In re-creating this special dish, I knew that lightening up the hollandaise sauce would not be easy. I am delighted to say that after countless trials with the help of a classically trained chef, my wonderful assistant Judy, a luxurious, yet healthy hollandaise sauce adorns this dish. It's hard to believe that anything that tastes this decadent is diet- friendly.

MAKES **2** TO **4** SERVINGS

Hollandaise Sauce (page 223)*

4 slices Canadian bacon

2 large eggs

2 large egg whites

4 light English muffins (like Thomas's 100-Calorie English Muffins)

* *You will only use one-half the hollandaise sauce for this recipe. You can double the recipe or serve the leftover hollandaise over potatoes or steamed vegetables.*

1. Make the hollandaise sauce according to directions. Keep warm by covering and placing back over the pot after water cools from simmering to warm. Brown the Canadian bacon in a large skillet over medium high heat and set aside. Split English muffins and ready halves for toasting.

2. Spray a medium non-stick skillet with non-stick cooking spray and place over medium heat. In a medium bowl, whisk together eggs, egg whites, a pinch of salt and pepper to taste. Start toasting English muffins. Pour egg mixture into heated skillet and push cooked egg to the center of the pan with a spatula, lifting if necessary, to allow uncooked egg to flow to the edges as you lightly stir, until eggs are softly cooked.

3. Place 1 or 2 toasted English muffin halves on each plate and top each with one slice Canadian bacon. Divide eggs among muffins and top each with 1½ tablespoons of hollandaise sauce. Sprinkle with chopped chives, if desired.

DARE TO COMPARE: An order of Eggs Benedict at IHOP serves up a heart-clutching 1,020 calories, a full day's worth of saturated fat, 2½ days' worth of cholesterol, and 3,140 mg of sodium.

NUTRITION INFORMATION PER SERVING (Each topped muffin half): Calories 165 | Carbohydrate 14g (Sugars 1g) | Total Fat 8g (Sat Fat 3.5g) | Protein 12g | Fiber 4g | Cholesterol 140mg | Sodium 420mg | Food Exchanges: 1½ Lean Meat, 1 Starch, 1 Fat | Carbohydrate Choices: 1 | Weight Watcher Plus Point Comparison: 3

Chicken Hash

HERE'S A DISH THAT TURNED ME into an anytime hash lover. While I had always thought of hash as a hearty breakfast dish (and a clever way to use up leftover meat and potatoes), I found myself digging into the leftovers of this recipe morning, noon, and night. Top or serve with your choice of eggs for breakfast or with a salad for a light lunch or dinner. (For an even more nutritious and colorful dish, try swapping in sweet potatoes or yams for the Yukon Golds.)

MAKES **4** SERVINGS

2 cups diced Yukon Gold potatoes

½ cup reduced sodium chicken broth, divided

2 teaspoons canola oil, divided

1 cup diced onion

¼ teaspoon paprika

½ teaspoon dried thyme

½ cup diced green peppers

½ cup diced red peppers

¾ teaspoon dried crushed sage leaves

¼ teaspoon black pepper (or more to taste)

½ teaspoon seasoned salt

2 cups diced cooked chicken breast

1 teaspoon chopped fresh parsley

1. Place potatoes in a medium microwave-safe bowl. Add ¼ cup chicken broth, cover, and microwave on high for 5 minutes. Drain and set aside. (Or use leftover potatoes.)

2. Heat 1 teaspoon of oil in a medium skillet over medium high heat. Add onion and cook 5 to 7 minutes or until softened and slightly browned. Add another teaspoon of oil to pan and add potatoes. Sprinkle with paprika and cook, stirring often, for 10 minutes or until potatoes are tender and well browned.

3. Crush thyme over potatoes and add peppers, sage, black pepper, and remaining ¼ cup chicken broth to the pan. Sauté for 2 to 3 minutes or until peppers soften and then add seasoned salt and chicken. Cook hash for another 2 to 3 minutes, tossing until chicken is hot and peppers tender.

4. Remove from heat and garnish with chopped parsley.

DARE TO COMPARE: A breakfast platter of corned beef hash and eggs at IHOP has 1,110 calories, 61grams of fat, 2,970 mg of sodium and 91grams of carb. To create a similar full-fledged breakfast plate, add two large eggs and 2 slices of light wheat toast to a serving of hash. It adds just 240 calories.

NUTRITION INFORMATION PER SERVING (1 cup): Calories 190 | Carbohydrate 19g (Sugars 4g) | Total Fat 5g (Sat Fat 0g) | Protein 19g | Fiber 3g | Cholesterol 50mg | Sodium 350mg | Food Exchanges: 2 Lean Meat, 1 Starch, 1 Vegetable | Carbohydrate Choices: 1 | Weight Watcher Plus Point Comparison: 5

Crispy Waffles with Creamy Maple Syrup

THIS RECIPE IS FOR THOSE OF YOU who asked if the pancake recipes in my book Eat What You Love *can be used to make waffles. Unfortunately, the answer is "no," as it takes a different mix of flour and fat to produce a light and crispy waffle. I'm happy to report, however, that this batter fills the bill. The creamy maple syrup is not to be missed.*

MAKES **4** SERVINGS

Waffles

¾ cup white whole-wheat flour

3 tablespoons cornstarch

2 teaspoons granulated sugar

½ teaspoon baking powder

¼ teaspoon baking soda

¼ teaspoon salt

¼ teaspoon ground cinnamon

1 cup low-fat buttermilk

2 tablespoons canola oil

1 large egg, beaten

1 teaspoon vanilla extract

Creamy Maple Syrup

½ cup sugar-free syrup

¼ cup low-fat evaporated milk

2 teaspoons granulated sugar

½ teaspoon vanilla extract

¼ teaspoon ground cinnamon

2 teaspoons butter or margarine

1. In a medium bowl, combine the first 7 batter ingredients (flour through cinnamon). In a separate bowl, whisk together the buttermilk, oil, egg, and vanilla. Pour over the flour mix and stir until well combined. Do not overmix. Let batter rest for 15 minutes.

2. To make the syrup, combine the first 5 syrup ingredients (syrup through cinnamon) in a small saucepan and cook for 2 to 3 minutes. Remove from heat and stir in butter.

3. Preheat the waffle iron and spray it with non-stick cooking spray. Ladle about 1 cup of batter or amount recommended for your waffle maker onto the iron. Close the waffle iron and cook until the steam subsides and the waffle is golden on both sides. Serve immediately, topping waffles with Creamy Maple Syrup.

NUTRITION INFORMATION PER SERVING (2 waffles plus 3 tablespoons syrup): Calories 260 | Carbohydrate 32g (Sugars 8g) | Total Fat 10g (Sat Fat 2g) | Protein 8g | Fiber 3g | Cholesterol 55mg | Sodium 410mg | Food Exchanges: 2 Starch, 2 Fat, ½ Lean Meat | Carbohydrate Choices: 2 | Weight Watcher Plus Point Comparison: 7

Wholesome Silver Dollar Hots

IF YOU LOVE PANCAKES but avoid them because you're trying to curb "the white stuff," this recipe is for you. I've pumped up the protein and whole grains in this nutritious, yet light-textured batter, to provide sustained energy while keeping blood sugar in check. As their name suggests, it's best to eat these pancakes while they're hot. Like a Swedish pancake, when hot, these tasty high protein pancakes literally melt in your mouth.

MAKES **4** SERVINGS

½ cup low-fat cottage cheese

½ cup light sour cream

2 large eggs

2 large egg whites

1 tablespoon granulated sugar

¼ teaspoon baking soda

¼ teaspoon salt

1½ cups white whole-wheat flour

1. Place cottage cheese and sour cream in a food processor or blender and blend until smooth. Transfer to a medium bowl. Beat in eggs and egg whites. Stir in sugar, baking soda, and salt. Add flour and stir until well combined. Do not overmix.

2. Spray a non-stick skillet or griddle with cooking spray and place over medium heat, then wipe out lightly with a paper towel. When hot enough for a drop of water to sizzle, spray again with cooking spray. Pour 1 tablespoon of batter per pancake into skillet and spread into a 2-inch circle. Cook the pancakes for 1 to 2 minutes on the first side or until golden on the bottom. Flip the pancakes and cook for an additional 1 to 2 minutes. Repeat with remaining batter and serve hot.

NUTRITION INFORMATION PER SERVING (6 pancakes): Calories 270 | Carbohydrate 33g (Sugars 6g) | Total Fat 6g (Sat Fat 3g) | Protein 16g | Fiber 4g | Cholesterol 115mg | Sodium 420mg | Food Exchanges: 2 Lean Meat, 2 Starch | Carbohydrate Choices: 2 | Weight Watcher Plus Point Comparison: 6

Strawberry Cheesecake Pancake Stacks

IF, LIKE ME, YOU FIND YOUR MOUTH WATERING at the thought of strawberry cheesecake pancakes, yet cringe at the thought of eating too many calories, I have you covered. This pancake stack, with a whopping 75% fewer calories and a fraction of the usual carbs, is pure pleasure. Quick-fix tip: make the cheesecake filling and strawberry topping to stuff and top your favorite frozen pancakes.

MAKES **4** SERVINGS

⅓ cup low fat cottage cheese

⅓ cup light cream cheese

¾ cup light whipped topping, thawed

3½ tablespoons granulated no-calorie sweetener, divided (or 5 packets)

1 cup unsweetened frozen strawberries, thawed

1 tablespoon no-sugar-added strawberry jam

1 cup all-purpose flour

¾ teaspoon baking powder

½ teaspoon baking soda

1 large egg

1 large egg white

1 cup low-fat buttermilk

¾ teaspoon vanilla extract

1. Using a food processor or blender, process the cottage cheese until smooth. Blend in cream cheese and 1 tablespoon (or 1½ packets) sweetener. Scoop into a small bowl and fold in whipped topping. Set aside. In another small bowl, combine strawberries, jam and 1 tablespoon (or 1½ packets) sweetener. Set aside.

2. In a medium bowl, combine the flour, 1½ tablespoons (or 2 packets) sweetener, baking powder, and baking soda. In a separate bowl, whisk together remaining ingredients. Pour into the dry ingredients and stir until well combined.

3. Spray a non-stick skillet or griddle with cooking spray and place over medium heat. Pour ¼ cup of batter per pancake into the skillet and spread into a 3-inch circle. Cook the pancake for 3 to 4 minutes on the first side or until golden on the bottom. Flip the pancakes and cook until done, about 2 to 3 minutes. Stack on a plate and cover to keep warm.

4. For each stacker, lay one pancake on a plate. Top with ⅓ cup cheesecake filling and then another pancake. Pour ¼ cup strawberry topping over the stack and dig in.

DARE TO COMPARE: A stack of IHOP New York Cheesecake pancakes has 1,100 calories, 44 grams of fat, 152 grams of carbohydrate and a crazy 2,430 mg of sodium.

NUTRITION INFORMATION PER SERVING: Calories 270 | Carbohydrate 38g (Sugars 10g) | Total Fat 7g (Sat Fat 3.5g) | Protein 11g | Fiber 2g | Cholesterol 65mg | Sodium 420mg | Food Exchanges: 2 Starch, ½ Fruit, 1 Lean Meat, 1 Fat | Carbohydrate Choices: 2 ½ | Weight Watcher Plus Point Comparison: 7

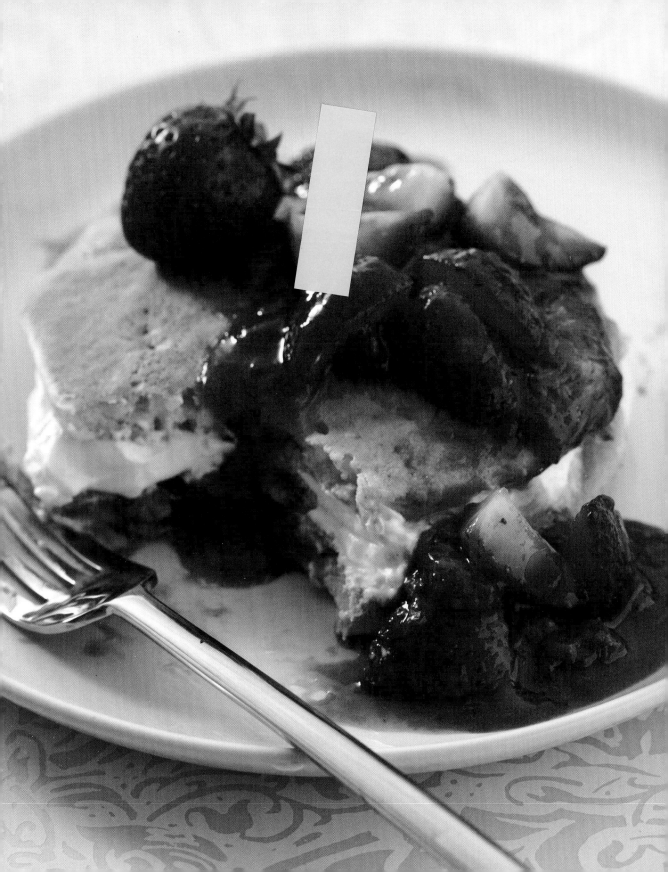

Berry Good Breakfast Sundaes

THIS SIMPLE, SCRUMPTIOUS BREAKFAST SUNDAE tastes more like a dessert—and that's fine with me! A quick trip to the microwave turns easy-to-keep-on-hand frozen berries into a delectable warm topping that's terrific when paired with cool and creamy cottage cheese or yogurt. You also have the option of adding nuts to top the "sundae." When is the last time you ate a delicious sundae with the satisfying protein of two eggs, four fabulous grams of fiber, and a mere 150 calories? So berry good.

MAKES **1** SERVING

½ cup low fat cottage cheese or Greek yogurt

1 tablespoon light sour cream

½ cup frozen blackberries or raspberries

2 teaspoons granulated no-calorie sweetener (or 1 packet)

2 teaspoons chopped almonds, optional

1. Mix cottage cheese or Greek yogurt with light sour cream and place in a small dish.

2. Place frozen berries in a small microwave-safe dish. Sprinkle with sweetener and microwave on high for 1 minute or until hot. Pour hot berry mix over cottage cheese or yogurt. Top with nuts, if desired.

Marlene Says: *Thick creamy Greek-style yogurt has more than twice the protein but only half the carbs of regular yogurt (as does cottage cheese). To make your own Greek yogurt, line a strainer with paper towels, place over a bowl, and pour 1 cup of regular low-fat yogurt into the lined strainer. Refrigerate until the yogurt is reduced by one-half.*

NUTRITION INFORMATION PER SERVING: Calories 150 | Carbohydrate 16g (Sugars 12g) | Total Fat 2.5g (Sat Fat 1.5g) | Protein 16g | Fiber 4g | Cholesterol 470mg | Sodium 470mg | Food Exchanges: 2 Lean Meat, 1 Fruit | Carbohydrate Choices: 2 | Weight Watcher Plus Point Comparison: 4

appetizers and small bites

Creamy Fruit Dip

Ooey Gooey Pizza Dip

Pan Fried Onion Dip

Susan's "Zero Point" Wonder Dip

More Baked Pita Chips

Seven Layer Greek Dip

Jalapeno Artichoke Party Squares

James' Pepperoni Pizza Puffs

Coconut Coconut Shrimp

Parmesan-Crusted Asparagus Straws

Awesome Nacho Quesadilla

Beef and Blue Quesadillas

Barbequed Chicken Flatbread Pizza

Cheesy Chili Nachos

By definition, appetizers are meant to be small bites that *whet the appetite*. But alas, in today's world of chain restaurants (where bigger is seen as better), the start of a meal is often anything but a little (or lite) bite. Quite honestly, I never cease to be amazed by the calorie and fat content of *popular restaurant appetizers*, such as the Chili Cheese Nachos at Applebee's (1,680 calories and 108 grams of fat) or their Sampler Platter (a whopping 2,590 calories, 50 grams of saturated fat and close to 7,000 milligrams of sodium—yes, that's 7,000 mg!). Even if you share these with a table of four, the numbers alone are enough to kill any appetite.

The appetizers and snacks we serve our family and guests do not always fare much better. *Creamy dips, chips, nachos*, and pizzas are often on our own entertaining menus, as are the fat and calories that come with them.

I am happy to say that this chapter changes all that—and oh, so deliciously. Here you will find appetizers and anytime *nibblers* that are "killer" in taste only. If you are a dip lover, you will be delighted to find five fantastic brand-new dips, ranging from my cool and Creamy Fruit Dip to a new must-try, my Ooey Gooey Pizza Dip. Served straight from the oven, it's *ooey, gooey,* easy, cheesy—and totally delicious. For family *snacking* with ease you can't beat my son James' Pepperoni Pizza Puffs or the Awesome (100 Calorie) Nacho Quesadillas—and, of course, you'll discover even more *crave-worthy* restaurant-inspired nibbles. To whet your appetite I offer you crispy Coconut Coconut Shrimp served with a *sweet and spicy* dipping sauce, super Chili Cheese Nachos piled high with quick-fix chili, and Barbecued Chicken Flatbread Pizza. Ready to eat?

For the Love of

GLUTEN-FREE FOOD

If you or someone you love is on a gluten-free diet, the good news is that many of nature's finest (and healthiest) foods, such as fruits, vegetables, meats, seafood, beans, nuts, and eggs—along with nutrient-rich dairy products and oil—are naturally gluten-free.

And while foods made with wheat-based flour (or barley or rye), like bread, cakes, and cookies can be challenging, luckily, today's vast array of gluten-free products has made it easier to cook and eat gluten-free. One of the easiest and least expensive ways to ensure meals and baked goods are good-for-you, great-tasting, and gluten-free is to prepare them yourself. Here are a few tips:

GLUTEN FREE MADE EASY

- For sandwiches use gluten-free bread or go "bunless" by wrapping sandwich fillings in lettuce leaves. Process toasted or stale gluten-free bread into breadcrumbs.

- Gluten-free pastas are easy to find and can be used anywhere I specify pasta. Alternately, pour pasta sauces over cooked rice, spaghetti squash, or baked potatoes.

- Most corn tortillas are gluten-free. Use them to make your own tortilla chips or look for 100% corn tortilla chips for scooping dips and making nachos.

- For thickening, cornstarch is naturally gluten-free with twice the thickening power of flour. Arrowroot is another option. For dredging, tapioca starch/flour works well.

- For pancakes, waffles, and baked goods, store-bought gluten-free flours and baking mixes are the easy way to go (taste and texture vary considerably). Pamela's brand is great for pancakes and muffins while Bob's Red Mill works beautifully in my Fresh Orange and Almond Cake (page 313).

- Xanthan gum can help with structure and texture when baking (as a protein, gluten provides structure in wheat-based flours). Use according to package directions.

- For better flavor, double extracts, bump up the spices, and consider flavorful add-ins like citrus zests, nuts, or chocolate chips when creating your own gluten-free goodies.

NOTE: *Experts agree that there is no need to avoid wheat if you do not have celiac disease or gluten sensitivity. A gluten-free diet does not guarantee weight loss or better health. Many gluten-free foods are higher in sugar, fat and calories, as well as lower in nutrients such as fiber, B vitamins and iron. Consult a physician or registered dietitian before starting a gluten-free diet.*

Creamy Fruit Dip

IT'S A GREAT HEALTHY OPTION to have a fruit tray at a party—even more so when it's served with a healthy dip. But most "healthy" dips are not as healthy as you think. Fruit dip recipes often start with sweetened yogurt and then add additional sweeteners, such as honey. The result is more added sugar in just a couple tablespoons of dip than in an entire serving of fruit! I start instead with unsweetened yogurt to blend a luscious dip with a fraction of the usual sugar, leaving plenty of room for sweet fruity dippers like fresh strawberries, melon, kiwi, and apple slices.

MAKES **10** SERVINGS

½ cup plain low-fat yogurt

½ cup low-fat cottage cheese

¼ cup low-fat sour cream

2 tablespoons granulated no-calorie sweetener (or 3 packets)

½ teaspoon lime zest

1. Using a food processor or immersion blender, blend the yogurt and cottage cheese until very smooth and creamy.

2. Spoon yogurt mix into a medium bowl (or serving bowl) and stir in sour cream, sweetener and lime zest until well blended. Refrigerate until ready to use.

NUTRITION INFORMATION PER SERVING (2 tablespoons): Calories 25 | Carbohydrate 2g (Sugars 2g) | Total Fat 1g (Sat Fat .5g) | Protein 2g | Fiber 0g | Cholesterol 5mg | Sodium 50mg | Food Exchanges: Free | Carbohydrate Choices: 0 | Weight Watcher Plus Point Comparison: 1

Ooey Gooey Pizza Dip

OOEY, GOOEY, CHEESY—AND EASY! This dip is just crazy good. My son James, who is not a dip fan, had one bite and immediately dug in for more. Not only can you whip up this decadent-tasting dip in mere minutes, you can even use it to eat more veggies. Add sautéed mushrooms or diced green peppers between the sauce and cheese for an extra boost of fiber and vitamins, or serve it with thick cuts of zucchini and sweet bell pepper in addition to the usual bread or pita chips, for extra healthy dipping. Who knew dip could be so good for you?

MAKES **10** SERVINGS

½ cup light cream cheese

½ cup nonfat sour cream

¾ teaspoon dried oregano

½ cup pizza sauce

1 cup shredded part-skim mozzarella cheese

½ cup grated Parmesan cheese

1. Preheat the oven to 350°F. In a small bowl, combine cream cheese, sour cream, and oregano. Stir until smooth.

2. Spread evenly into a 9-inch pie pan. Top with pizza sauce and then mozzarella cheese.

3. Sprinkle on the Parmesan cheese and bake for 15 minutes or until cheese is melted.

Marlene Says: *Calci-yum! A single serving of this cheesy dip delivers 20% of the daily recommended allowance for calcium.*

NUTRITION INFORMATION PER SERVING (3 tablespoons): Calories 90 | Carbohydrate 4g (Sugars 2g) | Total Fat 5g (Sat Fat 3g) | Protein 8g | Fiber 0g | Cholesterol 15mg | Sodium 270mg | Food Exchanges: 1 Medium Fat Meat | Carbohydrate Choices: 0 | Weight Watcher Plus Point Comparison: 2

Pan Fried Onion Dip

KISS THOSE SOUP MIX PACKETS and deli case tubs goodbye—here's your ▓▓▓ onion dip for entertaining. Adapted from Food Network star Ina Garten's Pan Fried Onio▓ ▓e, this makeover saves tons of calories—with even more layers of flavor. Caramelized onio▓ ▓ a sweet richness, while my add-ins of dried minced onion and soy sauce give the dip an ext▓ ▓ texture and flavor. Be sure to have lots of cool crunchy dippers, like baby carrots, red bell ▓▓▓ces and celery stalks, on hand.

MAKES ▓▓ ▓INGS

1 teaspoon canola oil

3 cups roughly chopped or sliced onions

1 teaspoon brown sugar

3 tablespoons light tub-style cream cheese

3 tablespoons light mayonnaise

1 cup light sour cream

1 teaspoon dried minced onion

¾ teaspoon reduced-sodium soy sauce

¼ teaspoon Worcestershire sauce

¼ teaspoon salt

¼ teaspoon black pepper

1. Heat the oil in a medium non-stick skillet over ▓▓▓gh heat. Stir in the onions, lower the heat to medium, cover, and cook for 10 minutes, stirring occasionally. (To quick start your onions cook them in the microwave for 5 minutes first.)

2. Stir in the brown sugar and continue to cook for another 7 to 10 minutes, stirring periodically, until onions are deep golden brown. Remove from heat.

3. In a medium bowl, mix the cream cheese and mayonnaise. Add the sour cream and then the remaining ingredients, including the warm caramelized onions.

4. Serve immediately, or place dip into a serving dish, cover, and put in refrigerator for 30 minutes to meld flavors and serve as a cool dip.

DARE TO COMPARE: With 230 calories and 23 grams of fat, Ina Garten's Pan Fried Onion Dip recipe has three times the calories and seven times the fat of my extra-layers-of-flavors adaption.

NUTRITION INFORMATION PER SERVING (3 tablespoons): Calories 70 | Carbohydrate 7g (Sugars 5g) | Total Fat 4g (Sat Fat 2g) | Protein 3g | Fiber 1g | Cholesterol 10mg | Sodium 140mg | Food Exchanges: 1 Vegetable, 1 Fat | Carbohydrate Choices: ½ | Weight Watcher Plus Point Comparison: 2

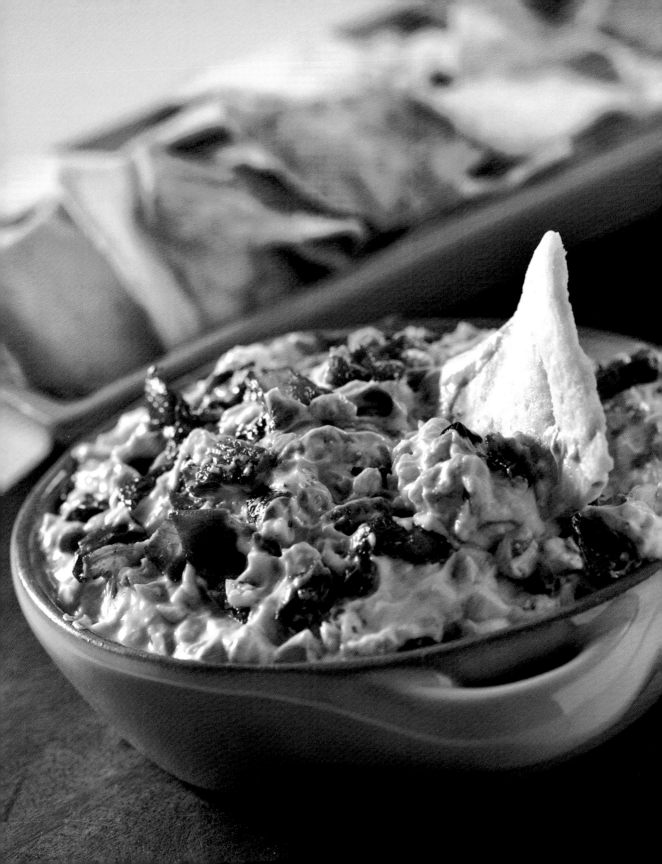

Susan's "Zero Point" Wonder Dip

LAST YEAR ONE OF MY VERY GOOD FRIENDS, Susan, made it her goal to lose weight. To help her get to her target weight—and her new fabulous figure—she used the Weight Watchers point system. Susan could barely contain her excitement when she shared with me her wonderful dip recipe —with zero points!* Serve it with crackers or crudité, or enjoy it the way I do, with scrambled eggs, grilled meat, or tucked into a pita with feta cheese for lunch. Any way you serve it, this dip is truly wonder–ful.

MAKES **14** SERVINGS

1 large or 2 small eggplants
(about 1½ pounds)

1 tablespoon olive oil

1 (15-ounce) can tomato sauce

2 cloves garlic, minced or pressed

1 green pepper, seeded and chopped

2 teaspoons ground cumin

¼ teaspoon cayenne

2 teaspoons sugar

1 teaspoon salt

¼ cup red wine vinegar

¼ cup chopped fresh cilantro

1. Dice the eggplant (including the skin), discarding ends.

2. In a large frying pan, heat the oil over medium high heat; add the eggplant, tomato sauce, garlic, green pepper, cumin, cayenne, sugar, salt, and vinegar. Cook, covered, over medium heat for 20 minutes. Uncover and simmer mixture over high heat, stirring, for an additional 10 to 15 minutes or until eggplant is very soft. Cover and chill at least 2 hours or until the next day.

3. Before serving, stir in the fresh cilantro.

Marlene Says: *A single serving is zero points (or basically a "free food"). If you want to count additional servings as "free" as well, I won't tell, and neither will your waistline.*

NUTRITION INFORMATION PER SERVING (¼ cup): Calories 25 | Carbohydrate 5g (Sugars 3g) | Total Fat 0g (Sat Fat 0g) | Protein 1g | Fiber 2g | Cholesterol 10mg | Sodium 290mg | Food Exchanges: 1 Vegetable | Carbohydrate Choices: 0 | Weight Watcher Plus Point Comparison: 0

More Baked Pita Chips

WITH SO MANY MORE GREAT DIPS, how could I go forgo the chips? This updated recipe includes a new trick that makes it easier-than-ever to separate the layers of pita bread. Instead of separating the bread into two thin rounds before I cut the chips, I now do so after the wedges are cut. (For heartier chips do not separate and double the calories.) I have also increased the yield of my original recipe and added a sweet new variation—Sugar Cinnamon Chips! They are really tasty, if a bit too addictive!

MAKES **8** SERVINGS

4 (8-inch) whole wheat or regular pita pockets

½ teaspoon salt or more to taste (kosher salt works nicely)

½ teaspoon paprika

¼ teaspoon garlic powder

Cooking spray

1. Preheat the oven to 350°F.

2. Stack 2 pita rounds and cut into eight wedges. Carefully separate each wedge into 2 pieces using a sharp knife to cut dough at widest end. Spray a baking sheet with cooking spray. Place the pita pieces on the sheet and spray with an even coating of the cooking spray. Mix the spices in a small bowl and sprinkle evenly with spice mixture.

3. Bake for 8 to 10 minutes or until pita is crisp and golden brown.

Marlene Says: *To make* **Sugar Cinnamon Pita Chips**, *substitute spices listed above with a mixture of 1 tablespoon granulated sugar, 2 tablespoons no-calorie granulated sweetener and 2 teaspoons of cinnamon. Spray pita chips with plain or butter-flavored cooking spray and bake as directed (adds 6 calories and 1 gram of carb per serving).*

NUTRITION INFORMATION PER SERVING (8 chips): Calories 85 | Carbohydrate 17g (Sugars 5g) | Total Fat 1g (Sat Fat 0g) | Protein 3g | Fiber 2g | Cholesterol 0mg | Sodium 300 mg | Food Exchanges: 1 Carbohydrate | Carbohydrate Choices: 1 | Weight Watcher Plus Point Comparison:2

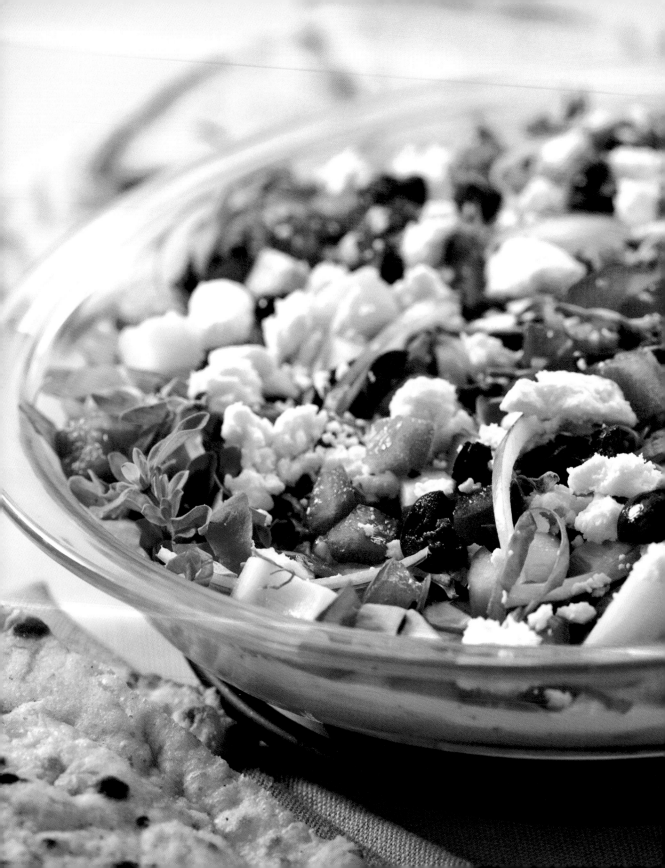

Seven Layer Greek Dip

EVERYTHING I LOVE ABOUT GREEK SALAD is in this dip. Similar in concept to a Seven Layer Mexican Dip, this dip gets a fresher and lighter twist by layering tasty veggies, Greek flavors, and healthy hummus. It comes together in no time, can hang out in the fridge until ready to serve, and when arranged in a pie plate, this beauty of a dip is super-portable for party travel.

MAKES **10** SERVINGS

1 (8-ounce) container hummus

¾ cup light sour cream

1 cup chopped fresh spinach

¾ cup chopped, seeded tomatoes

½ cup chopped, peeled, seeded cucumber

¼ cup slivered red onion

¼ cup crumbled reduced-fat feta cheese

3 kalamata olives, chopped

1. Spread the hummus evenly across the bottom of a 9-inch pie or serving plate. Spread the sour cream over the hummus. Sprinkle on the spinach, then the tomatoes, cucumber, onion, and feta cheese, topping with chopped kalamata olives. If desired, garnish around the edges with chopped parsley.

2. Cover with plastic wrap or foil, place in refrigerator, and chill until serving time.

NUTRITION INFORMATION PER SERVING (1/3 cup): Calories 80 | Carbohydrate 6g (Sugars 2g) | Total Fat 5g (Sat Fat 1.5g) | Protein 4g | Fiber 1g | Cholesterol 5mg | Sodium 85mg | Food Exchanges: ½ Carbohydrate, 1 Fat | Carbohydrate Choices: ½ | Weight Watcher Plus Point Comparison: 2

Jalapeño Artichoke Party Squares

THESE CROWD-PLEASING SQUARES are easy-fix party food at its best! Ready-to-use crescent rolls make the crust a snap to prepare, and the creamy jalapeño artichoke dip that adorns it is always a hit. I often make the dip an hour or two ahead of time and then finish the assembly just before guests arrive. For a milder dip, use fewer jalapeño peppers or swap them out entirely for canned green chilies. Another great add-in is lump crabmeat. Simply stir in one-half cup with the artichokes.

MAKES **32** SERVINGS

1 can refrigerated reduced-fat crescent rolls

⅓ cup light mayonnaise

⅓ cup low-fat yogurt

⅓ cup light tub-style cream cheese

1 (14-ounce) can water-packed artichoke hearts, drained and finely chopped,

or 1 (10-ounce) package frozen artichoke hearts, thawed and finely chopped

3 tablespoons finely chopped jalapeño peppers, or to taste

½ cup + 2 tablespoons shredded Parmesan cheese, divided

¼ teaspoon garlic powder

⅛ teaspoon salt

⅛ teaspoon black pepper

1. Preheat oven to 375°F. Lightly spray a 13 x 9-inch baking dish with non-stick cooking spray.

2. Unroll the crescent dough and place in the baking dish. Press the dough onto the bottom of the baking dish, pinching to close any perforations in dough. Prick dough all over with a fork. Bake for 10 minutes or until it begins to brown.

3. While dough is pre-baking, whisk together the mayonnaise, yogurt and cream cheese in a medium bowl until smooth. Add the remaining ingredients (including ½ cup Parmesan) and mix well.

4. Remove crust from oven, spread the dip mixture evenly over the dough, sprinkle the remaining 2 tablespoons cheese, return to the oven, and bake for an additional 5 to 7 minutes or until bottom of crust is well browned and dip is hot. Remove from the oven and let cool for 5 minutes. Cut 8 times across length and 4 times across width for 32 bite-sized squares.

DARE TO COMPARE: The super-popular Chunky Artichoke Dip with Jalapeños at my local club store inspired me to create this recipe. A two tablespoon serving of the dip has twice the calories and almost four times the fat of each Party Square. If you want to enjoy the dip by itself, make and serve it on the same day.

NUTRITION INFORMATION PER SERVING (1 square): Calories 45 | Carbohydrate 5g (Sugars 1g) | Total Fat 2.5g (Sat Fat 1g) | Protein 2g | Fiber 1g | Cholesterol 20mg | Sodium 135mg | Food Exchanges: ½ Starch | Carbohydrate Choices: 0 (1 for 2 to 3 squares) | Weight Watcher Plus Point Comparison: 1

James' Pepperoni Pizza Puffs

FRESH FROM THE OVEN, these puffs are irresistible yet so easy to make that my son James has been known to whip them up for his friends (who promptly gobble them up!). Much like a popover, they puff up beautifully while baking and deliver all the pizza flavor you love in one airy, eggy, gooey bite. And while teenage boys don't have to worry about calories, you won't need to either, as these have just 45 calories per delectable puff.

MAKES **12** SERVINGS

¾ cup reduced-fat baking mix

1 teaspoon dried oregano

1 teaspoon dried basil

¼ teaspoon garlic powder

¾ cup low-fat milk

2 large eggs

2 egg whites

1 cup shredded part skim mozzarella cheese

30 slices turkey pepperoni, chopped in ¼-inch pieces (about 1½ ounces)

Pizza sauce, optional

1. Preheat the oven to 375°F. Lightly spray a 24-cup mini-muffin tin with non-stick baking spray.

2. Place baking mix, oregano, basil, and garlic powder in a medium bowl. Slowly whisk in milk, mixing well to remove any lumps. Whisk in the eggs and egg whites, mixing until well combined. Stir in shredded mozzarella cheese.

3. Pour the egg mixture evenly into the prepared muffin tins, filling each about ¾ full. Sprinkle each muffin with about ½ teaspoon of the chopped pepperoni.

4. Bake for 12 to 15 minutes or until the center is lightly browned. Cool in the pan before removing. Serve warm with optional pizza sauce on the side for dipping.

NUTRITION INFORMATION PER SERVING (1 pizza bite)**:** Calories 45 Carbohydrate 3g (Sugars 1g) | Total Fat 2g (Sat Fat 1g) | Protein 3g | Fiber 0g | Cholesterol 30mg | Sodium 130mg | Food Exchanges: ½ Lean Meat (2 bites = 1 Lean Meat, ½ Starch) | Carbohydrate Choices: 0 | Weight Watcher Plus Point Comparison: 1

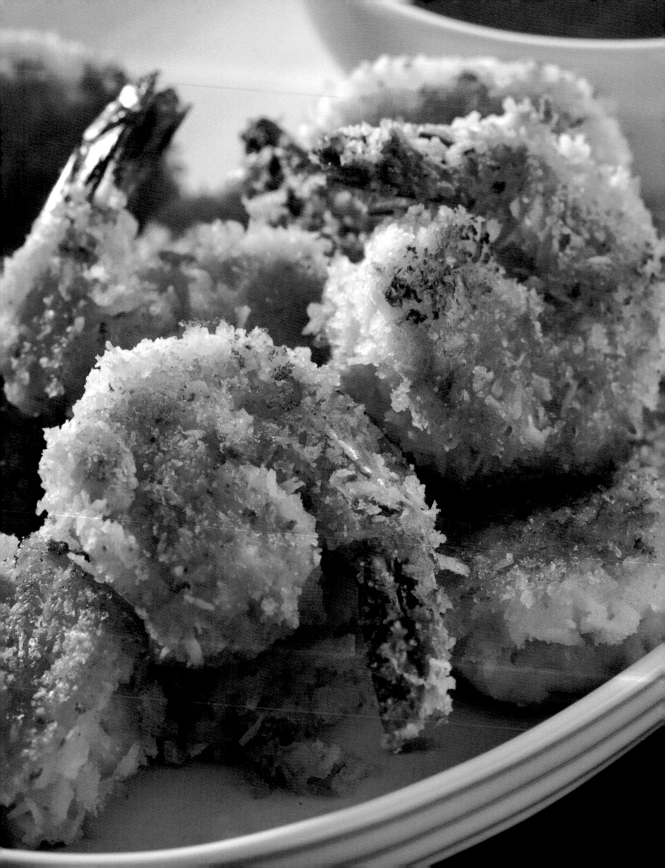

Coconut Coconut Shrimp

CRISPY, SWEET, COCONUT SHRIMP is an undisputed star among restaurant appetizers. All it takes is one bite to know that anything that tastes so good can't be healthy! Thus, creating a healthier version was no easy feat. In fact, I almost gave up when my first attempts weren't on par with the real (fried) thing. Then I had a revelation. I swapped out the customary egg white that most folks use to make the crumbs adhere to the shrimp for something stickier, creamier and far more flavorful. Voila! Coconut Coconut Shrimp—crispy and sweet as the "real" thing (served with a spicy Asian dipping sauce).

MAKES **8** SERVINGS

½ cup unsweetened shredded coconut

¾ cup panko breadcrumbs

¼ cup dry breadcrumbs

½ cup reduced-fat buttermilk

2 tablespoons light mayonnaise

½ teaspoon coconut extract

1 pound large or extra-large shrimp (about 24 per pound), peeled and deveined

1 tablespoon natural rice vinegar

¾ teaspoon reduced-sodium soy sauce

6 tablespoons no-added-sugar marmalade

3 tablespoons pineapple juice

½ teaspoon red pepper flakes

1. Preheat oven to 425°F. Spray a baking sheet with non-stick cooking spray.

2. In a wide, shallow bowl, mix together the coconut, panko, and dry breadcrumbs.

3. In a separate medium bowl, whisk together the buttermilk, light mayonnaise, and coconut extract. Dip each shrimp into the milk mixture and then into the crumb mixture to coat. Place coated shrimp onto prepared baking sheet. Spray shrimp well with cooking spray. (Tip: popping the shrimp into the freezer for 15 minutes will help hold crumbs in place.)

4. Bake for 15 minutes and then broil for 1 minute to lightly brown (watch carefully).

5. To prepare sauce, place all of the ingredients in a small measuring cup and stir. Microwave on high power for 30 to 60 seconds until warm. Stir again. Serve with shrimp.

DARE TO COMPARE: An order of coconut shrimp at Red Lobster has a hefty 784 calories, a far cry from the 165 calories per serving these crunchy beauties contain (they are just 33 calories each, including the dipping sauce!).

NUTRITION INFORMATION PER SERVING (3 Shrimp + Sauce): Calories 165 | Carbohydrate 18g (Sugars 3g) | Total Fat 6g (Sat Fat 4g) | Protein 12g | Fiber 1g | Cholesterol 90 mg | Sodium 230 mg | Food Exchanges: 1½ Lean Meat, 1 Starch | Carbohydrate Choices: 1 | Weight Watcher Plus Point Comparison: 5

Parmesan-Crusted Asparagus Straws

FOR ELEGANCE WITH EASE, look no further than this delicious appetizer. Made light and crisp with panko breadcrumbs, this dish is crunchy, creamy, and fresh— all in one appealing bite. Whether you are throwing a cozy dinner party or a big backyard bash, the "straws" look beautiful served on a simple white platter. This recipe also doubles nicely as a vegetable side. I find the straws a great complement to grilled meats, especially juicy steak. For an extra pop of flavor, serve 'em with Honey Mustard Dressing (page 162).

MAKES **6** SERVINGS

1 pound medium
asparagus
(about 18 to 20 spears)

2 tablespoons light
mayonnaise

2 large egg whites

1 teaspoon Dijon mustard

½ cup panko breadcrumbs

3 tablespoons grated
Parmesan cheese

¼ teaspoon seasoned salt

¼ teaspoon cayenne
pepper

Honey Mustard Dressing,
optional (page 162)

1. Preheat oven to 400°F. Place a wire rack on top of a baking sheet and spray with cooking spray. Wash and dry asparagus spears. Break off or trim tough ends and set aside.

2. In a small bowl, gently whisk together the mayonnaise, egg whites, and mustard until well combined. Pour mixture into a wide, shallow bowl (large enough so asparagus can lay flat). In another wide shallow pan, combine breadcrumbs, cheese, seasoned salt, and cayenne pepper.

3. Dip asparagus spears into the egg white mixture to coat evenly (I do four to six at a time). Transfer spears to the crumb mixture and with clean hands sprinkle crumbs evenly over the spears. Transfer to a wire rack. Repeat with remaining spears.

4. Lightly spray spears with cooking spray and bake until well browned and crisp-tender, about 15 to 18 minutes, turning spears midway. Serve with Honey Mustard Dressing, if desired.

NUTRITION INFORMATION PER SERVING (about 3 straws): Calories 60 | Carbohydrate 7g (Sugars 2g) | Total Fat 2g (Sat Fat .5g) | Protein 4g | Fiber 2g | Cholesterol 5mg | Sodium 180mg | Food Exchanges: 1 Vegetable, ½ Fat | Carbohydrate Choices: ½ | Weight Watcher Plus Point Comparison: 1

Awesome Nacho Quesadilla

*I DON'T OFTEN REFER TO THINGS as "awesome," but I'm making an exception here. Like many people, my boys like to grab an order of nachos when we attend sporting events. You may be familiar with this type of snack: tortilla chips are loaded into a plastic dish adorned with wells for nacho sauce and salsa. Ordering this snack can be costly, though, both in money and calories (a whopping 1,100!). Well, this 5-minute recipe recreates **all** the flavor of those nachos—with just 100 slim calories—and does so using healthy, easy-to-keep-on-hand ingredients. Honestly. Eat one, eat two. Enjoy them as an appetizer, a snack, or as part of meal. They are awesome!*

MAKES **1** SERVING

1 (6-inch) corn tortilla

1 tablespoon prepared salsa

1 slice 2% milk American cheese singles, torn into 4 pieces

Jarred jalapeño slices (optional to taste)

Salt (optional)

1. Spray a small non-stick skillet with non-stick cooking spray and place over medium high heat. Add tortilla to pan and heat for 30 seconds.

2. Spread salsa on one half of tortilla and cover with pieces of cheese. Scatter jalapeño slices over cheese and fold empty half of tortilla over filling to cover. Press down on quesadilla with a spatula. When bottom is browned, spray top lightly with cooking spray and flip to brown other side. Sprinkle with salt for more of a "chip" effect, if desired.

3. Quesadilla is ready when sides are brown and cheese is melted. (Caution: cheese "sauce" is hot. Let cool a minute before digging in.)

Marlene Says: *I was really excited to discover that 2% American cheese slices melt perfectly to create instant "nacho sauce." Nonfat slices will not work in this recipe, nor will regular grated cheese.*

NUTRITION INFORMATION PER SERVING (1 quesadilla): Calories 100 | Carbohydrate 14g (Sugars 4g) | Total Fat 3g (Sat Fat 1.5g) | Protein 5g | Fiber 1g | Cholesterol 10mg | Sodium 390mg | Food Exchanges: 1 Starch, 1 Lean Meat | Carbohydrate Choices: 1 | Weight Watcher Plus Point Comparison: 3

Beef and Blue Quesadillas

THIS UPTOWN QUESADILLA has a wonderful flavor combination found in traditional steakhouse fare—sweet caramelized onions, robust beef and tangy blue cheese. Despite being healthy, and as easy to make as a humble cheese quesadilla, these will please even your most discerning guests.

MAKES **4** SERVINGS

1½ cups sliced onion

2 teaspoons Worcestershire sauce

2 rounded tablespoons light cream cheese

4 (8-inch) reduced-carb high fiber flour tortillas

3 ounces sliced lean roast beef, chopped

2 tablespoons crumbled blue cheese

Black pepper to taste

1. Spray a medium skillet with non-stick cooking spray and place over medium low heat. Add onions, cover, and cook for 7 to 10 minutes, stirring occasionally. When onions are softened and browned, add 1 tablespoon of water and Worcestershire sauce to pan. Cook for 1 to 2 more minutes or until onions are soft and caramelized. Remove from pan and set aside.

2. Place two tortillas on work surface and spread 1 tablespoon cream cheese on each. Place half the roast beef, half the caramelized onions, and 1 tablespoon blue cheese on each, and season with freshly ground black pepper. Top with remaining two tortillas.

3. Wipe out onion pan, spray with non-stick cooking spray, and place over medium heat. Place one quesadilla in the pan and heat for about 2 minutes or until the bottom is golden brown. Carefully flip and cook for another 1 to 2 minutes. Cook second quesadilla.

4. Cut each quesadilla into 8 wedges before serving.

Marlene Says: *Reduced-carb tortillas taste great and have the added bonus of more fiber with fewer carbohydrates and calories. Mission and La Tortilla Factory are two brands to look for.*

NUTRITION INFORMATION PER SERVING (one-half Quesadilla or 2 wedges): Calories 150 | Carbohydrate 18g (Sugars 4g) | Total Fat 4.5g (Sat Fat 2g) | Protein 10g | Fiber 8g | Cholesterol 15mg | Sodium 520 mg | Food Exchanges: 1 Lean Meat, 1 Starch, 1 Fat | Carbohydrate Choices: 1 | Weight Watcher Plus Point Comparison: 3

Barbecued Chicken Flatbread Pizza

BEFORE CALIFORNIA PIZZA KITCHEN, who would have thought BBQ chicken could work as a pizza topping? Nowadays, just about every pizza joint offers a barbecued option. We love to eat pizza when we watch sports and find this pizza a perfect snack for game day. For true CPK authenticity, I use smoked gouda, but smoked provolone or mozzarella or even regular reduced-fat pizza blend cheese works fine. A winning move I don't recommend you change is the Ranch dressing. It's the final drizzle that puts this pizza over the top.

MAKES **10** SERVINGS

1 tablespoons olive oil

1 medium red onion, sliced

¼ cup barbecue sauce

1 fresh jalapeño, sliced (optional)

2 cups shredded chicken breast

1 cup smoked gouda cheese, shredded

1 (12-ounce) can refrigerated pizza dough

¼ cup fresh cilantro, minced

3 to 4 tablespoons reduced-fat Ranch dressing (optional)

1. Preheat oven to 450°F.

2. Heat the oil in a medium skillet over medium high heat. Add the onion and cook for 7 to 10 minutes or until slightly caramelized. Set aside.

3. Spray a large baking sheet with non-stick cooking spray. Working with the pizza dough, roll out until you get an even thickness of about ¼-inch. Place on the prepared baking sheet and place in oven. Bake for 10 minutes. Remove from oven and top with barbecue sauce, spreading over entire dough. Evenly spread chicken, cheese, jalapeños, and caramelized onions on sauce.

4. Bake for about 15 to 25 minutes or until the crust is golden brown and crisp. Sprinkle with cilantro and drizzle with Ranch dressing.

Marlene Says: *Ready-to-go pizza crust dough makes this recipe quick and easy, but feel free to make your own or use my Homemade Pizza Dough recipe on page 206. I find a jelly-roll pan (about 17 x 12 inches) works great.*

NUTRITION INFORMATION PER SERVING (1 square or 1/10 pizza): Calories 200 | Carbohydrate 23g (Sugars 3g) | Total Fat 6g (Sat Fat 2.5g) | Protein 13g | Fiber 0g | Cholesterol 35mg | Sodium 280mg | Food Exchanges: 1½ Starch, 1½ Lean Meat | Carbohydrate Choices: 1½ | Weight Watcher Plus Point Comparison: 5

Cheesy Chili Nachos

WHO CAN RESIST CHILI CHEESE NACHOS? Staggeringly high in fat, sodium and calories, this appetizer is usually a diet killer, but not here. With this lightened version you can still enjoy the great taste of meaty chili atop crunchy tortilla chips, complete with melted cheese sauce—only now, without a side of guilt. Speaking of sides, feel free to add guacamole, more salsa, light sour cream, or even more vegetables.

MAKES **4** SERVINGS

8 ounces lean ground turkey

¾ cup diced onion

½ cup diced red bell pepper

1½ teaspoons chili powder

1 teaspoon cumin

Pinch of cayenne pepper

½ cup fire-roasted tomatoes

½ cup canned black beans, rinsed and drained

3 ounces reduced-fat tortilla chips (about 25 chips)

2 teaspoons margarine or butter

2 teaspoons all-purpose flour

½ cup reduced-sodium chicken broth

Pinch of garlic powder

1 cup shredded reduced-fat cheddar cheese

1. Spray a medium skillet with non-stick cooking spray and place over medium high heat. Add ground turkey, onion, and red bell pepper to pan, breaking meat apart with a spoon. Cook until meat is browned and vegetables are soft, about 10 minutes.

2. Stir in chili powder, cumin and cayenne pepper. Stir in tomatoes and ½ cup water. Reduce heat to low, cover, and cook for about 10 minutes, stirring occasionally. Stir in beans and heat until warmed. Cover to keep warm and remove from heat.

3. In a small saucepan over low heat, melt margarine and flour and whisk until smooth. Add chicken broth and garlic powder and bring to a boil, stirring continuously for about 1 minute. Remove from heat and whisk in cheese one-half cup at a time.

4. Spread chips out onto a serving platter. Spoon chili mixture evenly onto chips and then drizzle cheese mixture over chili. Top with your favorite garnishes and serve.

DARE TO COMPARE: A single order of Chili Cheese Nachos at Applebee's serves up 1,680 calories, 107 grams of fat, 133 grams of carbohydrates, and 3,850 mg sodium!

NUTRITION INFORMATION PER SERVING (about 6 loaded chips): Calories 160 | Carbohydrate 12g (Sugars 4g) | Total Fat 7g (Sat Fat 2g) | Protein 13g | Fiber 3g | Cholesterol 45mg | Sodium 260mg | Food Exchanges: 2 Lean Meat, 1 Starch | Carbohydrate Choices: 1 | Weight Watcher Plus Point Comparison: 4

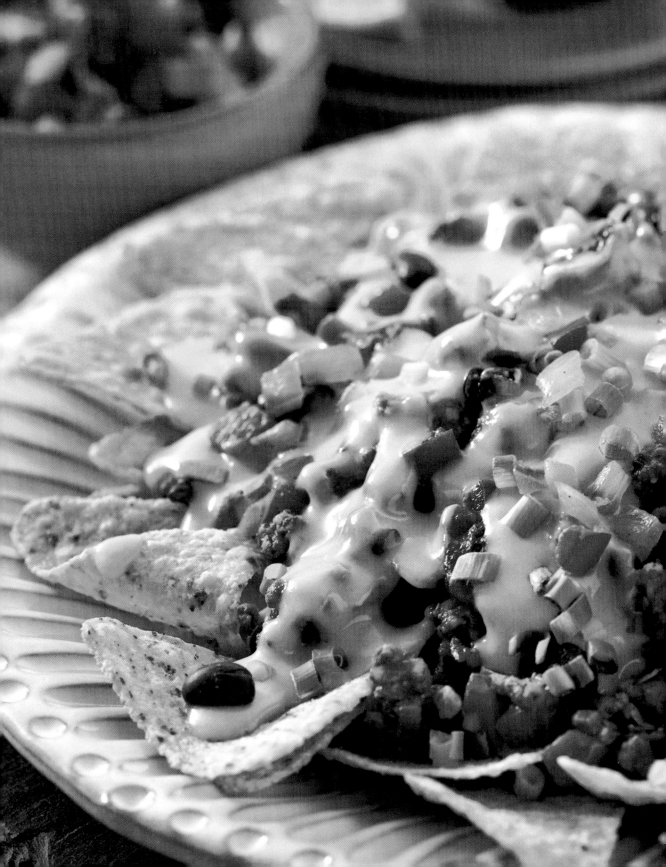

super soups and sensational sandwiches

New England Clam Chowder

Chicken Pot Pie Soup

Chicken Enchilada Soup

The Shadows Hearty Lentil Soup

15-Minute Roasted Red Pepper Bisque

Very Veggie Soup

Loaded Baked Potato Soup

Cincinnati Chili

Buffalo Chicken Salad Sandwich

Tuna Salad with a Twist

Grilled Cheese and Tomato Soup Sandwiches

Deli-licious French Dip Thinwich

Knife & Fork Chicken Caesar "Salad" Sandwich

Western Chicken Bacon Cheese Sandwiches

Totally Terrific Turkey Burgers

Outside-In Southwest Turkey Cheddar Burger

Stuffed Black and Blue Steak Burgers

Short-Cut Caramelized Onions

Brand New Reuben Sandwich

ome things just naturally go together, and when it comes to food there is no better combination than a *tasty* sandwich and a hot bowl of soup. This chapter highlights these two favorite foods with more *sensational* recipes for *everyday sandwiches* and *quick-fix soups*. (P.S. Mixing and matching is absolutely encouraged!)

First up are seven brand-new super soups and one chili recipe guaranteed to *soothe* your appetite and *warm* your soul. Of course, like all my soup recipes, each retains all the great flavor of traditional soup recipes but with less fat and sodium and fewer calories (see page 116). The perfect example is my *ultra-quick* 20-Minute Roasted Red Pepper Bisque, made with canned or jarred roasted red peppers and a splash of nonfat half-and-half for a creamy *rich-tasting* bisque (with just 85 calories per cup). For other *hearty* meals-in-a-bowl, look no further than The Shadows Hearty Lentil Soup with its smoky sausage flavor, thick and *creamy* Chicken Pot Pie Soup, or my take on Chili's zesty Chicken Enchilada Soup.

Like many, I consider sandwiches the *perfect fast-fix meal*. The ones you will find in this chapter are great alone or as an accompaniment to the lighter soups. *Flavorful and fun* to eat, my sandwiches—and that includes the burgers—are missing only one thing: excess calories! You asked for more *burgers* and I've complied. Be sure to check out the Totally Terrific Turkey and Stuffed Black and Blue Steak Burgers! If you *love deli* sandwiches, I think you'll be delighted with my Brand New Reuben, and for the *ultimate* soup & sandwich combo, bite into a comforting Grilled Cheese and Tomato Soup Sandwich (no bowl—or spoon—required). (P.S. You'll find two more *tempting* soup and chili *recipes*, including Wendy's-Style Chili, in the Slow Cooker Chapter.)

SALT

Here is a simple fact: Salt makes food taste better. In addition to adding its own crave-worthy flavor, salt helps other ingredients in a recipe shine by curbing bitterness and elevating sweet and sour flavors. Salt can add texture or enhance color and is sensational at slowing and preventing spoilage. Of course, not everything about salt is wonderful. Studies show that when eaten in excess the sodium in salt can contribute to high blood pressure, increasing the risk of heart disease and stroke.

Because restaurant meals are often sky high in sodium, the easiest way to keep sodium levels in check is to cook at home. Wholesome recipe ingredients such as fresh and frozen fruit and vegetables, grains, and lean meats are naturally low in sodium. In low-salt or reduced-salt dishes, you can pump up the flavor by adding more herbs and spices; if you're watching sodium content, add the salt last, as the finishing touch. (Fun fact: Foods that pack a spicy or sweet punch require less sodium!)

Rinsing and draining canned beans and vegetables reduces the sodium content by up to 50%, but many of today's most convenient ingredients, such as canned broths and tomato products, including jarred marinara sauce, cannot be rinsed or drained. This chart demonstrates how nearly identical products vary in sodium content. Be a savvy shopper by comparing food labels to keep sodium in check.

Product	Serving size	Mg Sodium
TOMATO PASTE		
Contadina *(Plain)*	2 T	20
Hunts *(Plain)*	2 T	105
Contadina *(with roasted garlic)*	2 T	300
DICED TOMATOES		
Del Monte *(No Salt Added)*	1 cup	100
Del Monte *(Plain)*	1 cup	320
O Organic *(Recipe-ready)*	1 cup	1300
MARINARA		
Prego Heart Smart	½ cup	360
Prego Traditional	½ cup	480
Newman's Own Cabernet	½ cup	590
Marlene's All-Purpose *(page 181)*	½ cup	220

TIP: *A delicious way to counteract the effect of sodium in your diet is to eat more potassium. Foods high in potassium include potatoes, tomatoes, oranges, bananas, spinach, Swiss chard and all types of beans.*

New England Clam Chowder

ALSO KNOWN AS BOSTON CLAM CHOWDER, this is the creamy, rich-beyond-belief style of clam chowder. My lighter (but still rich-tasting) version comes by way of a chef colleague who had the clever idea of using carb-conscious turnips to stud the soup instead of potatoes. She assured me that I would hardly notice because of all the rich flavors in the soup, and she was right. If you prefer to use potatoes, simply follow the instructions and add 15 calories and 4 grams of carb per serving to the nutritional content.

MAKES **5** SERVINGS

2 slices of lean center cut bacon

½ medium onion, chopped

2 celery stalks, chopped

1 large turnip or 1 medium potato, peeled and cubed

3 tablespoons flour (preferably Wondra), divided

2 (6-ounce) cans chopped clams

1 (8-ounce) bottle clam juice

1 cup low-fat milk

½ teaspoon dried thyme

½ teaspoon each garlic powder and onion powder

¼ teaspoon salt, optional

¼ teaspoon black pepper

¼ cup nonfat half-and-half

1. In a medium soup pot over medium high heat, cook the bacon until crisp. Remove from the pot, crumble, and set aside.

2. Add the onion, celery, and turnips (or potatoes) to the pot. Cook, stirring occasionally, for 5 minutes or until the onions are soft. Sprinkle in 2 tablespoons of flour and cook for 1 minute.

3. Drain the canned clams and add the juice, along with the bottled clam juice and milk, to the pot. Crush the thyme into the soup with your fingers. Add the garlic powder, onion powder, salt, if desired, and pepper. Bring the soup to a boil, reduce to a simmer, cover, and cook for 10 minutes or until soup has thickened and turnips are tender (for potatoes, add 5 minutes).

4. Stir remaining tablespoon of flour into the half-and-half. Add to the soup along with the canned clams and crumbled bacon, and cook for 2 to 3 minutes or until thickened. Adjust salt and pepper, if desired.

DARE TO COMPARE: If you love clam chowder served in a bread bowl, consider this: the average bread bowl filled with clam chowder has 1150 calories, 3,000 mg of sodium, and close to an *entire day's worth* of carbs.

NUTRITION INFORMATION PER SERVING (1 cup): Calories 145 | Carbohydrate 14g (Sugars 9g) | Total Fat 2g (Sat Fat 1g) | Protein 13g | Fiber 2g | Cholesterol 35mg | Sodium 420mg | Food Exchanges: 1½ Lean Meat, 1 Starch | Carbohydrate Choices: 1 | Weight Watcher Plus Point Comparison: 3

Chicken Pot Pie Soup

LIKE ITS NAMESAKE, this creamy soup is pure comfort food. My husband enjoys it with saltines (crushed over the top to create a "crust"), but it's also fun to splurge and serve it with real pastry crust. To do so, lay a single sheet of refrigerated pie dough on a flat surface and cut out six 3¾-inch rounds (discard scraps). Place the dough rounds on a baking sheet, prick them lightly with a fork, brush with milk for extra browning, if desired, and then bake at 425°F for 12 to 15 minutes. Place a crust round on top of each bowl of soup just before serving.*

MAKES **6** SERVINGS

1 teaspoon canola oil

½ small onion, chopped

2 stalks celery, chopped

1 large potato, peeled and cubed

1 cup sliced mushrooms

¾ teaspoon dried thyme

1 teaspoon garlic powder

1 (12-ounce) bag frozen mixed vegetables (or 2½ cups)

4 cups reduced-sodium chicken broth

scant ½ teaspoon black pepper

1 (12-ounce) can low-fat evaporated milk

⅓ cup instant flour (like Wondra)

2 cups diced cooked chicken

1. Heat the oil in large soup pot over medium heat. Add the onions and celery and sauté for 4 to 5 minutes. Add potatoes and mushrooms and continue to cook another 2 minutes. Using your fingers, crush in the thyme and sprinkle garlic salt over the vegetables, stir, and cook for one minute.

2. Add the frozen vegetables to the pot along with broth, salt, and pepper. Bring to a simmer, cover, and cook for 15 to 18 minutes or until potatoes are tender (soup will look heavy in vegetables at this point).

3. Mix together the milk and flour and add to the pot along with the chicken. Simmer on low for 3 to 5 minutes, stirring until soup is thickened (if soup is too thick add a bit of water).

DARE TO COMPARE: Splurge with the crust, if you please. A 10-ounce Marie Callender's frozen white chicken pot pie contains 640 calories, 38 grams of fat, 56 carbs, and 1,100 mg of sodium.

* *A crust round adds 110 calories, 7 grams of fat, and 12 grams of carbohydrate.*

NUTRITION INFORMATION PER SERVING (1½ cups): Calories 230 | Carbohydrate 30g (Sugars 9g) | Total Fat 3g (Sat Fat 1g) | Protein 22g | Fiber 4g | Cholesterol 10mg | Sodium 470 mg | Food Exchanges: 2 Lean Meat, 2 Vegetable, 1 Starch, ½ Low-Fat Milk | Carbohydrate Choices: 2 | Weight Watcher Plus Point Comparison: 6

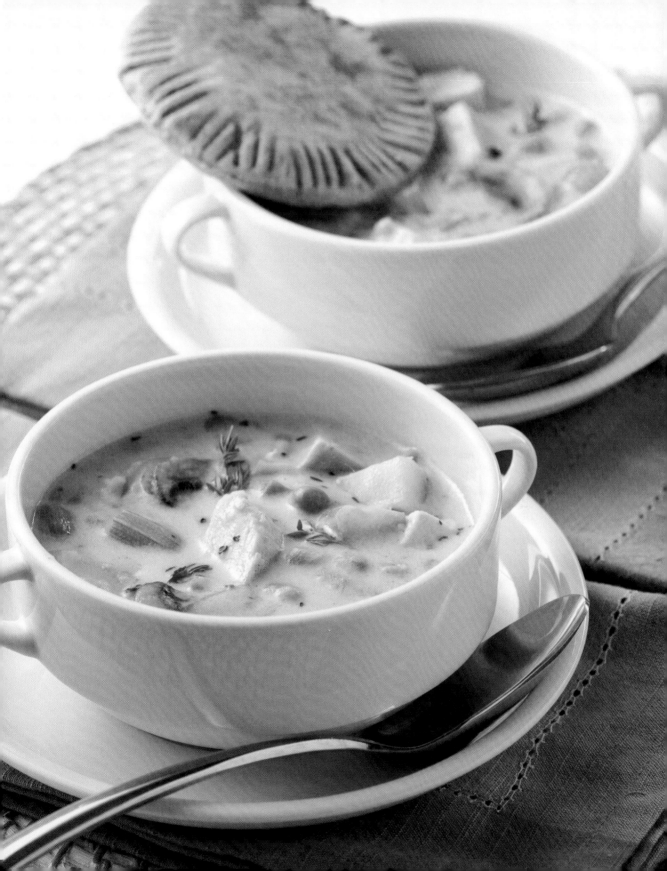

Chicken Enchilada Soup

THIS SOUP WAS INSPIRED by the ever popular Chicken Enchilada soup at Chili's Bar & Grill. With a more vibrant taste and healthier stats, the winning combination of enchilada sauce, chili powder and cumin, blended with chicken and melted cheese, will have you licking the spoon after every bite. It's delicious alone and ideal as part of a Mexican buffet or paired with my Awesome Nacho Quesadilla (page 109), Quick 'n Healthy Taco Salad (page 164) or Simple Southwest Tilapia (page 274). For a main meal this recipe makes four 1½-cup servings.

MAKES **6** SERVINGS

1 teaspoon oil

½ cup diced onion

½ teaspoon minced garlic

3 cups reduced-sodium chicken broth

¾ cup enchilada sauce

¼ cup plus 2 tablespoons cornmeal

1 teaspoon chili powder

½ teaspoon ground cumin

2 cups shredded cooked chicken

4 slices 2% milk American cheese singles

Diced tomato, lime wedges, cilantro (optional)

1. Heat the oil in a medium soup pot over medium heat. Add the onion and sauté for 3 to 4 minutes or until translucent. Add the garlic and sauté until soft, another 1 to 2 minutes.

2. Add the chicken broth, 1 cup water and enchilada sauce, and bring to a low boil.

3. In a small bowl, whisk together the cornmeal and ¾ cup water. Add cornmeal mixture, chili powder and cumin to the pot. Let simmer until thickened, 4 to 5 minutes, stirring occasionally.

4. Add the chicken and cheese and simmer over low heat for an additional 10 minutes. Serve with diced tomatoes, chopped cilantro and wedges of lime, if desired.

Marlene Says: *Leftover enchilada sauce keeps for weeks in the refrigerator when stored in a sealed container. For more flavorful tortillas, tacos or burritos, make a filling by combining enchilada sauce with any leftover meat. It's also a great substitute for salsa as a condiment for eggs, quesadillas, or my Chile Relleño Casserole (page 83).*

NUTRITION INFORMATION PER SERVING (1 cup): Calories 135 | Carbohydrate 12g (Sugars 2g) | Total Fat 3g (Sat Fat 1g) | Protein 15g | Fiber 2g | Cholesterol 0mg | Sodium 620 mg | Food Exchanges: 2 Lean Meat, 1 Starch | Carbohydrate Choices: 1 | Weight Watcher Plus Point Comparison: 3

The Shadows Hearty Lentil Soup

WHEN COOL WEATHER HITS, nothing is more warming than a steaming bowl of soup. For as long as I can remember, my mother warmed us up with this legendary sausage and lentil soup from The Shadows, a German restaurant in San Francisco. Even though the restaurant is long gone, this robust and comforting soup lives on—and after one taste you'll know why. Rich with the smoky flavor of sausage and hearty with tender lentils, this easy-to-throw-together soup always satisfies.

MAKES **4** SERVINGS

1 teaspoon canola oil

½ medium onion, finely chopped

2 stalks celery, chopped

1 clove garlic, minced

1 large carrot, peeled and chopped

1 cup brown or green lentils, rinsed, picked over, and drained

1 (14-ounce) can, or 2 cups, reduced-sodium beef broth

½ teaspoon liquid smoke

6 ounces turkey kielbasa sausage

¼ teaspoon salt

1 tablespoon tomato paste

1 tablespoon red wine vinegar

¼ cup chopped fresh parsley

1. Heat the oil in a large soup pot over medium heat. Add the onion and celery and cook for 5 minutes or until slightly softened. Add the garlic and cook another two minutes.

2. Add the carrots, lentils, beef broth, 4½ cups water, and liquid smoke. Bring to a boil, reduce heat and simmer 20 to 30 minutes, partially covered, until lentils are soft but not mushy, stirring occasionally.

3. Slice sausage link in half horizontally and then into half-moon slices. Add to pot with salt, tomato paste and vinegar, and simmer for 10 minutes.

4. Ladle into bowls and sprinkle each bowl with 1 tablespoon parsley.

Marlene Says: *When it comes to adding a source of nutritious fiber to your diet you can't beat lentils, which have a whopping 15 grams of fiber in every cup. Lentils are also a great source of B vitamins, iron, and protein.*

NUTRITION INFORMATION PER SERVING (1½ cups) **:** Calories 270 | Carbohydrate 36g (Sugars 6g) | Total Fat 5g (Sat Fat 1.5g) | Protein 20g | Fiber 14g | Cholesterol 30mg | Sodium 645mg | Food Exchanges: 3 Lean Meat, 2 Starch | Carbohydrate Choices: 2 | Weight Watcher Plus Point Comparison: 6

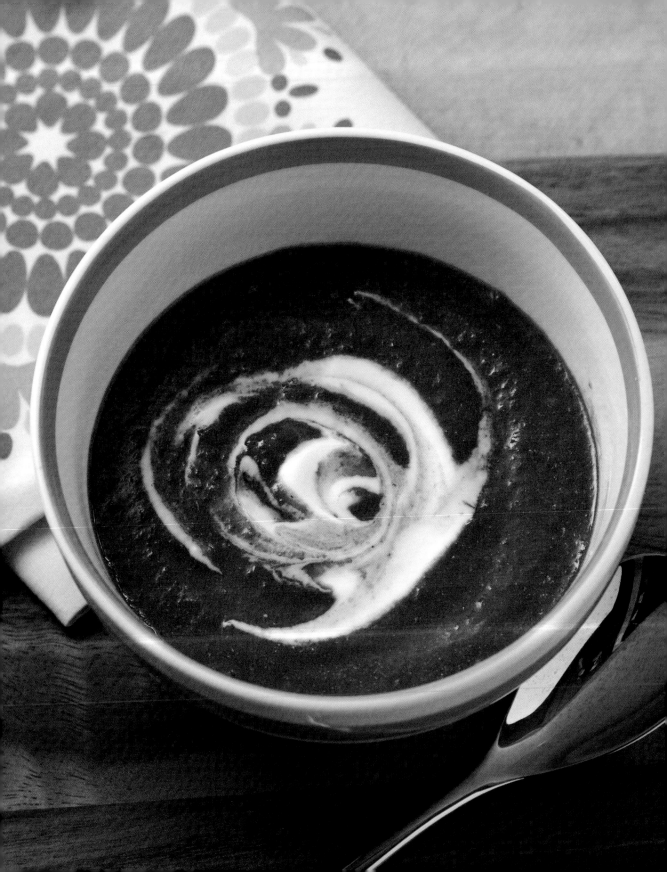

15-Minute Roasted Red Pepper Bisque

SO SPEEDY, SO SKINNY, SOOO GOOD! It's hard to believe that you can make a restaurant-quality soup in just 15 minutes—but you can. Using canned or jarred roasted red peppers makes this recipe extra quick but it's also easy to make your own roasted red peppers (see "Marlene Says" below). Enjoy a cup of this amazing soup with a casual lunchtime salad or sandwich or as a wonderful starter to a special-occasion entrée or meal.

MAKES **6** SERVINGS

2 teaspoons canola oil

1 garlic clove, minced

1 small shallot, diced

2 cups roasted red peppers (about two 15-ounce jars)

1 tablespoon tomato paste

2 (14-ounce) cans, or 4 cups, reduced-sodium chicken broth

1 teaspoon sugar

1 teaspoon paprika (smoked, if possible)

Pinch of cayenne

Pinch of salt

½ cup nonfat half-and-half

2 teaspoons cornstarch

Light sour cream (optional)

1. Heat the oil in large soup pot over medium heat. Add the garlic and shallots and sauté 3 to 4 minutes or until shallots are softened. Add the peppers, tomato paste, broth, sugar, paprika, cayenne, and salt, and bring to a boil. Reduce heat and let simmer for 10 minutes.

2. In small bowl, whisk together the half-and-half and cornstarch. Set aside.

3. Transfer the soup to a blender, or use an immersion blender to puree soup, while slowly adding the half-and-half mixture. Blend until smooth. If using a blender, return the pureed soup to the pot. Bring the bisque to a low simmer for 1 to 2 minutes until thickened and warm. Serve garnished with sour cream, if desired.

Marlene Says: *To make your own roasted red peppers, slice the sides off the peppers, leaving the core behind. Lay the pepper slices skin side up on a baking sheet and broil until the skin is completely blackened, about 15 minutes. Remove from the oven and place pepper slices in a sealed bag. Let sit 15 minutes, remove peppers from bag, and peel off the loosened skin.*

NUTRITION INFORMATION PER SERVING (1 cup): Calories 85 | Carbohydrate 12g (Sugars 4g) | Total Fat 2g (Sat Fat 0g) | Protein 4g | Fiber 2g | Cholesterol 0mg | Sodium 390mg | Food Exchanges: 2 Vegetable | Carbohydrate Choices: 1 | Weight Watcher Plus Point Comparison: 2

Very Veggie Soup

THIS TASTY SOUP GIVES YOU A BIG VEGGIE BANG for your buck. I love how versatile this recipe is: it's jam-packed with nutrients, and I can use fresh produce in the warmer months and the convenience of frozen in the off season. (Yes, frozen veggies are just as nutritious as fresh, as they are picked and quickly frozen at their flavor peak.) For a heartier soup, add ½ cup of quick-cooking barley or rice in Step 2, along with an additional ½ cup of water.

MAKES **8** SERVINGS

2 teaspoons olive oil

½ medium onion, chopped

1 stalk celery, chopped

1 tablespoon finely minced garlic

2 medium carrots, peeled and cut into rounds

1 medium zucchini, chopped

1 cup fresh or frozen green beans (¾-inch length)

½ cup fresh or frozen corn kernels

1 teaspoon Italian seasoning

2 (14-ounce) cans, or 4 cups, reduced-sodium chicken broth

1 (14.5-ounce) can diced fire-roasted tomatoes

⅛ teaspoon salt, or more, to taste

¼ teaspoon pepper

8 teaspoons Parmesan cheese (optional)

1. Heat the oil in a large soup pot over medium heat. Add the onion and celery and cook for 5 minutes or until slightly softened. Add the garlic, carrots, zucchini, green beans and corn. Sprinkle on the Italian seasoning and cook for 3 to 4 more minutes while stirring.

2. Add the stock, increase heat, and bring to a simmer. Add the fire-roasted tomatoes, salt and pepper. Reduce the heat to low, cover, and simmer for 20 minutes or until vegetables are tender and flavors have melded. Adjust salt and pepper to taste. Dust each serving with 1 teaspoon Parmesan cheese, if desired.

Marlene Says: *Researchers at Pennsylvania State University found that people who ate broth-based (or low-fat cream-based) soups once or twice a day were more successful in losing weight and keeping it off than those who ate the same number of calories in snack foods.*

NUTRITION INFORMATION PER SERVING (1 cup): Calories 60 | Carbohydrate 9g (Sugars 5g) | Total Fat 1g (Sat Fat 0g) | Protein 3g | Fiber 2g | Cholesterol 0mg | Sodium 440mg | Food Exchanges: 2 Vegetable | Carbohydrate Choices: ½ | Weight Watcher Plus Point Comparison: 1

Loaded Baked Potato Soup

WHEN I ASKED MY READERS what flavors they liked in their potato soup, their answer was a resounding, "Everything!" So in order to please everyone I created this ultra-fast fully loaded soup that brings on extra flavor without extra calories, sodium or fat. I personally had an "aha" moment when I added all of the bacon, cheese and sour cream **into** the soup, but if you are a baked potato soup purist, use them as toppings.

MAKES **6** SERVINGS

1½ pounds russet potatoes (about 2 large)

2 slices center cut bacon, chopped

½ cup onion, finely diced

2 garlic cloves, minced

½ teaspoon dried thyme

2 (14-ounce) cans, or 4 cups, reduced-sodium chicken broth

½ cup low-fat milk

½ cup nonfat half-and-half

2 tablespoons flour, preferably Wondra

¼ teaspoon salt or more to taste

½ teaspoon black pepper

¼ cup shredded reduced-fat cheddar cheese

¼ cup light sour cream

Chopped green onion tops or chives

1. Microwave the potatoes on high for 10 minutes or until fork tender.

2. While potatoes are "baking," place a large soup pot over medium high heat and cook the bacon until crisp. Add the onion and cook for 3 to 4 minutes or until slightly softened. Add the garlic, crush the thyme in with your fingers, and cook for one minute. Stir in the chicken broth and milk. Cut potatoes in half and scoop flesh into the soup. Mash the potato with a spoon (or potato masher) and simmer for 5 minutes.

3. Ladle soup into a blender, or use an immersion blender, and puree the soup until smooth. Return to the pot. Whisk together the half-and-half and flour. Add to the soup and bring to a low boil, stirring constantly, until thickened. Add the salt and pepper to taste.

4. Stir the cheddar cheese and sour cream into the soup, or reserve, and top each bowl with 2 teaspoons each cheese and sour cream. Garnish with green onion tops.

DARE TO COMPARE: A typical bowl of baked potato soup fully loaded with cream, butter, and salt packs over 400 calories, 30 grams of fat, and 1,000 mg of sodium.

NUTRITION INFORMATION PER SERVING (1 cup): Calories 165 | Carbohydrate 22g (Sugars 5g) | Total Fat 4g (Sat Fat 1.5g) | Protein 10g | Fiber 2g | Cholesterol 5mg | Sodium 380mg | Food Exchanges: 1½ Starch, ½ Lean Meat | Carbohydrate Choices: 1 ½ | Weight Watcher Plus Point Comparison: 4

Cincinnati Chili

HAVING LIVED IN OHIO, my boys grew up eating at Skyline Chili, where the chili is served "5-ways." (See "Marlene Says" below for my 5-way guide.) Cocoa and cinnamon are usually considered baking spices in American cooking, but here, like in Cincinnati, they work their magic in a crowd-pleasing chili you can use as a base and serve "any way" your family desires.

MAKES **5** SERVINGS

1 pound lean ground beef

2 cups chopped onion

2 cloves garlic, chopped

4 teaspoons chili powder

1½ teaspoons dried oregano

1½ teaspoons unsweetened cocoa powder

¾ teaspoon ground cinnamon

½ teaspoon cumin

⅛ teaspoon allspice

1 tablespoon cider vinegar

2 teaspoons brown sugar

1 (14.5 ounce) can tomato sauce

1 cup reduced-sodium chicken broth

1. Heat a large skillet over medium high heat. Add the beef, onion, and garlic, breaking up the meat with a fork. Cook until the meat has mostly browned, about 7 to 8 minutes.

2. Add the chili powder, oregano, cocoa powder, cinnamon, cumin, and allspice and cook until fragrant, about 1 minute.

3. Stir in the remaining ingredients. Reduce heat to low and simmer for 15 to 18 minutes. (While chili is simmering, cook spaghetti and have it ready to build your 2-, 3-, 4- or 5-way!)

Marlene Says: *There are 5-ways to order up Cincinnati Chili: The 1-way is plain chili; a 2-way is chili served over spaghetti; 3-way is chili over spaghetti topped with cheese; 4-way is topped with either beans or chopped red onions; and 5-way gets you spaghetti topped with chili, beans, onions, and cheese! Whew.*

NUTRITION INFORMATION PER SERVING (1 generous cup chili): Calories 200 | Carbohydrate 16g (Sugars 8g) | Total Fat 7g (Sat Fat 3g) | Protein 25g | Fiber 4g | Cholesterol 60mg | Sodium 520mg | Food Exchanges: 3½ Lean Meat, 2 Vegetables | Carbohydrate Choices: 1 | Weight Watcher Plus Point Comparison: 6

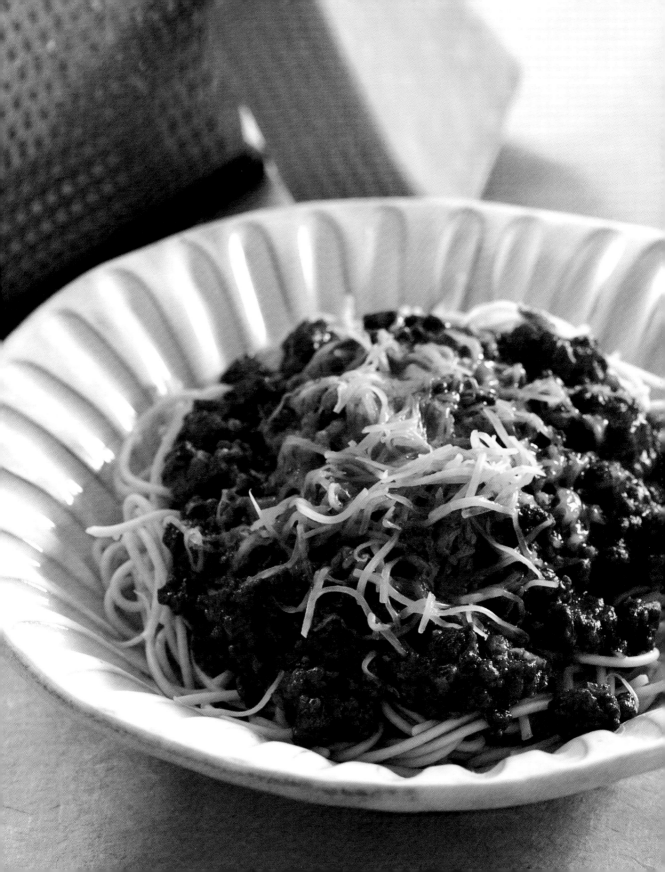

Buffalo Chicken Salad Sandwich

WHILE VISITING NAPA VALLEY last summer, my husband and I ventured into a family-run deli whose deli case was filled with exceptional salads prepared with fresh, local ingredients. When I asked which was the most popular, the chef promptly pointed to his Buffalo Chicken Salad. While not exactly packed with all local ingredients, the salad was, like this one, jam-packed with flavor. Be sure to finish the sandwiches with the grated carrot. It adds great color and texture and is a wonderful sweet complement to the savory chicken salad.

MAKES **4** SERVINGS

2 cups cubed cooked chicken breast

2 tablespoons hot sauce, divided

½ cup diced celery

3 tablespoons light mayonnaise

3 tablespoons low-fat plain yogurt

¼ teaspoon onion powder

¼ teaspoon garlic powder

2 tablespoons crumbled blue cheese

½ cup grated carrot

4 large lettuce leaves, washed and dried

8 slices light white or wheat bread

1. Place the chicken in a large bowl. Add 1 tablespoon of the hot sauce and mix well. Stir in celery.

2. In a small bowl, mix together the light mayonnaise, yogurt, onion powder, and garlic powder. Stir in the blue cheese and add it to the chicken. Stir well to combine. Add remaining hot sauce to taste.

3. To assemble the sandwiches, place the lettuce on four slices of the bread. Scoop ½ cup of chicken salad onto each of the lettuce leaves. Top chicken salad with 2 tablespoons of grated carrot and a remaining slice of bread.

Marlene Says: *Equal parts light mayonnaise and low-fat plain yogurt meld together beautifully as a replacement for full fat mayonnaise. The taste is wonderful and the savings in fat and calories is amazing. Six tablespoons of full-fat mayonnaise has 600 calories. Six tablespoons of a 50/50 combination of light mayonnaise and low-fat plain yogurt has just 135 calories!*

NUTRITION INFORMATION PER SERVING (1 sandwich): Calories 220 | Carbohydrate 24g (Sugars 3g) | Total Fat 6g (Sat Fat 1.5g) | Protein 21g | Fiber 6g | Cholesterol 5mg | Sodium 460mg | Food Exchanges: 3 Lean Meat, 1½ Starch | Carbohydrate Choices: 1½ | Weight Watcher Plus Point Comparison: 6

Tuna Salad with a Twist

WHEN IT COMES TO CONVENIENT, healthy, protein-rich foods, it's hard to beat canned tuna. Here good old tuna salad gets a wakeup call with garlicky "aioli" (a fancy French term for garlic mayonnaise). Add a twist of lemon and a spoonful of capers and the result is a creamy, tangy, tuna sandwich delight that's as easy to make as reaching into the pantry.

MAKES **2** SERVINGS

1 (6-ounce) can waterpacked albacore tuna, drained and rinsed

1½ tablespoons light mayonnaise

1½ tablespoons low-fat plain yogurt

2 teaspoons lemon juice

1 teaspoon lemon zest

½ clove garlic

1 teaspoon capers, optional

2 large lettuce leaves

2 slices light white bread or 1 pita pocket

½ small red onion, sliced into rings

1. In a medium bowl, mix together the mayonnaise, yogurt, lemon juice, lemon zest, garlic and capers, if desired. Flake the tuna into the bowl and mix gently.

2. Place the lettuce on two slices of bread. Pile half the tuna mixture onto each slice and top with sliced red onion and the remaining bread slices.

Marlene Says: *This tasty tuna mix is as versatile as it is delicious— pack it into a pita, scoop it up with whole grain crackers, stuff it into a tomato, or toss it with your favorite greens.*

NUTRITION INFORMATION PER SERVING (1 sandwich): Calories 250 | Carbohydrate 21g (Sugars 6g) | Total Fat 6g (Sat Fat 1g) | Protein 25g | Fiber 6g | Cholesterol 10mg | Sodium 540mg | Food Exchanges: 3 Lean Meat, 1 Starch, ½ Fat | Carbohydrate Choices: 1 | Weight Watcher Plus Point Comparison: 5

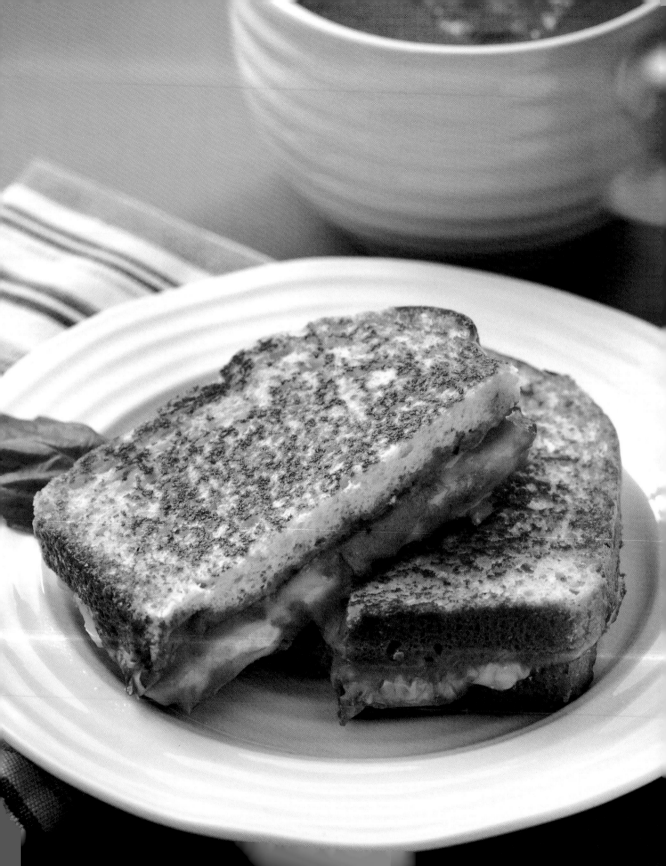

Grilled Cheese and Tomato Soup Sandwiches

NOTHING GOES TOGETHER quite like grilled cheese and tomato soup. This super fun recipe cleverly combines the two so you get the soothing taste of creamy tomato soup in your melted cheese sandwich. You'll never have to bother "dunking" again. Talk about your ultimate comfort food sandwich—this is a must-try!

MAKES **4** SERVINGS

¼ cup light cream cheese

2 tablespoons tomato paste

1 tablespoon finely chopped fresh basil (or ½ teaspoon dried)

¼ teaspoon granulated sugar

¼ teaspoon black pepper

¼ teaspoon garlic powder

4 2% milk American cheese singles or sharp cheddar cheese slices

8 slices light white bread

1. Place the cream cheese, tomato paste, basil, sugar, garlic powder, and black pepper in a small bowl and mix thoroughly to combine.

2. Spread 1 rounded tablespoon of the tomato spread on half of the slices of bread. Top with a slice of cheese and close sandwich with remaining bread.

3. Spray a non-stick skillet with cooking spray and heat over medium high heat. Place sandwich in the hot skillet and cook for about 2 to 3 minutes or until the underside is golden brown. Flip the sandwich and cook for 2 to 3 more minutes or until cheese is melted and underside is golden brown.

Marlene Says: *To make a Grilled Pizza Sandwich, substitute part-skim mozzarella cheese and swap out the basil for oregano. To make a Grilled Cheese and Tomato Waffle Sandwich, place the prepared sandwich in your waffle iron and cook until golden brown.*

NUTRITION INFORMATION PER SERVING (1 sandwich): Calories 170 | Carbohydrate 21g (Sugars 1g) | Total Fat 4.5g (Sat Fat 2g) | Protein 14g | Fiber 4g | Cholesterol 10mg | Sodium 530mg | Food Exchanges: 2 Lean Meat, 1½ Starch | Carbohydrate Choices: 1 ½ | Weight Watcher Plus Point Comparison: 4

Deli-licious French Dip Thinwich

THIS SKINNY, LOWER-SODIUM RE-CREATION of the classic French Dip is a first-rate lesson in smart shopping. Start by picking up 50% less sodium beef broth and lean roast beef (which has less sodium than most packaged brands) from the deli counter, and finish with a package of the newest bread sensation –"thin" sandwich rolls (with a mere 100 calories and an impressive 5 grams of fiber each). To make this sandwich extra special, top it with Short-Cut Carmelized Onions (page 140).

MAKES **2** SERVINGS

¾ cup reduced sodium beef broth

⅛ teaspoon dried thyme

⅛ teaspoon ground black pepper

1 tablespoon sherry

½ teaspoon dried minced onion

Pinch of sugar

2 100-calorie sandwich thins

4 ounces very thinly sliced lower sodium deli roast beef

2 ¾-ounce slices of Provolone or Swiss cheese (optional)

1. To make the warm au jus, place the broth, thyme, pepper, sherry, onion, and sugar in a medium-sized microwave-safe shallow bowl and microwave on high for 1½ to 2 minutes or until very hot.

2. Remove the bowl from microwave and roll the roast beef slices in the au jus, letting them remain in the liquid for about 30 seconds to warm.

3. Remove the meat from the au jus, letting the excess drip back into the bowl, and divide the meat evenly between the two thinwiches. Top with cheese, if desired, close buns, and pour the remaining jus into two dipping cups and serve alongside the sandwiches.

DARE TO COMPARE: A regular French Dip sub with Swiss Cheese at Arby's has a modest 450 calories, but packs over 2,000 mg of sodium. Add an order of hard-to-resist curly fries and watch the total sodium balloon to over 3,500 mg.

NUTRITION INFORMATION PER SERVING (1 sandwich): Calories 190 | Carbohydrate 21g (Sugars 2g) | Total Fat 3g (Sat Fat 1g) | Protein 16g | Fiber 5g | Cholesterol 35mg | Sodium 480 mg | Food Exchanges: 2 Lean Meat, 1 Starch | Carbohydrate Choices: 1 | Weight Watcher Plus Point Comparison: 4

Knife & Fork Chicken Caesar "Salad" Sandwich

GRAB A KNIFE AND FORK AND GET READY to enjoy a sandwich in a league of its own. Tender white meat chicken is layered with warm Everyday Garlic Toast (page 235), cool shredded lettuce, and homemade Caesar dressing, making this royal sandwich as fit for the dinner table as it is for lunch.

MAKES **2** SERVINGS

2 tablespoons plain yogurt

1 tablespoon light mayonnaise

2 teaspoons lemon juice

½ teaspoon Dijon mustard

½ teaspoon Worcestershire

½ teaspoon minced garlic

3 tablespoons grated Parmesan cheese, divided

3 teaspoons olive oil

2 slices Everyday Garlic Toast (page 235)

2 (4-ounce) boneless skinless chicken breasts

⅛ teaspoon garlic salt

Fresh black pepper, to taste

1 tablespoon sweet vermouth, optional

2 cups mixed greens or chopped romaine

1. In a small bowl, whisk together the first six ingredients (yogurt through garlic) along with 2 tablespoons of the Parmesan cheese and 1 teaspoon oil. Set aside.

2. Prepare 2 slices of garlic toast per recipe. Set aside.

3. Wrap the chicken breasts in plastic wrap, pound thin (between ⅜- and ¼-inch thick). Season with the garlic salt and black pepper. Heat the oil in a medium non-stick skillet over medium high heat. Add the chicken and cook for 4 minutes on each side or until well browned and almost cooked through. Add the sweet vermouth (or water) and cover. Place garlic toast in oven. Remove the cover on the chicken after 3 minutes and cook off any excess liquid. Check garlic toast after 5 minutes and remove from oven when golden brown.

4. Place a piece of garlic toast on each of two plates. Top each with chicken and then lettuce. Pour Caesar dressing over each and garnish with remaining tablespoon of cheese and fresh cracked pepper.

NUTRITION INFORMATION PER SERVING: Calories 320 | Carbohydrate 15g (Sugars 3g) | Total Fat 13g (Sat Fat 2g) | Protein 34g | Fiber 2g | Cholesterol 80mg | Sodium 680mg | Food Exchanges: 4½ Lean Meat, 1 Starch, ½ Vegetable, 1 Fat | Carbohydrate Choices: 1 | Weight Watcher Plus Point Comparison: 8

Western Chicken Bacon Cheese Sandwiches

THIS IS ONE OF MY FAMILY'S FAVORITE sandwiches. When Carl's Junior first introduced the Western Bacon Charbroiled Chicken Sandwich, they called it a classic in the making—and they were right. While the restaurants no longer sell the sandwich it really doesn't matter because this version offers the same great taste satisfaction with less than half the calories, one-third the fat and carbs, and more fiber and protein than the original, for a fraction of the price.

MAKES **4** SERVING

4 slices center cut bacon

4 boneless, skinless chicken breasts (about 1 pound)

Salt and pepper to taste

4 slices reduced fat cheddar cheese

4 whole wheat hamburger buns

4 large green or red lettuce leaves

4 thick slices tomato

½ small red onion, sliced, if desired

¼ cup barbecue sauce

1. Place the bacon on a paper towel and microwave 4 to 5 minutes or until desired crispness.

2. Pound the chicken breasts until about ½-inch thick, season with salt and pepper and set aside. Spray a large non-stick skillet with cooking spray or heat a grill until hot. Add the chicken to the pan or grill and cook for 3 to 4 minutes on each side or until browned and just cooked through.

3. Top each breast with slice of cheese. Add 2 teaspoons of water to the skillet and quickly cover to melt the cheese.

4. Heat buns on grill or in microwave. Place one lettuce leaf, one tomato slice, and sliced red onion (if desired), on each bun. Add chicken breast, barbecue sauce and bacon, and then close with the top half of the bun.

DARE TO COMPARE: The ever-popular Western Bacon Cheese-burger has 720 calories, 34 grams of fat (14 of them saturated), 70 grams of carb, and 1,460 mg of sodium.

NUTRITION INFORMATION PER SERVING (1 sandwich): Calories 320 | Carbohydrate 25g (Sugars 5g) | Total Fat 10g (Sat Fat 4g) | Protein 37g | Fiber 4g | Cholesterol 80mg | Sodium 420mg | Food Exchanges: 5 Lean Meat, 1½ Starch | Carbohydrate Choices: 1½ | Weight Watcher Plus Point Comparison: 8

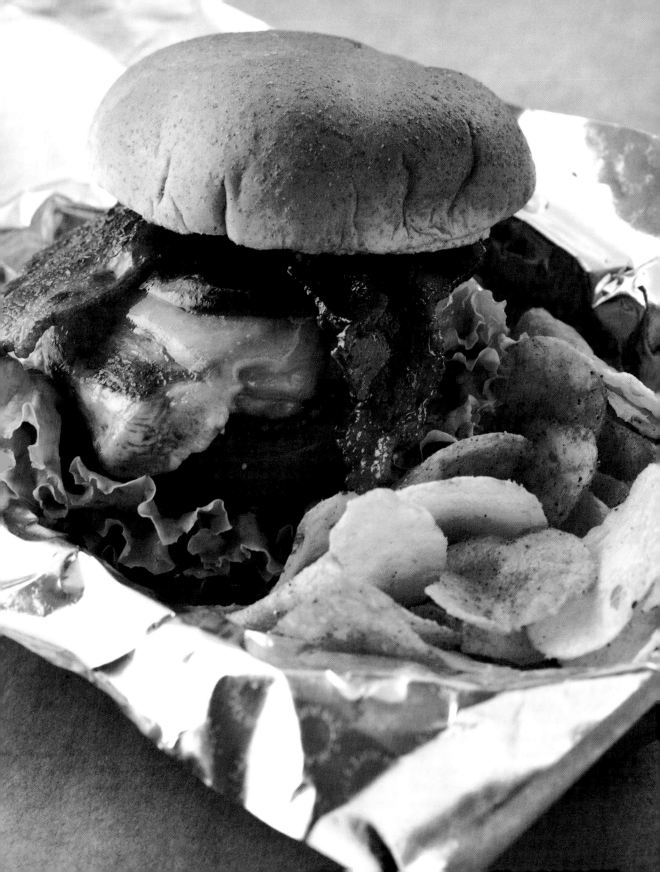

Totally Terrific Turkey Burgers

THE PROBLEM WITH MOST TURKEY BURGERS is that they are either healthy, but don't really taste good—or they're tasty, but not really healthy (restaurant turkey burgers clock in at about 1,000 calories!). To cook up a totally terrific lean turkey burger every time is not hard, it just takes a few tricks. Trick number one: start with the right meat (see "Marlene Says" below). Trick number two: add egg and breadcrumbs to the meat for extra moistness. Trick number three: add seasonings to seal the deal for a turkey burger that puts a plain hamburger to shame! Here I share my basic turkey burger mix, but feel free to alter the seasonings to your own taste. Oregano will add an Italian flair; a touch of Worcestershire or Montreal steak seasoning, Steakhouse style; and a sprinkling of chili powder and cumin, Southwestern sass.

MAKES **5** SERVINGS

1¼ pounds lean ground turkey

3 tablespoons breadcrumbs

1 green onion, finely minced

1 large egg white

½ teaspoon garlic salt

⅛ teaspoon black pepper

Lettuce leaves

Sliced tomatoes

5 white whole-grain hamburger buns (like Pepperidge Farm brand)

1. In a large bowl, mix together the turkey, breadcrumbs, green onion, egg white, garlic salt, and black pepper until all ingredients are thoroughly incorporated.

2. Evenly separate the turkey mixture into 5 balls and flatten well to form burger patties.

3. Heat a grill or spray a non-stick grill pan with cooking spray and place over medium high heat. Add the patties to the pan and cook the turkey burgers about 4 minutes per each side or to 165°F.

4. Place lettuce leaves and sliced tomatoes on warmed buns. Top with turkey burger, your favorite condiments, and top half of bun.

Marlene Says: *Ninety-three percent lean turkey breast offers the best blend of good health and great taste with 68% less fat than regular ground beef. Eighty-five percent lean ground turkey includes dark meat and a whopping 68% of its calories actually come from fat, while healthy 99% lean ground turkey is simply too lean to produce a moist burger. Jennie-O is the brand I use.*

NUTRITION INFORMATION PER SERVING (1 burger): Calories 290 | Carbohydrate 18g (Sugars 2g) | Total Fat 10g (Sat Fat 2.5g) | Protein 29g | Fiber 2g | Cholesterol 90mg | Sodium 510mg | Food Exchanges: 4 Lean Meat, 1 Starch | Carbohydrate Choices: 1 | Weight Watcher Plus Point Comparison: 8

Outside-In Southwest Turkey Cheddar Burger

WARNING: ONCE YOU SERVE THIS SCRUMPTIOUS BURGER at your next BBQ you may have to make it at every cookout from now until eternity. Adding breadcrumbs ensures that this is the most flavorful and moist turkey burger possible. After the first bite releases the oozing, fiery, cheesy goodness from the center of this burger your guests will consider you a star grill master.

MAKES **4** SERVINGS

1 (4-ounce) can fire-roasted diced green chilies, divided

½ cup reduced-fat shredded sharp cheddar cheese

1 pound lean ground turkey

3 tablespoons dry breadcrumbs

½ teaspoon ground cumin

2 tablespoons grated onion

½ teaspoon garlic salt

½ teaspoon black pepper

4 whole wheat hamburger buns

4 large lettuce leaves, washed and dried

1 large tomato, sliced

Avocado slices, optional

1. Drain the chilies. Measure out ¼ cup into a small bowl and combine with the cheese. Set aside.

2. Pour the remaining chilies into a large bowl. Add the turkey, breadcrumbs, and all of the spices. Mix gently to combine. Separate the mixture into 4 balls. Divide each ball in half and flatten to form two thin 4-inch patties. Sprinkle one-fourth of the chile-cheese mixture onto the center of each patty, leaving about a ¾-inch border free of cheese. Top with the remaining patties. Pinch the edges together to seal the cheese and flatten patties to even thickness (for best results, chill the burgers before cooking).

3. Heat a grill or grill pan over medium high heat. Add the patties and cook for 3 to 4 minutes on each side or until cooked through. Remove and let sit for 2 minutes.

4. Warm the buns, add lettuce leaf, sliced tomato, burger to each bun. Top with tomato and avocado slices, if desired.

Marlene Says: *An easy way to form these burgers is to place two patties side-by-side on a 8 x 12-inch sheet of wax paper. Top one patty with cheese, then lift the wax paper to flip the plain patty on top of it. Pinch edges together and continue as described in Step 3 above.*

NUTRITION INFORMATION PER SERVING (1 burger): Calories 305 | Carbohydrate 25g (Sugars 1g) | Total Fat 12g (Sat Fat 3.5g) | Protein 28g | Fiber 6g | Cholesterol 95mg | Sodium 760 | Food Exchanges: 4 Lean Meat, 1½ Starch | Carbohydrate Choices: 1½ | Weight Watcher Plus Point Comparison: 8

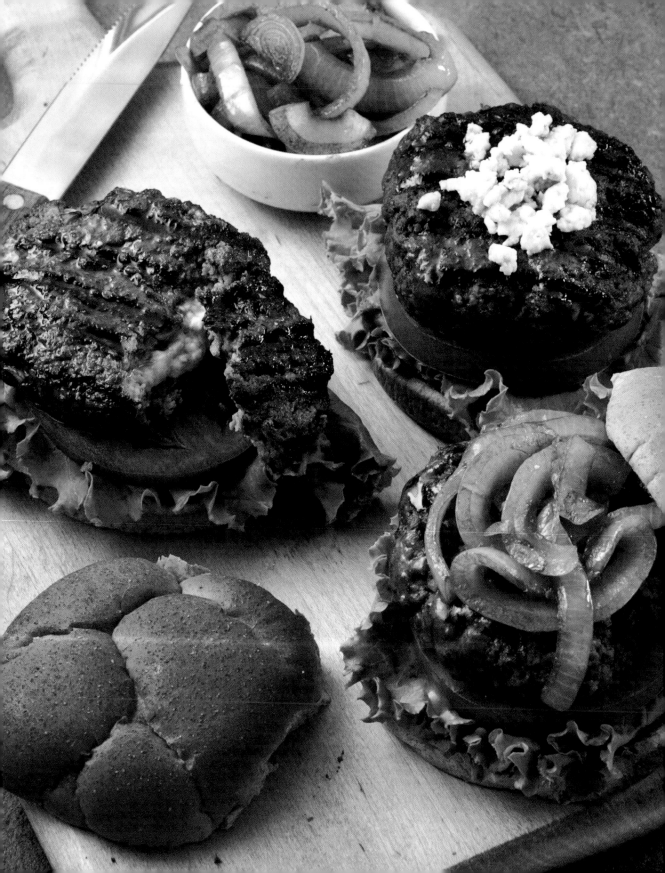

Stuffed Black and Blue Steak Burgers

IF YOUR DREAM IS TO HAVE THE FLAVOR of a steakhouse steak on a bun, this is your burger. With mushrooms to keep it juicy and a burst of tangy blue cheese tucked in the middle, this deluxe burger doesn't disappoint. To take this burger over the top, toast the buns and add a layer of Shortcut Caramelized Onions (page 140). No time to stuff it, no problem! Simply make and shape the steak burgers, grill 'em, and top with blue cheese.

MAKES **4** SERVINGS

½ cup minced fresh mushrooms

3 tablespoons dry breadcrumbs

½ teaspoon black pepper

1 teaspoon garlic salt

1 pound lean ground beef

¼ cup crumbled blue cheese

Black pepper to taste

4 whole wheat hamburger buns

4 large lettuce leaves, washed and dried

1 large tomato, sliced

1. Place the mushrooms in a large microwave-safe bowl and cook on high for 1 minute. Remove and let cool slightly. Add the breadcrumbs, pepper, garlic salt and ground beef. Mix together with a fork until all ingredients are thoroughly incorporated.

2. Evenly separate the beef mixture into 4 balls. Divide each ball in half and flatten to form two 4-inch patties. Sprinkle 1 tablespoon of blue cheese in the center of the patties, leaving about a ¾-inch border free of cheese. Top with the remaining patties and pinch the edges together to seal the cheese (for best results, chill the burgers for one hour before cooking).

3. Heat a grill or grill pan over medium high heat. Add the patties and cook for 3 to 4 minutes on each side or until cooked through. Remove and let sit for 2 minutes.

4. Warm the bun and add a lettuce leaf, slice of tomato, burger and caramelized onions, if desired, to the bottom half. Cover with top half and enjoy.

DARE TO COMPARE: Typical of most restaurant blue cheese burgers, a Black & Blue Cheeseburger from the local burger joint will set you back 780 calories. Tucked inside are also 47 grams of fat (19 of them saturated) and 1,400 mg of sodium.

NUTRITION INFORMATION PER SERVING (1 burger): Calories 360 | Carbohydrate 24g (Sugars 1g) | Total Fat 16g (Sat Fat 7g) | Protein 32g | Fiber 5g | Cholesterol 55mg | Sodium 700mg | Food Exchanges: 4½ Lean Meat, 1½ Carbohydrate, 1 Fat | Carbohydrate Choices: 1½ | Weight Watcher Plus Point Comparison: 9

Short-cut Caramelized Onions

IF YOU LOVE CARAMELIZED ONIONS, you are really going to love this recipe. Sweet, buttery soft caramelized onions elevate everything from eggs and casseroles to pasta and pizza. One of my favorite uses for them is as a condiment for sandwiches and burgers. The only downside of caramelized onions is the time and attention usually required to make them. Not anymore. Here, a quick 5-minute start in the microwave, a pinch of salt, and a touch of vinegar shortcuts the cooking time to as little as 15 minutes!

MAKES **8** SERVINGS

8 cups thinly sliced onions (about 2 large onions)

1 teaspoon canola oil

Pinch of salt

1 teaspoon water

1 teaspoon balsamic vinegar

1. Place the onions in a microwave-safe bowl and cover with plastic wrap. Cook on high for 5 minutes. Remove and set aside.

2. Heat the oil in a large non-stick skillet over medium heat. Add the onions and salt and cook for 5 minutes, stirring occasionally, until they are well softened. Add 1 teaspoon of water and 1 teaspoon of balsamic vinegar to the pan, scraping the bottom of the pan while stirring. Continue to stir onions until nicely browned, about 5 to 8 minutes longer.

Marlene Says: *Onions are amazingly healthy. Low in calories and virtually fat-free (like their cousin, garlic), they have been shown to improve immunity, reduce certain types of cancer, help control blood sugar, and lower blood pressure.*

NUTRITION INFORMATION PER SERVING (¼ cup): Calories 45 | Carbohydrate 9g (Sugars 0g) | Total Fat .5g (Sat Fat 0g) | Protein 1g | Fiber 2g | Cholesterol 0mg | Sodium 25mg | Food Exchanges: 1½ Vegetable | Carbohydrate Choice: ½ | Weight Watcher Plus Point Comparison: 1

Brand New Reuben Sandwich

EVEN THOUGH THE REUBEN SANDWICH is heralded as a New York deli creation, every Nebraskan knows that Omaha grocer Reuben Kulakofsky was the actual inventor of this now-classic masterpiece. No matter where you order it, though, there is no confusion that this tasty combination of Russian dressing, sauerkraut and cured beef can wreak havoc on even the most liberal of diets. Feel free to claim this very tasty better-for-you Reuben as your very own.

MAKES **2** SERVINGS

1½ tablespoons light mayonnaise

1½ tablespoons low-fat plain yogurt

1 tablespoon ketchup

1 teaspoon pickle relish

4 slices rye bread

2 slices reduced-fat Swiss cheese

10 slices or 3.5 ounces thin pastrami

¼ cup sauerkraut, rinsed, drained and squeezed dry

1. In small bowl, whisk together the mayonnaise, yogurt, ketchup, and relish. Set aside.

2. Spread each slice of bread with 1 tablespoon of the dressing. Cut cheese slices in half. Top two of the slices of bread with a piece of cheese, then half the pastrami, two tablespoons of sauerkraut, and another piece of cheese. Top sandwiches with remaining bread.

3. Spray a large non-stick skillet with cooking spray and heat over medium heat. Place the sandwiches in the skillet and cook for 3 to 4 minutes or until underside is golden brown.

4. Lift the sandwiches out of the way, spray the skillet again with cooking spray, and flip the sandwiches. Cook for 3 more minutes or until the underside is golden brown and the cheese is melted.

Marlene Says: *When it comes to bread and keeping your blood sugar in check, rye is your guy. A study published in the American Journal of Clinical Nutrition found that rye bread triggers even less of an insulin response than many whole wheat breads, making it a healthy, high fiber, low-glycemic index selection.*

NUTRITION INFORMATION PER SERVING (1 sandwich): Calories 270 | Carbohydrate 32 g (Sugars 6g) | Total Fat 8g (Sat Fat 2.5g) | Protein 17g | Fiber 4g | Cholesterol 10mg | Sodium 880mg | Food Exchanges: 2½ Lean Meat, 2 Starch, ½ Fat | Carbohydrate Choices: 2 | Weight Watcher Plus Point Comparison: 7

best dressed salads

Side Salads

Good Ol' Iceberg with Classic French Dressing

Green Leafy Salad with Green Goddess Dressing

Mixed Greens with Everyday Balsamic Vinaigrette

Lime-Cottage Cheese Jell-O Salad

Classic Spinach Salad with Bacon Dressing

Creamy Ranch Slaw

Potluck Peanut Slaw

Farmer's Market Potato Salad

Corn and Tomato Salad

Super Spinach and Orzo Pasta Salad

Entrée Salads

Almost Everything Chopped Salad

Apple, Chicken, and Walnut Salad with Raspberry Vinaigrette

Crispy Chicken Salad with Honey Mustard Dressing

Anything Goes Asian Spinach Salad

Quick 'n Healthy Taco Salad

According to an article in the *Wall Street Journal*, the average American eats salad at mealtimes only about 36 times a year. Fewer than half of all Americans *eat* a leaf salad at home each week. As a registered dietitian and, more importantly, as a true salad lover, I am confident that the recipes in this chapter will *inspire you* and yours to make, and *eat, more salads*.

With so many wonderful ingredients to choose from, I love developing *healthy* salad recipes, but I also find it surprisingly challenging. While it's easy to combine bagged greens and bottled reduced-calorie dressing (and that's okay), it is quite another task to create easy, healthy, *crave-worthy* salads—especially when they include bacon, cheese, and nuts—and flavorful *sweet* and *creamy* dressings that we all *love*. But I am proud to say that I have done it; I am delighted to present you with fifteen incredible *healthy* salads (bacon, cheese, and nuts included!).

A few of my *favorite* new side salads are the *lovely* Green Leafy Salad with luscious Green Goddess Dressing (which doubles nicely as a dip), Classic Spinach Salad with Bacon Dressing (only 75 calories!), and the old-fashioned, but *never out of style*, Lime Cottage Cheese Jell-O Salad. On the entrée side, the flavor's big and the fat and calorie savings are even *bigger* in memorable lunch and *dinner salads* that I dare you not to love. Let me tempt you with the fit and fresh Apple, Chicken and Walnut Salad, or the *super-satisfying* Crispy Chicken Salad with Honey Mustard Dressing, or the filling Almost Everything Chopped Italian Salad, which combines cubed turkey, salami, cheese, garbanzo beans, tomatoes, lettuce, and fresh basil with an Italian-style dressing for, well, *a bit of everything*.

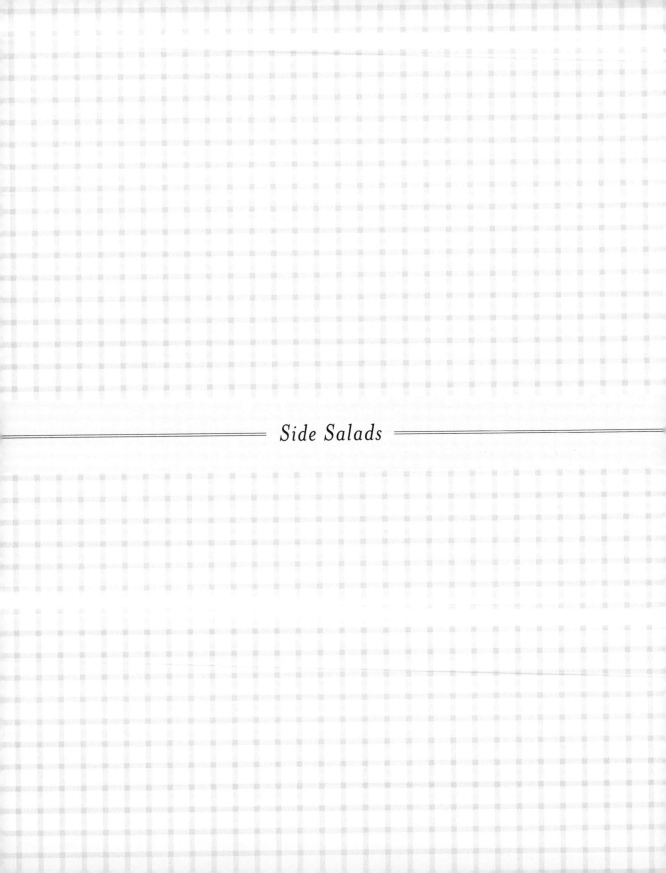

Side Salads

Good Ol' Iceberg with Classic French Dressing

WHEN I WAS GROWING UP, green salad meant iceberg lettuce. Today, good ol' iceberg is often pushed aside in favor of darker leafy greens. While iceberg may have fewer nutrients, it still provides fiber, along with that satisfying cool crispy crunch you can't get from other salad greens. Here I pair it with carrots, cucumbers, tomatoes and the true star, a crowd-pleasing "Catalina-style" French dressing. (Note: You will use only half of the dressing for this recipe. The rest will keep for up to 2 weeks in the refrigerator.)

MAKES **4** SERVINGS

Dressing

¾ teaspoon cornstarch

¼ cup cider vinegar

3 tablespoons canola oil

3 tablespoons tomato paste

3 tablespoons granulated no-calorie sweetener (or 4 packets)

1 teaspoon Worcestershire sauce

¼ teaspoon garlic powder

¼ teaspoon onion powder

½ teaspoon prepared mustard

¼ teaspoon salt

Scant ¼ teaspoon black pepper

Salad

4 cups chopped iceberg lettuce

½ cup grated carrot

1 cucumber, peeled and sliced

2 medium tomatoes, cut into wedges

1. For the dressing, whisk together ½ cup water and cornstarch in a small saucepan. Bring to a simmer and cook over low heat 3 to 4 minutes, stirring, until mixture thickens slightly and clears. Remove from heat and set aside. Whisk together remaining dressing ingredients in a medium bowl. Add the cornstarch mixture and whisk again until smooth.

2. For the salad, in a large bowl combine the lettuce and carrot and toss lightly.

3. Add the cucumber slices and tomato wedges and lightly toss with dressing.

NUTRITION INFORMATION PER SERVING (1½ cups): Calories 70 | Carbohydrates 6g (Sugar 2g) | Total Fat 5g (Sat Fat .5g) | Protein 1g | Fiber 2g | Cholesterol 0mg | Sodium 100mg | Food Exchanges: 1 Vegetable, 1 Fat | Carbohydrate Choices: ½ | Weight Watcher Plus Point Comparison: 2

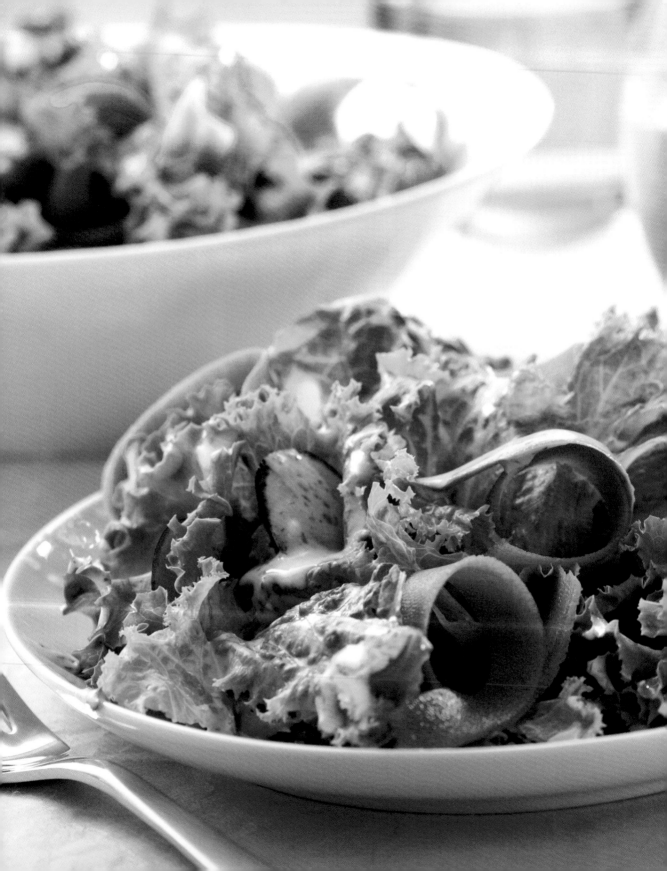

Green Leafy Salad with Green Goddess Dressing

REMEMBER WHEN GREEN GODDESS DRESSING was queen? Well, I think it's time for a come-back (with a healthy twist). With the perfect blend of fresh herbs, vibrant green color and creamy base, Green Goddess dressing is also fabulous as a dip. To serve it with your favorite veggies just add half of the milk. Speaking of its green color, if you don't have chives on hand, chopped green onion tops are a fine substitute.

MAKES **6** SERVINGS

Dressing

¼ cup light mayonnaise

¼ cup plain low-fat yogurt

⅓ cup 1% milk

¼ cup chopped fresh parsley, packed

2 tablespoons chopped chives

¼ teaspoon dried tarragon

1 tablespoon white wine or cider vinegar

¼ teaspoon garlic powder

⅛ teaspoon black pepper

⅛ teaspoon salt

½ teaspoon anchovy paste (optional)

Salad

9 cups torn green leaf lettuce, about 1 head

3 carrots

6 radishes

1. For the dressing, combine all of the ingredients in a blender (or deep bowl if you're using an immersion blender) and blend briefly just until smooth. Set aside.

2. For the salad, peel the carrots and trim off the ends. With a vegetable peeler, starting from the top, lightly peel strips to form wide, thin ribbons. Place the carrot strips in a bowl of ice water and set aside. Slice the radishes and add slices to ice water.

3. When ready to serve, drain the carrot and radish slices. Place 1½ cups of lettuce on each plate. Top the lettuce with 4 to 5 carrot curls and 4 to 5 radish slices. Drizzle 2 tablespoons of the dressing over each salad.

Marlene Says: *Green Goddess Louie Salads offer a delicious twist on a classic favorite. Top salad greens with shrimp or crab, asparagus, tomato and egg wedges and dressing.*

NUTRITION INFORMATION PER SERVING (1 salad): Calories 60 | Carbohydrate 7 g (Sugars 4g) | Total Fat 3g (Sat Fat 0g) | Protein 3g | Fiber 2g | Cholesterol 5mg | Sodium 210mg | Food Exchanges: 1 Vegetable, ½ Fat | Carbohydrate Choices: 1 | Weight Watcher Plus Point Comparison: 1

Mixed Greens with Everyday Balsamic Vinaigrette

THIS SIMPLE SALAD IS TOO EASY AND TOO GOOD not to share. It's my easy weeknight go-to salad, with my favorite all-purpose dressing. While I often switch up the greens (and veggies) depending on what's on hand, the balsamic vinaigrette stays put. This versatile dressing can also be used as a marinade for chicken or beef or drizzled onto hot or cold vegetables.

MAKES **4** SERVINGS

Dressing

2 tablespoons balsamic vinegar

2 tablespoons virgin or extra virgin olive oil

2 tablespoons water

1 clove garlic, minced

1 teaspoon Dijon mustard

1 tablespoon grated Parmesan cheese

Pinch of salt

Pinch of pepper

Salad

5 cups bagged mixed greens

1 cup cherry tomatoes

Fresh pepper to taste

Parmesan cheese (optional)

1. For the dressing, whisk together or vigorously shake all of the dressing ingredients. Adjust salt and pepper to taste.

2. For the salad, place mixed greens and tomatoes in a large bowl. Add dressing and toss. Top with fresh ground pepper to taste and garnish with shaved Parmesan cheese, if desired. (I usually top my salad with a few thin shavings of Parmesan cheese. It adds about 15 calories and one additional gram each of protein and fat.)

DARE TO COMPARE: Because of the oil, vinaigrette dressings tend to have even *more* calories than their creamy counterparts. A typical restaurant serving of balsamic dressing can have as many as 360 calories and 40 grams of fat.

NUTRITION INFORMATION PER SERVING (1½ cups): Calories 80 | Carbohydrate 5g (Sugars 3g) | Total Fat 7g (Sat Fat 0g) | Protein 2g | Fiber 1g | Cholesterol 0mg | Sodium 100mg | Food Exchanges: 1 Vegetable, 1 Fat | Carbohydrate Choices: ½ | Weight Watcher Plus Point Comparison: 2

Lime-Cottage Cheese Jell-O® Salad

GELATIN SALADS NEVER GO OUT OF STYLE. While its heyday may have been in the 1950s, over 300 million boxes of Jell-O® gelatin are sold in the US each year—and plenty of it still makes its way into salads. What I love about this salad (besides its creamy, fruity, dessert-like taste) is that it proves how making small changes in a traditional recipe can make a big difference. While its nutritional content previously made it a buffet no-no for much of my family, it's now a can-do for everyone. That's always in style.

MAKES 12 SERVINGS

1 package (8-serving size) sugar-free lime gelatin

1 cup boiling water

2 tablespoons fresh lemon juice

1 (8-ounce) can crushed pineapple, packed in unsweetened juice

1 cup low-fat cottage cheese

3 cups light whipped topping, thawed

1. Place the gelatin and boiling water in a medium bowl and whisk for 2 minutes or until gelatin is dissolved. Stir in lemon juice and pineapple with its juice. Refrigerate until the mixture begins to thicken and has a syrupy consistency, about 30 minutes.

2. Place the cottage cheese in a small food processor and process until smooth, or put it in a deep bowl if you're using an immersion blender.

3. Gently fold the cottage cheese and whipped topping into the thickened gelatin mixture. Pour mixture into a 9 x 13-inch pan and refrigerate until set, about an hour.

Marlene Says: *The original recipe that inspired this (made with regular lime gelatin and heavy whipping cream) had triple the calories and carbs and five times the fat! This slim salad offers a lot of bang for your calorie buck.*

NUTRITION INFORMATION PER SERVING (1 square): Calories 80 | Carbohydrate 8g (Sugars 5g) | Total Fat 3g (Sat Fat 2.5g) | Protein 3g | Fiber 0g | Cholesterol 0mg | Sodium 105mg | Food Exchanges: ½ Carbohydrate, ½ Fat | Carbohydrate Choices: ½ | Weight Watcher Plus Point Comparison: 2

Classic Spinach Salad with Bacon Dressing

WHO CAN RESIST SPINACH SALAD with warm bacon dressing? You might want to after reading my "Dare to Compare," but you won't have to when armed with this better-than-ever recipe for Classic Spinach Salad, with just 75 calories per serving! (P.S. Turn this into a waist-whittling meal for two by dividing the salad in half and topping each with 3 ½ ounces grilled shrimp, chicken, or sliced steak.)

MAKES **4** SERVINGS

3 slices center-cut lean bacon

¼ cup diced red onion

3 tablespoons cider vinegar

1 tablespoon sugar

¼ teaspoon liquid smoke

⅛ teaspoon salt

⅛ teaspoon black pepper

1 teaspoon cornstarch

1½ cups sliced mushrooms

8 to 10 cups cleaned spinach

½ cup thinly sliced red onion

Fresh black pepper, optional

1. In a medium non-stick sauté pan, cook the bacon over medium heat until crisp. Transfer the bacon to a paper-towel-lined plate, crumble, and set aside.

2. Add the diced onion to the drippings in the pan. Cook onion for 3 to 4 minutes or until softened. Add vinegar, 3 tablespoons water, sugar, liquid smoke, salt, and black pepper, and stir, scraping the pan to incorporate drippings. Bring to a low boil. Mix cornstarch with 1 tablespoon of water and add to pan. Cook, while stirring, until thickened and clear. Add mushrooms to skillet, and sauté for 1 to 2 minutes, tossing until they soften slightly and are coated with the dressing.

3. In a large bowl, combine the spinach and onion. Pour hot dressing over spinach mixture and lightly toss. Sprinkle with bacon and fresh black pepper, if desired. Serve immediately.

DARE TO COMPARE: Like other spinach salads, the Bacon and Spinach Salad at Trader Joe's appears rather healthy—until you read the label! With 880 calories, over 75 grams of fat and 1,500 mg of sodium in each container, it's anything but.

*Healthy tip: read the label on the package **before** you eat what's inside.*

NUTRITION INFORMATION PER SERVING (about 1½ cups): Calories 75 | Carbohydrate 9g (Sugars 5g) | Total Fat 1.5 g (Sat Fat 1) | Protein 3g | Fiber 2g | Cholesterol 5mg | Sodium 105mg | Food Exchanges: 1 Vegetable | Carbohydrate Choices: ½ | Weight Watcher Plus Point Comparison: 1

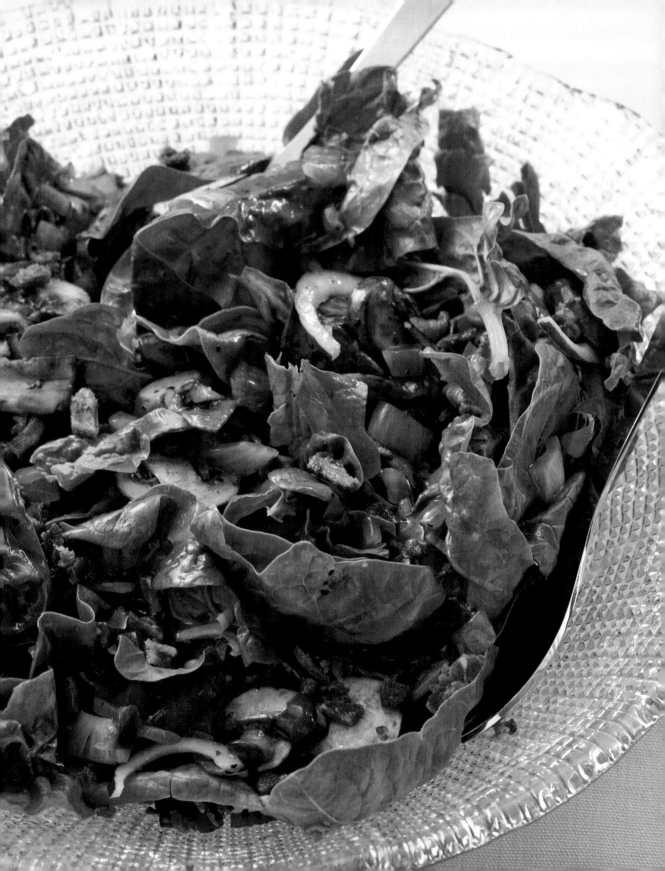

Creamy Ranch Slaw

THIS TASTY SLAW WILL BE THE HIT OF THE PARTY. Graced with creamy Ranch-style dressing, it's studded with everyone's favorite Ranch dressing dippers—celery and carrots—for a creamy, crunchy combination that's hard to beat. Serve it at home or pack it up and tote it to your next get-together and watch it disappear.

Dressing

½ cup light mayonnaise

⅓ cup plain low-fat yogurt

⅓ cup low-fat milk

1 tablespoon cider vinegar

¾ teaspoon onion powder

¾ teaspoon garlic powder

¼ teaspoon salt

¼ teaspoon black pepper

Salad

6 cups shredded green cabbage

3 stalks celery, chopped (about 1½ cups)

2 medium carrots, peeled and chopped

3 tablespoons minced fresh parsley

1. For the dressing, whisk together all the dressing ingredients in a small bowl.

2. For the slaw, in a large bowl, combine the cabbage, celery, and carrots. Pour dressing over the salad and toss. Add parsley and toss lightly once more.

Marlene Says: *The creamy, crunchy texture of this salad is best when freshly dressed. The salad mix can be made up to one day in advance and held in the refrigerator. The dressing can be made up to 3 hours before serving. Once you toss the salad with the dressing, it's best to serve it within 2 hours.*

NUTRITION INFORMATION PER SERVING (¾ cup): Calories 60 | Carbohydrate 8g (Sugars 4g) | Total Fat 4g (Sat Fat .5g) | Protein 2g | Fiber 2g | Cholesterol 5mg | Sodium 240mg | Food Exchanges: 1 Vegetable, 1 Fat | Carbohydrate Choices: ½ | Weight Watcher Plus Point Comparison: 2

Potluck Peanut Slaw

HANDS-DOWN, THIS IS THE SIMPLEST, EASIEST, BEST-TASTING peanut dressing I've ever created! You'll want to use this sweet, tangy, salty, creamy sauce on everything from pasta to shrimp— it's that good. Here I pair it with an abundance of shredded raw veggies for a unique and pretty slaw worthy of any potluck, but plain old cabbage and carrots (or a bag of ready-to-eat coleslaw mix) works fine too. Be ready to share this recipe because you'll be asked for it time and time again.

MAKES **8** SERVINGS

Dressing

¼ cup rice wine vinegar

3 tablespoons creamy peanut butter

1 tablespoon hoisin sauce

1 teaspoon sesame oil

Red pepper flakes, to taste

Salad

5 cups shredded green cabbage

2 medium zucchini, shredded, about 2 cups

2 medium yellow squash, shredded, about 2 cups

2 medium carrots, shredded

½ cup thinly sliced green onions

Chopped peanuts, optional

Fresh cilantro, optional

1. For the dressing, in a blender combine vinegar, peanut butter, hoisin, 2 tablespoons water, and sesame oil and process until smooth.

2. For the slaw, in a large bowl, combine the cabbage, zucchini, squash, carrots, and green onion. Pour dressing over cabbage mixture and toss well to coat.

3. Cover and place in the refrigerator. Serve chilled, topped with optional chopped peanuts and/or cilantro.

NUTRITION INFORMATION PER SERVING (1 cup): Calories 70 | Carbohydrate 8g (Sugars 4g) | Total Fat 4g (Sat Fat 1g) | Protein 3g | Fiber 3g | Cholesterol 0mg | Sodium 75mg | Food Exchanges: 1 Vegetable, 1 Fat | Carbohydrate Choices: ½ | Weight Watcher Plus Point Comparison: 2

Farmer's Market Potato Salad

THIS DELICIOUS FARM-FRESH potato salad will have your guests sitting up and taking notice. Roasting the potatoes rather than boiling them adds another layer of flavor that combines perfectly with crunchy celery and the tangy, slightly creamy mustard dressing. Corn, zucchini and basil add a fresh burst of summer. If you are a potato-mayo salad fan, look for my Red, White and Blue Potato Salad in Eat What You Love *(page 188), or better yet, make them both for an extra special backyard celebration.*

MAKES **6** SERVINGS

Salad

1½ pounds red potatoes cut into large (about 2-inch) chunks

1½ teaspoons olive oil

2 medium zucchini, sliced lengthwise, then cut in half

2 cups sliced red onion (about 1 small)

½ cup corn, fresh or frozen/ thawed

1 cup cherry tomatoes, halved

½ cup chopped celery

Dressing

2 tablespoons Dijon mustard

2 tablespoons cider vinegar

1 tablespoon oil

2 tablespoons fresh basil, chopped

¾ teaspoon seasoned salt or more to taste

½ teaspoon ground black pepper

1. Preheat the oven to 425°F. Spray a baking sheet with cooking spray.

2. Place the potatoes and 1 teaspoon of the oil in a medium bowl and toss. Pour potatoes onto the baking sheet in a single layer and spray lightly with cooking spray. Bake for 10 minutes, stir the potatoes, and bake another 10 minutes.

3. While the potatoes are baking, place the zucchini and onions in the bowl and toss with ½ teaspoon oil. After 20 minutes, remove the potatoes from the oven, stir, and push to one side of the pan. Add zucchini, onions and corn. Return to the oven for another 10 to 15 minutes or until potatoes are tender. Remove from oven and allow to cool slightly.

4. Combine dressing ingredients in a small bowl and whisk to combine. Place the cooked vegetables in a large bowl with tomatoes and celery. Pour the dressing over the vegetables and toss. Serve immediately or refrigerate to let the flavors meld.

NUTRITION INFORMATION PER SERVING (1 cup): Calories 160 | Carbohydrate 26g (Sugars 4g) | Total Fat 6g (Sat Fat 0g) | Protein 3g | Fiber 3g | Cholesterol 0mg | Sodium 310mg | Food Exchanges: 1 Starch, 1 Vegetable, 1 Fat | Carbohydrate Choices: 1½ Weight Watcher Plus Point Comparison: 5

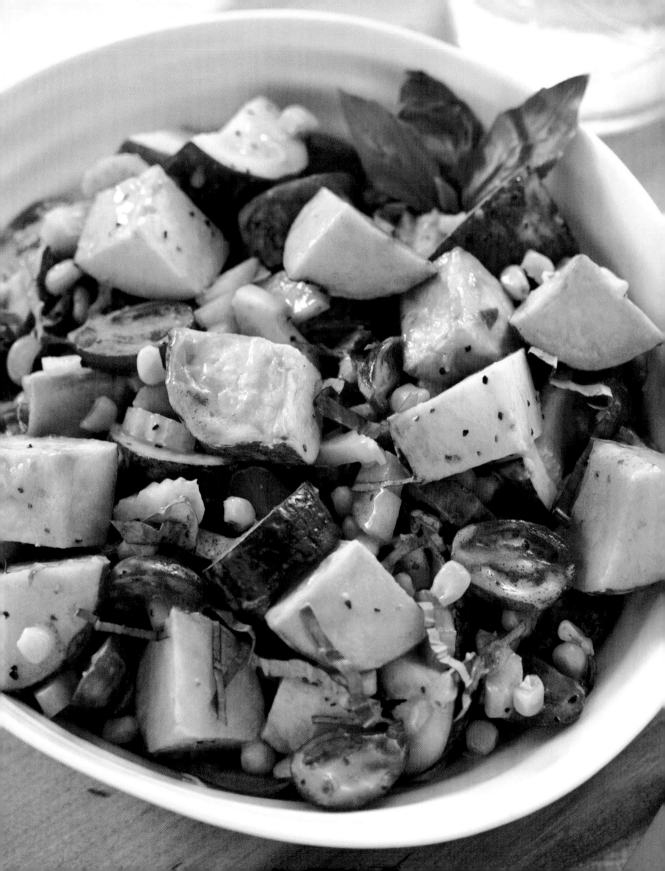

Corn and Tomato Salad

THIS SALAD BOASTS AN ARRAY OF COLORS, textures and flavors from summer's cream of the crop. It's also a great way to use leftover corn on the cob. Equally delicious when served cold, at room temperature, or warm, enjoy it as a salad or as a side dish to grilled steak, chicken or seafood. In colder months, you can still savor the taste of summer by using frozen corn, which is packaged at the peak of its flavor.

MAKES **8** SERVINGS

Dressing

¼ cup white wine vinegar

2 tablespoons water

3 tablespoons olive oil

1 teaspoon Dijon mustard

2 tablespoons sugar or granulated no-calorie sweetener (or 3 packets)

1 teaspoon minced garlic (1 clove)

¼ teaspoon seasoned salt

⅛ teaspoon black pepper

Salad

2½ cups frozen corn niblets, thawed, or 5 ears of corn, kernels stripped from the cob

1 medium zucchini, diced

½ small red onion, diced, about ½ cup

½ medium red bell pepper, diced

2 medium Italian tomatoes, cored, seeded and diced

1. For the dressing, in a small bowl, whisk all the ingredients together.

2. In a large bowl combine the corn, zucchini, onion and bell pepper. Pour the dressing over and toss lightly. Add the tomatoes and toss lightly. Refrigerate for 30 minutes to let flavors meld. This dish holds well for two to three days.

Marlene Says: *For a healthy twist, substitute 1¼ cups frozen shelled edamame for half of the corn (adds 3 grams protein, 1 gram fiber and 20 calories).*

NUTRITION INFORMATION PER SERVING (⅔ cup): Calories 80 | Carbohydrate 12g (Sugars 7g) | Total Fat 3g (Sat Fat 1g) | Protein 2g | Fiber 2g | Cholesterol 0mg | Sodium 40mg | Food Exchanges: ½ Starch, 1 Vegetable | Carbohydrate Choices: 1 | Weight Watcher Plus Point Comparison: 2

Super Spinach and Orzo Pasta Salad

IF YOU ARE LOOKING FOR A SUPER VERSATILE, super-satisfying pasta salad, this salad fits the bill. Featuring the rice-sized pasta, orzo, it works beautifully as a picnic-friendly side, a buffet salad, or even a warm side dish. Toss in some shrimp or chicken and you have a light, yet filling, entrée salad. Bonus: it can be served immediately, at room temperature, cold out of the fridge, warmed, or even reheated the next day.

MAKES **6** SERVINGS

¾ cup orzo

1 teaspoon plus 1 tablespoon plus olive oil

2 tablespoons red wine vinegar

½ teaspoon Dijon mustard

½ teaspoon dried oregano

½ teaspoon dried basil

¼ teaspoon salt

¼ teaspoon pepper

2 cups fresh spinach, julienned

¼ cup chopped soft sun-dried tomatoes (not oil-packed)

1 cup cherry tomatoes, halved

1. Cook the pasta according to package directions, drain, and rinse. Place orzo in a large bowl, toss with 1 teaspoon olive oil, and set aside to cool.

2. To make the dressing, in a medium bowl whisk together 1 tablespoon olive oil, vinegar, mustard, oregano, basil, salt, and pepper.

3. Add the dressing, spinach, sun-dried and cherry tomatoes to the orzo and toss lightly to combine.

Marlene Says: *The blend of pasta and spinach makes this a great side dish for grilled chicken, meat, or fish. To serve it warm, mix the dressing and other ingredients with just cooked, hot orzo and serve immediately.*

NUTRITION INFORMATION PER SERVING (about ⅔ cup): Calories 140 | Carbohydrate 24g (Sugars 2g) | Total Fat 3g (Sat Fat 0g) | Protein 5g | Fiber 2g | Cholesterol 0mg | Sodium 170mg | Food Exchanges: 1½ Starch, 1 Vegetable | Carbohydrate Choices: 1½ | Weight Watcher Plus Point Comparison: 4

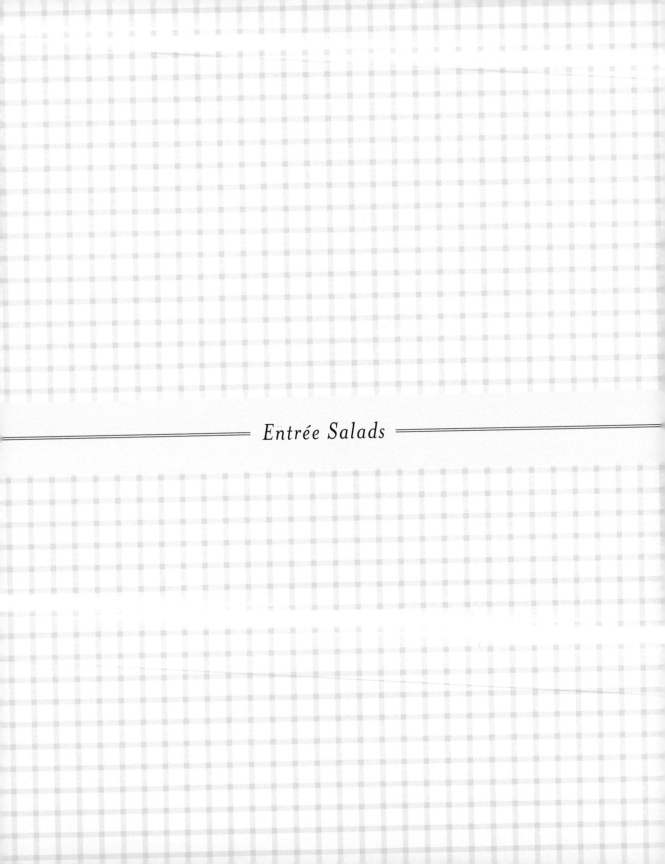

Entrée Salads

Almost Everything Chopped Salad

AT CALIFORNIA PIZZA KITCHEN, this type of salad is known as "The Original Chopped" salad. With two kinds of meat, cheese, beans, lettuce and a killer dressing, it's a salad that tastes like it has everything! This tasty knock-off also gives you "everything"—except the excessive fat and calories. For a mere 330 calories, you get salami, chicken, mozzarella, Parmesan, tomatoes, romaine and the same type of decadent-tasting dressing that will make you forget about the original Original.

Dressing

2 tablespoons Dijon mustard

2 tablespoons red wine vinegar

2 tablespoons extra virgin olive oil

3 tablespoons grated Parmesan cheese

½ teaspoon dried oregano

1 garlic clove, minced

⅛ teaspoon salt

Salad

1 cup canned garbanzo beans, drained and rinsed

2 cups chopped cooked skinless chicken or turkey breast

¼ cup light salami, about 6 large slices (like Gallo brand)

¾ cup shredded part skim mozzarella cheese

2 medium tomatoes, seeded and diced

4 cups chopped romaine lettuce

¼ cup fresh slivered basil

1. For the dressing, in a medium bowl or lidded container, place the ingredients plus 2 tablespoons water. Whisk, or cover and shake well, to combine.

2. For the salad, in a large bowl, place the garbanzos, chicken or turkey, salami, and mozzarella. Pour half of the dressing over the salad and toss gently to combine. Add the tomatoes, lettuce and basil. Pour on the remaining dressing and toss lightly to coat.

DARE TO COMPARE: Think salads are healthy? An Original Chopped Salad at California Pizza Kitchen has 987 calories, almost a day's worth of saturated fat and over 2,000 mg of sodium!

NUTRITION INFORMATION PER SERVING (1½ cups): Calories 330 | Carbohydrate 15g (Sugars 2g) | Total Fat 16g (Sat Fat 4g) | Protein 31g | Fiber 5g | Cholesterol 80mg | Sodium 810 mg | Food Exchanges: 4 Lean Meat, 1 Starch, 2 Fat | Carbohydrate Choices: 1 | Weight Watcher Plus Point Comparison: 8

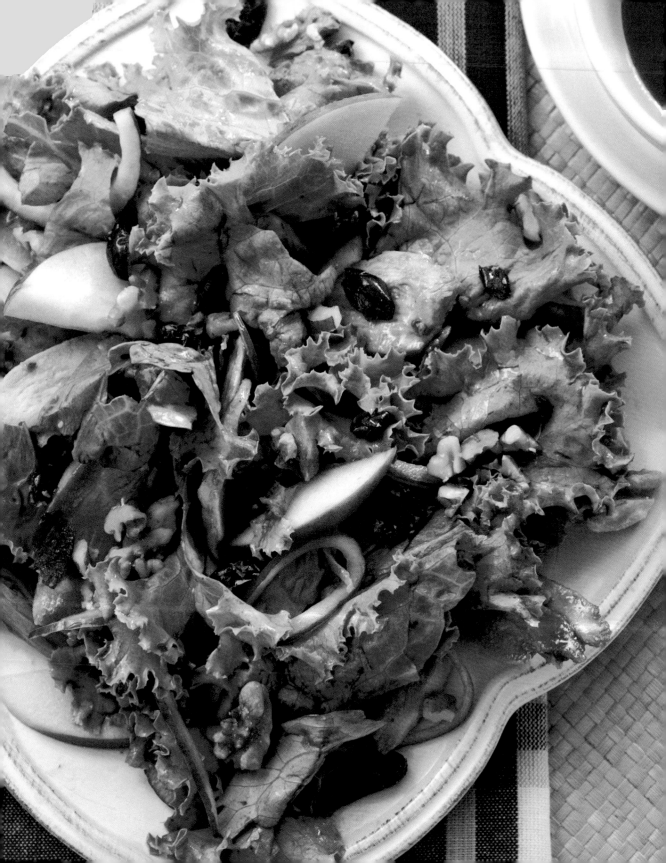

Apple, Chicken, and Walnut Salad with Raspberry Vinaigrette

*THE ADDITION OF FRUIT AND NUTS is the best thing that's happened to s___ ___ oil and vinegar. While the duo **are** healthier replacements for ingredients such as bacon an___ ___ it's possible to overdo even a good thing (see my "Dare to Compare" below). With a tast___ ___ of fruit, nuts, lean chicken breast and reduced-fat raspberry vinaigrette, this good-for-you ___ ___ bo hits just the right spot.*

MAKES ___ GS

Dressing

3 tablespoons rice wine vinegar

1½ tablespoons olive oil

4 tablespoons sugar-free raspberry jam

2 teaspoons Dijon mustard

1 tablespoon lime juice

⅛ teaspoon black pepper

Pinch of salt

Salad

8 cups chopped green leaf lettuce

1 large Fuji apple, cored and sliced

½ small red onion, thinly sliced

2 cups chopped cooked skinless chicken breast

2 tablespoons dried cranberries

¼ cup chopped walnuts

1. For the dressing, in a small bowl, vigorously whis___ ___ gredients together until smooth.

2. In a large bowl, combine the lettuce, apple, and onion. Pour the dressing over the salad and toss lightly to coat. Add the chicken and lightly toss again.

3. Portion the salad onto four plates. Top evenly with the cranberries and walnuts.

DARE TO COMPARE: A typical Apple, Chicken, and Walnut Salad at your neighborhood restaurant can set you back as much as 1,000 calories and contains up to an entire day's worth of fat and sodium. No wonder studies show a heavy correlation between dining out and weight gain.

NUTRITION INFORMATION PER SERVING: Calories 230 | Carbohydrate 16g (Sugars 5g) | Total Fat 12g (Sat Fat 1g) | Protein 19g | Fiber 3g | Cholesterol 45mg | Sodium 170mg | Food Exchanges: 3 Lean Meat, 1 Vegetable, 1 Fat, ½ Fruit | Carbohydrate Choices: 1 | Weight Watcher Plus Point Comparison: 6

Crispy Chicken Salad with Honey Mustard Dressing

THIS IS FOR THE KIND READER who asked me to please make over her favorite (incredibly fattening) salad. Note: The Honey Mustard Dressing is a stand-out. Please feel free to use it anywhere you choose. It keeps well in the fridge for several days and has just 50 calories, 5 grams of carbohydrate and 3 grams of fat per 2 tablespoon serving.

MAKES **2** SERVINGS

Dressing

¼ cup light mayonnaise

¼ cup light sour cream

2 tablespoons prepared mustard

1 tablespoon cider vinegar

1 tablespoon honey

Salad

2 (4-ounce) skinless, boneless chicken breasts

6 tablespoons panko breadcrumbs, finely crushed

2 tablespoons flour, divided

¼ teaspoon seasoned salt

¼ teaspoon black pepper

1 teaspoon canola oil

1 large egg white, beaten

4 cups chopped romaine

¼ cup shredded carrots

4 tablespoons reduced-fat cheddar cheese

1 large tomato, cut into wedges

1. For the dressing, whisk together all ingredients with 2 tablespoons of water.

2. Preheat oven to 400°F. Wrap the chicken breasts in plastic and place on a cutting board and gently pound until ¼-inch thick.

3. Place the panko crumbs in a wide flat bowl along with 1 tablespoon flour and the spices. Add oil and mix until well combined. Coat the chicken breasts with remaining flour, dip into egg white, and coat with crumb mixture. Put chicken on a baking pan and place in oven. Bake for 15 to 20 minutes or until golden brown and center is cooked.

4. To assemble salad, mix together the romaine lettuce and carrots and place on 2 plates. Sprinkle each with 2 tablespoons cheese. Arrange tomato wedges on the edges of plates and drizzle salads with 2 tablespoons dressing. Slice chicken breasts into ½-inch slices and lay across tops of the salads. Drizzle chicken with 1 tablespoon dressing.

NUTRITION INFORMATION PER SERVING: Calories 340 | Carbohydrate 25g (Sugars 7g) | Total Fat 12g (Sat Fat 2.5g) | Protein 34g | Fiber 3g | Cholesterol 90mg | Sodium 610mg | Food Exchanges: 4 Lean Meat, 1 Starch, 1 Vegetable, 1 Fat | Carbohydrate Choices: 1 ½ | Weight Watcher Plus Point Comparison: 9

Anything Goes Asian Spinach Salad

*ON A RECENT LUNCH DATE WITH MY MOM (who happens to **love** Asian chicken salad), I noted the popular Asian chicken salad on the menu was offered multiple ways. Inspired, I thought I would offer you multiple ways in which to enjoy my version of this popular salad. Not a spinach fan? Feel free to swap it out for chopped romaine. Feeling fishy? Top it with salmon. Want extra crunch? Add a tablespoon of almonds. It's the sweet and tangy Asian dressing that is the mainstay of the salad—other than that, anything goes!*

MAKES **2** SERVINGS

Dressing

2 tablespoons rice vinegar

4 teaspoons granulated no-calorie sweetener (or 2 packets)

1 tablespoon reduced-sodium soy sauce

1 tablespoon sesame oil

½ teaspoon grated ginger

½ teaspoon Dijon mustard

Salad

3 cups spinach or chopped romaine

1 cup snow peas or sugar snap peas (about 3 ounces)

½ cup shredded carrot

¼ cup red onion, thinly sliced

½ small Fuji apple, cut into medium cubes

8 ounces chicken, salmon or shrimp, grilled

1. To make the dressing, in a small bowl whisk together the vinegar, sweetener, soy sauce, oil, ginger and mustard.

2. For the salad, in a medium bowl, toss the spinach, peas, carrot, onion, and apple. Pour the dressing over the salad mixture and toss lightly.

3. Arrange the salad on two plates and top each salad with 4 ounces of the grilled protein of your choice.

NUTRITION INFORMATION PER SERVING (1 salad with chicken): Calories 250 | Carbohydrate 14g (Sugars 0g) | Total Fat 10g (Sat Fat 1g) | Protein 27g | Fiber 4g | Cholesterol 10mg | Sodium 470mg | Food Exchanges: 3 Lean Meat, 2 Vegetable, 1 Fat | Carbohydrate Choices: 1 | Weight Watcher Plus Point Comparison: 6

Quick 'n Healthy Taco Salad

ONCE YOU REALIZE HOW UNHEALTHY most taco salads are, it's tough to enjoy eating one without a side of guilt. By ditching the usual fried tortilla bowl and swapping in more fresh vegetables and leaner meat, I was able to substantially lower the fat in this Tex-Mex favorite. The creamy cilantro dressing replaces the guilt with a big side of yum!

MAKES **4** SERVINGS

Dressing

⅓ cup light sour cream

⅓ cup low-fat yogurt

½ cup chopped cilantro, loosely packed

2 tablespoons lime juice (about 1 lime)

⅛ teaspoon garlic salt

Salad

1 medium red bell pepper, diced

¾ pound lean ground beef

½ teaspoon chili powder

¾ cup salsa

6 cups chopped romaine lettuce

2 green onions, sliced

¾ cup low-fat Mexican blend cheese

2 medium tomatoes, cut into wedges

Reduced fat tortilla strips, optional

1. For the dressing, combine all the ingredients in a blender and blend until smooth.

2. For the salad, spray a large non-stick skillet with cooking spray and place over medium heat. Add diced pepper and sauté 3 to 4 minutes or until slightly softened. Add the beef and chili powder to the pan and sauté 5 to 6 minutes or until meat is well browned. Stir in the salsa and cook for one minute to combine. Remove from heat.

3. To assemble, place 1½ cups chopped lettuce on each of four plates. Top each salad with ¾ cup of the meat mixture. Sprinkle on ¼ of the green onions, 3 tablespoons cheese, and 3 table-spoons of dressing. Garnish with tomato wedges and optional tortilla strips, if desired.

DARE TO COMPARE: I am happy to say "adios" to the Taco Salad with Beef served at On the Border restaurant with its 1,280 calories, 85 grams fat, and 2,250 mg of sodium!

NUTRITION INFORMATION PER SERVING (one salad): Calories 280 | Carbohydrate 11g (Sugars 6g) | Total Fat 14g (Sat Fat 7g) | Protein 27g | Fiber 3g | Cholesterol 45mg | Sodium 460mg | Food Exchanges: 3 Lean Meat | Carbohydrate Choices: ½ | Weight Watcher Plus Point Comparison: 7

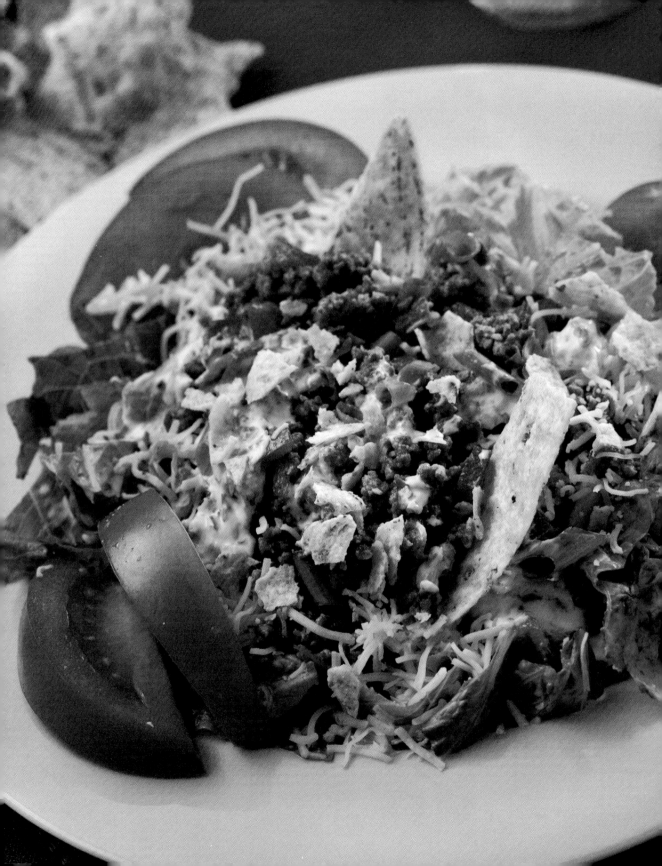

slow cooker favorites

Chicken Chili Verde

Barbecued Pulled Pork

Italian Stuffed Peppers

Chicken at the Ready

Lazy Day Lasagna

Creamy King Ranch Casserole

Wendy's-Style Chili

Stephen's Beef Stew

Fast Fix Ratatouille

Boston Baked Beans

Creamy Slow Cooker Cheesecake Sundaes

Italian Bean and Bacon Soup

Marlene's All-Purpose Marinara Sauce

I'm in love—with my slow cooker! What's not to love about coming home at the end of a long day and having a *delicious dinner ready to eat?* Or being able to entertain friends and family effortlessly with food that practically serves itself? I must admit that slow cooking is relatively new to me. While I've owned a slow cooker for years, and I've even developed a few *terrific* recipes using it, I just never used it regularly. So when I set out to create an entire chapter of healthy *family-friendly* slow-cooker recipes (which, of course, also had to be easy and taste great!), I knew I had my work cut out for me.

The truth is, slow cookers, like all cooking appliances, are better suited for some types of dishes than others. While Asian stir-fry dishes rely on short cooking times and high heat, stews, chilis, soups and *slowly braised* meats are perfectly suited to *moist slow cooking.* This chapter reflects on what really works well when cooked "slow." See page 168 for my tips for easy slow-cooker success.

An unexpected new family favorite in my home is the Lazy Day Lasagna. *My boys both love it* and I make it regularly (leftovers are terrific). My usual lasagna (and the entire day it took to make it) is a thing of the past—relinquished now to only the most special of occasions. *Quick-fix chicken dishes* like Chicken Chili Verde and Creamy King Ranch Casserole make for fabulous weeknight meals and Stephen's Sunday Stew, with its *flavorful* sauce and *fork-tender meat,* is the perfect one-pot Sunday dinner. Slow cookers are also exceptional for producing high-quality everyday basics, like Chicken at the Ready and Marlene's All-Purpose Marinara. Slow-cooker desserts, well, they're also a *delightful* surprise. Slow Cooker Apples are *meltingly tender,* while Creamy Cheesecake Sundaes (yes, in a slow cooker) are a unique crowd-pleasing treat.

For the Love of

SLOW COOKERS

The promise of slow cooking is that it is easy and effortless. Simply throw a handful of ingredients into a ceramic crockpot, leave for the day, and return to a fabulous meal. I am happy to report that it's absolutely possible—but it takes the right recipe and a bit of slow cooker smarts. Here are eight tips on how to achieve slow cooker success:

1. Cooking slow is a moist-heat method of cooking at very low temperatures. Foods that cook best quickly with very high heat, like steak and stir fries, are not as well-suited to slow cooking.

2. Reducing the amount of liquid is required for slow cooking. Due to the moist sealed environment, a rule of thumb is that slow cooker recipes require 50% less liquid. Thin sauces and extra liquid can be thickened if needed with cornstarch or flour at the end of cooking.

3. On average, the HIGH setting cooks twice as fast as LOW. For many recipes, including soups and sauces, the choice is yours. Tough meats cook up most tender when cooked on LOW (and slower), while many desserts are best on HIGH. It's best to follow recipe instructions.

4. Canned and frozen products are convenient, but it's the addition of fresh, flavorful ingredients that make slow-cooked food taste great!

5. Know your slow cooker. They're not uniformly calibrated the way ovens are (LOW on one slow cooker can be HIGH on another!). The first time you make a recipe, check for doneness at the halfway point to calibrate time. Don't check too often, however, as it slows cooking.

6. As a general rule, pack your slow cooker one-half to three-fourths full, for the best results. Medium slow cookers are 3 to 4½ quarts in capacity, while large ones hold 5 to 7 quarts. Most slow cookers hold between 4 and 6 quarts. The recipes in this book were tested with a 6-quart.

7. Onions and aromatics, such as garlic, add great flavor to slow-cooked foods, as do herbs and spices. Slow-cooking can mute flavors, so I often double the amount of spices when I slow-cook.

8. To convert slow cooker recipes to the stovetop, each hour on the stovetop is equal to approximately 6 hours on LOW or 3 hours on HIGH.

Chicken Chili Verde

THIS SOUTHWESTERN-STYLE STEW IS SATISFYING, flavorful and perfect for the slow cooker – just combine the ingredients in the crockpot and forget about it until dinnertime. Here I use economical, boneless skinless chicken thighs that cook up melt-in-your-mouth tender. My secret trick is to mix in cornmeal at the end of the cooking process. It thickens the chili quickly and smoothly and kicks up the great Southwestern-style flavor. I guarantee this dish will have your family saying "Olé!" every time they eat it.

MAKES **8** SERVINGS

2¼ pounds boneless skinless chicken thighs, visible fat removed, cut into 1-inch pieces

1 medium onion, diced

2 cloves garlic, minced

1 cup water

1 (12 ounce) jar salsa verde

1 (7-ounce) can diced green chilies

1 (15-ounce) can reduced-sodium white beans, rinsed and drained

4 teaspoons chili powder

1 teaspoon ground cumin

¼ teaspoon salt or to taste

1 tablespoon cornmeal

1. Heat a 4- to 6-quart slow cooker on high for five minutes. Add the first 9 ingredients (chicken through cumin) to the slow cooker and stir to combine.

2. Cover and cook for 6 to 8 hours on low or 3 to 4 hours on high.

3. Remove the cover and shred the chicken with two forks. Stir in the salt and the cornmeal, let sit for five minutes or until thickened to desired consistency, stir again, and serve.

Marlene Says: *For authentic Mexican flair, replace the water with one cup of your favorite beer. The chicken in this recipe can also be used to fill tacos, enchiladas or burritos.*

NUTRITION INFORMATION PER SERVING (1 cup): Calories 240 | Carbohydrate 16g (Sugars 4g) | Total Fat 5g (Sat Fat 1.5g) | Protein 29g | Fiber 3g | Cholesterol 105mg | Sodium 630mg | Food Exchanges: 4 Lean Meat, 1 Starch | Carbohydrate Choices: 1 | Weight Watcher Plus Point Comparison: 5

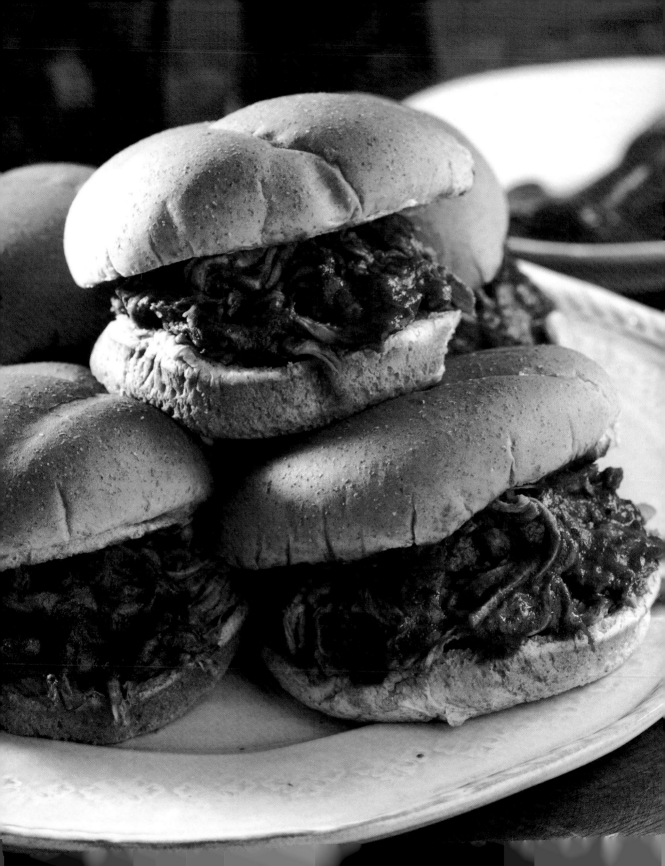

Barbecued Pulled Pork

I LOVE DISCOVERING NEW WAYS to create delicious healthy recipes, so after successfully preparing this recipe with a pork loin roast, I decided to give it a try with pork tenderloin. The result, thanks to the slow cooker, is moist, tender, falling-apart deliciousness, from the leanest cut of pork you can buy. The lip-smacking cherry cola barbecue sauce takes it over the top to pulled pork perfection.

MAKES 10 SERVINGS

2½ pounds pork tenderloin, trimmed

1 medium onion, finely chopped

2 medium cloves garlic, chopped

12 ounces diet cherry cola, divided

¾ cup low-sugar ketchup

3 tablespoons tomato paste

2 tablespoons vinegar

2 tablespoons molasses

2 tablespoons Worcestershire sauce

1½ teaspoons paprika

1 teaspoon dry mustard

¼ teaspoon black pepper

1. Place the tenderloins in a 4- to 6-quart slow cooker, along with the onions, garlic, and ½ cup cola. Cover and cook for 6 to 8 hours on low or 3 to 3½ hours on high, or until meat pulls apart when tested with a fork.

2. Pour the rest of the cola, along with the remaining ingredients, into a small saucepan. Whisk together and cook over medium heat for 10 to 15 minutes or until reduced by about one-third (you should have about 1½ cups). Set aside.

3. Transfer the cooked pork to a cutting board. Using two forks, shred the meat by pulling it apart, and set aside. Drain the liquid from the slow cooker, reserving ½ cup. Return the pork and reserved liquid back to the slow cooker.

4. Re-warm the barbecue sauce, if necessary, and pour it over the pulled pork, tossing gently to coat. Serve on buns of your choice.

Marlene Says: *There are so many healthy bun choices these days. My family likes Pepperidge Farms' soft Whole Grain White Hamburger Buns. They have a slim 100 calories, just 18 grams of carb and 2 grams of fiber.*

NUTRITION INFORMATION PER SERVING (½ cup pulled pork): Calories 170 | Carbohydrate 11g (Sugars 5g) | Total Fat 3.5g (Sat Fat 1g) | Protein 22g | Fiber 1g | Cholesterol 65mg | Sodium 310mg | Food Exchanges: 2½ Lean Meat, 1 Carbohydrate | Carbohydrate Choices: 1 Weight Watcher Plus Point Comparison: 4

Italian Stuffed Peppers

ITALIAN COMFORT FOOD MEETS A MIDWEST CLASSIC in this tasty twist on traditional stuffed peppers. Ground turkey and turkey sausage help keep these lean, and brown rice adds a boost of fiber, but it's the steam of the slow cooker that works its magic, resulting in beautiful, perfectly cooked peppers with a moist meaty filling that's hearty, yet healthy.

MAKES **6** SERVINGS

6 medium green bell peppers

6 ounces (about 2 links) mild Italian turkey sausage

1 pound lean ground turkey

1 cup cooked brown rice (like Uncle Ben's Fast and Natural)

½ cup diced onion

1 garlic clove, minced

¼ cup chopped fresh parsley

¼ cup chopped fresh basil

½ teaspoon dried oregano (or 2 tablespoons fresh)

2 tablespoons grated Parmesan or Romano cheese

¼ cup Italian breadcrumbs

1 large egg

½ teaspoon black pepper

1 (26-ounce) jar marinara sauce

¼ teaspoon red pepper flakes (optional)

1. Cut the tops off the peppers and dice the tops into small pieces. Set aside. Core, stem, and seed the peppers.

2. Remove the casings from the sausage links and place the sausage into a large bowl. Add the next 11 ingredients (turkey through black pepper), 2 tablespoons marinara, and half the reserved diced pepper tops. Using your hands or a spoon, gently mix the ingredients. Stuff the peppers with the meat mixture and place peppers upright in a 4 quart or larger slow cooker (it's fine to stack the peppers).

3. Add red pepper flakes to the remaining marinara and pour it over the peppers. Add ¾ cup water to the sauce jar or container, give it a swirl to clean out any remaining sauce, and pour into a 4- to 6-quart slow cooker. Toss in the remaining chopped pepper. Cook for 3 to 4 hours on high or until the peppers are tender, but not mushy. Remove peppers and serve topped with sauce.

NUTRITION INFORMATION PER SERVING (1 stuffed pepper): Calories 310 | Carbohydrate 26g (Sugars 7g) | Total Fat 11g (Sat Fat 3g) | Protein 25g | Fiber 4g | Cholesterol 115mg | Sodium 660mg | Food Exchanges: 3 Lean Meat, 1 Starch, 1 Vegetable, 1 Fat | Carbohydrate Choices: 1½ | Weight Watcher Plus Point Comparison: 8

Chicken at the Ready

THIS CHICKEN RECIPE IS ONE OF THE MOST PRACTICAL recipes I have in my repertoire. Make it once and you have tender, ready-to-use chicken all week long. Use it in any recipe calling for chopped or shredded cooked chicken, such as my Chicken Pot Pie Soup (page 118), Almost Everything Chopped Salad (page 159) or Chicken Fettuccine Alfredo (page 200). Getting chicken "ready" has never been easier.

MAKES ABOUT **4 CUPS** COOKED CHICKEN

4 fresh or frozen boneless, skinless chicken breasts, about 8 ounces each

1 cup water

1. Place the fresh or frozen chicken breasts in the slow cooker. Cover and cook for 6 to 8 hours on low or 3 to 4 hours on high or until chicken is cooked through and tender (frozen chicken breasts will take the longer cooking time).

2. For shredded meat, use two forks and shred meat while it is still hot. Alternately, cut into bite-sized cubes. Place chicken in an air-tight container and let cool. Store in the refrigerator until ready to use.

Marlene Says: *To make Mexican Chicken at the Ready, add 1 to 1½ cups of your favorite salsa and ½ teaspoon of cumin. Shred the meat and use it in tacos, burritos, tostadas, and quesadillas.*

NUTRITION INFORMATION PER SERVING (½ cup): Calories 130 | Carbohydrate 0g (Sugars 0g) | Total Fat 3g (Sat Fat 0g) | Protein 24g | Fiber 0g | Cholesterol 70mg | Sodium 120mg | Food Exchanges: 3½ Lean Meat | Carbohydrate Choices: 0 | Weight Watcher Plus Point Comparison: 3

Lazy Day Lasagna

IF YOU'RE SKEPTICAL about cooking lasagna in a slow cooker, have no fear—it's as easy as layering the ingredients and walking away. This recipe will have your lasagna pan gathering dust. The Italian purist in me was happy to find that traditional lasagna noodles bake up beautifully without boiling them first, and my boys were delighted to eat this for dinner and again as tasty leftovers. Try it with my All-Purpose Marinara Sauce (page 181) and check below for my meat lasagna variation.

MAKES **6** SERVINGS

15 ounces low-fat ricotta cheese

1½ cups low-fat cottage cheese

6 tablespoons grated Parmesan cheese

¾ teaspoon dried oregano, divided

1 (24- to 28-ounce) jar marinara sauce (or about 3 cups)

7 traditional lasagna noodles, uncooked

⅔ cup shredded part-skim mozzarella cheese, divided

1. In a medium bowl, combine the ricotta, cottage cheese, 2 tablespoons water, ¼ cup Parmesan cheese, and ½ teaspoon oregano. Mix thoroughly.

2. Place the marinara sauce in a medium bowl or large measuring cup. Add ½ cup water (unless the marinara is already fairly thin) to the empty sauce jar or container, give it a swirl, and add to the marinara sauce. Spread ½ cup of the sauce on the bottom of a 4- to 6-quart slow cooker.

3. Place half the lasagna noodles over the sauce, breaking the noodles to fit (don't worry if small spaces are uncovered). Cover the noodles with half of the cheese mixture (about 1½ cups), then top with 1 cup sauce. Repeat.

4. Top with the remaining noodles, cover with the remaining sauce, and sprinkle on the mozzarella, the remaining oregano and Parmesan. Cook for 3 to 3½ hours on low or until fork tender. Turn off heat and let sit at least 15 minutes before serving.

Marlene Says: *For Beefy Slow Cooker Lasagna, brown ½ pound lean ground beef with ½ teaspoon garlic powder and 1 teaspoon crushed fennel seeds. After spreading ½ cup of marinara on the bottom of the slow cooker, add beef to remaining marinara and continue as directed (adds 55 calories and 2 grams fat).*

NUTRITION INFORMATION PER SERVING (one-sixth of the lasagna or 1 generous cup): Calories 320 | Carbohydrate 35g (Sugars 12g) | Total Fat 8g (Sat Fat 7g) | Protein 24g | Fiber 2g | Cholesterol 35mg | Sodium 690mg | Food Exchanges: 3 Lean Meat, 2 Carbohydrate, ½ Fat | Carbohydrate Choices: 2 | Weight Watcher Plus Point Comparison: 8

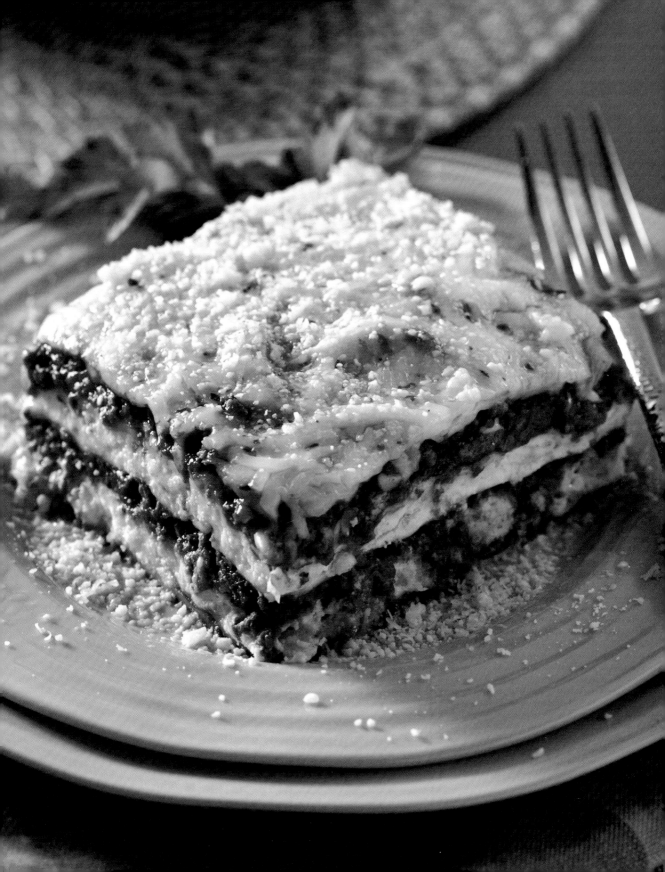

Creamy King Ranch Casserole

CREAMY IS INDEED "KING" in this smooth and sassy variation of the traditional Texas casserole. Make it mild, medium, or hot by adjusting the heat level of the chilies and the amount of added Tabasco. Using light sour cream keeps the calories in check, while elevating the flavorful sauce to its creamy best. This dish is destined to become a family favorite.

MAKES **4** SERVINGS

1 (10 ¾ ounce) can reduced-fat cream of chicken soup

1 (4.5 ounce) can diced green chilies, undrained

4 tablespoons all-purpose flour, divided

1 to 2 teaspoons green Tabasco sauce

½ teaspoon dried oregano

½ teaspoon ground black pepper

1 large onion, halved and sliced

3 medium carrots, peeled and sliced diagonally into ¼-inch pieces

1 tender medium celery stalk, sliced diagonally into ¼-inch pieces

1 pound chicken tenders (8 pieces)

3 tablespoons light sour cream

Salt to taste

¼ cup chopped cilantro, optional

1. In a medium bowl, stir together the soup, chilies, 3 tablespoons flour, Tabasco, oregano, and pepper. Combine the onion, carrots and celery in the bottom of a 4- to 6-quart slow cooker. Arrange the chicken tenders on top and spread the soup mixture over, distributing it evenly with a rubber spatula.

2. Cover and cook for 4 hours on low or 2 to 2½ hours on high until the chicken is tender and the sauce is bubbling. Remove the chicken to a warmed serving dish. Stir the last tablespoon of flour into the sour cream, stir into the sauce, and cook with the cover off until the sauce thickens. Adjust salt to taste.

3. Spoon the sauce and vegetables over the chicken. If desired, sprinkle with the cilantro before serving.

Marlene Says: *For an even richer-tasting sauce, substitute 3 tablespoons of light cream cheese for the sour cream and flour in Step 2 (adds 10 calories and 1 gram of fat per serving).*

NUTRITION INFORMATION PER SERVING (2 tenders and ¾ cup of sauce): Calories 260 | Carbo-hydrate 24g (Sugars 9g) | Total Fat 5g (Sat Fat 1g) | Protein 29g | Fiber 4g | Cholesterol 80mg | Sodium mg 680 | Food Exchanges: 3 ½ Lean Meat, 1 Starch, 1 Vegetable | Carbohydrate Choices: 1 ½ | Weight Watcher Plus Point Comparison: 6

Wendy's®-Style Chili

WHEN I THINK SLOW COOKER, I think chili. This recipe fills the bill with an all-American-tasting chili fashioned after the one served at Wendy's restaurants. Browning the meat after mixing it with a slice of bread may seem unusual, but after umpteen tries, I found it was the perfect way to ensure stovetop quality, color, and texture (a rarity for lean slow cooker chilis). Offer it with all your favorite chili toppers and watch it disappear.

MAKES **10** SERVINGS

1 pound 90% lean ground beef

1 piece whole-wheat bread

1 (28-ounce) can diced tomatoes with juice

1 (8-ounce) can tomato sauce

2 medium red bell peppers, coarsely chopped

1 large onion, chopped

3 medium stalks celery, diced small

4 to 5 tablespoons chili powder

1 tablespoon ground cumin

½ teaspoon garlic salt

½ teaspoon ground black pepper

1 can (15 to16 ounces) red kidney beans, rinsed and drained

1 can (15 to16 ounces) pinto beans, rinsed and drained

1. Tear the bread into small pieces in a large bowl. Moisten with 2 tablespoons water and mash with a fork. Add the beef and mix with your hands until blended.

2. Spray a large non-stick skillet with cooking spray and set over medium high heat. Crumble in the ground beef and cook, stirring often, until the pink color is gone, 6 to 7 minutes. Transfer to a 4- to 6-quart slow cooker.

3. Add the tomatoes and their juices, the tomato sauce, bell peppers, onion, celery, chili powder, cumin, garlic salt and pepper, and mix well. Gently stir in the beans.

4. Cover and cook for 8 hours on low or 4 hours on high, stirring once halfway through, if you can. If chili looks a little saucy to your taste, uncover and let stand for 10 to 15 minutes before serving.

Marlene Says: *Yes, you need 4 to 5 tablespoons of chili powder. Slow-cooked foods require more spice, as the long cooking process can break down flavors. Four tablespoons gives you a mild chili powder flavor. Five tablespoons is my personal preference.*

NUTRITION INFORMATION PER SERVING (1 cup): Calories 190 | Carbohydrate 25g (Sugars 4g) | Total Fat 5g (Sat Fat 1.5g) | Protein 16g | Fiber 7g | Cholesterol 15mg | Sodium 440mg | Food Exchanges: 2 Lean Meat, 1 Starch, 1 Vegetable | Carbohydrate Choices: 1½ | Weight Watcher Plus Point Comparison: 5

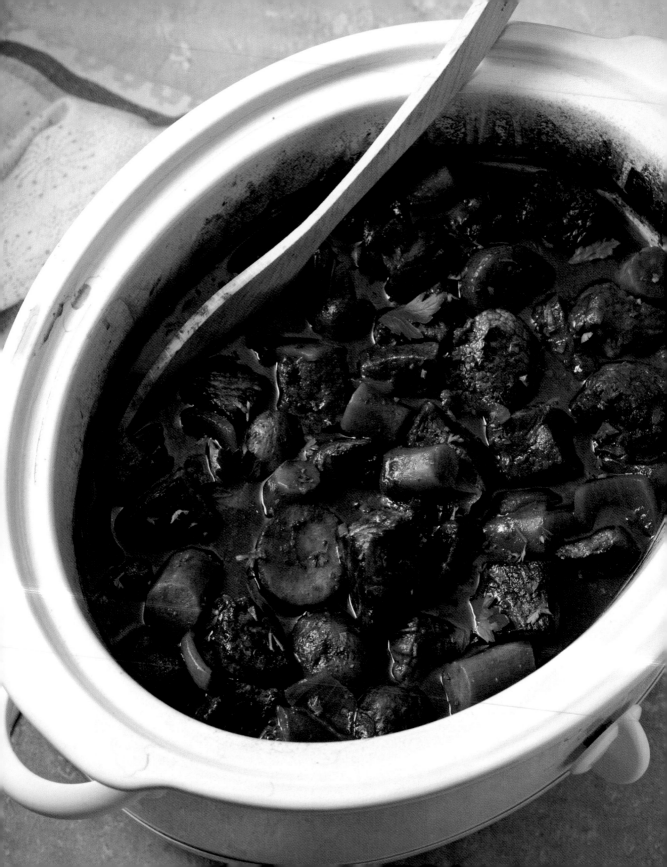

Stephen's Beef Stew

IN THIS STEW WORTHY OF SUNDAY supper status, "low-and-slow" tenderizes lean stewing meat so it is fork tender. The tender meat and sweet tomato-based sauce had my son Stephen declaring this his favorite dish the first time he ate it; I relish the fact that once the meal is loaded in the slow cooker, I get the afternoon off! My favorite way to finish this meal is with a side of fresh green beans and a nice green salad.

MAKES **8** SERVINGS

1½ pounds small white or red potatoes, peeled and halved

1 pound carrots, peeled and cut crosswise into ¾-inch slices

2½ pounds lean beef stew meat, well-trimmed

1 medium onion, chopped (about 1 cup)

1 (6-ounce) can tomato paste

2 tablespoons brown sugar

2 tablespoons Worcestershire sauce

2 tablespoons cider vinegar

½ teaspoon salt or celery salt

¼ teaspoon black pepper

1 tablespoon cornstarch

1. Place the potatoes and carrots in a 5- to 7-quart slow cooker. Top with the beef and onions.

2. In a small bowl, whisk together the tomato paste, 2 cups water, brown sugar, Worcestershire sauce, vinegar, salt and pepper, and pour over the meat and vegetables. Cover and cook on low for 8 to 9 hours or on high for 4 to 5 hours or until the meat is fork tender.

3. In a small bowl, whisk the cornstarch together with 1 tablespoon of water. Using a slotted spoon, move the meat and vegetables to one side of the cooker, and stir the cornstarch mixture into the liquid in the cooker. Cover and cook on high for 10 minutes or until sauce is slightly thickened.

Marlene Says: *This hearty stew is packed with heart-healthy potassium. Studies show potassium may help counteract the negative effects of salt in your diet and may help to lower blood pressure.*

NUTRITION INFORMATION PER SERVING (1 generous cup): Calories 340 | Carbohydrate 33g (Sugars 10g) | Total Fat 10g (Sat Fat 3.5g) | Protein 30g | Fiber 5g | Cholesterol 90mg | Sodium 490mg | Food Exchanges: 3½ Lean Meat, 2 Vegetable, 1 Starch, ½ Fat | Carbohydrate Choices: 2 | Weight Watcher Plus Point Comparison: 9

Italian Bean and Bacon Soup

THIS SIMPLE (SUPER SKINNY) RUSTIC ITALIAN-STYLE SOUP fills the belly and heals the soul. The barley virtually disappears in the cooking but it gives the soup additional body, more nutrition, and a richer feel. You can substitute a 6-ounce bag of baby spinach or kale for the Swiss chard (cook the spinach for just 15 minutes), add a few drops of liquid smoke to the chicken broth, or mix in a bit of chicken for a heartier meal.

MAKES **10** CUPS

½ pound (1 ¼ cups) dry Great Northern beans

2 slices center cut bacon, cut crosswise into 1-inch pieces

2 large garlic cloves, peeled and thinly sliced

1 medium onion, chopped

3 medium carrots, peeled and sliced ¼-inch thick

2 medium celery stalks, sliced ¼-inch thick

4 cups or 2 (14-ounce) cans reduced-sodium chicken broth

½ cup pearl barley

4 sprigs fresh rosemary, plus 1 tablespoon coarsely chopped, divided

½ teaspoon salt

½ teaspoon pepper

8 cups loosely packed, stemmed Swiss chard leaves, chopped

1. Pick over the beans, rinse, soak overnight, and drain. Add to a 4- to 6-quart slow cooker.

2. In a small skillet, cook the bacon over medium heat, stirring often, for 2 minutes, just until the fat starts to render. Add the onion and garlic, stirring often and reducing the heat, if necessary, for 3 to 4 minutes or until the bacon is lightly crisp and the garlic is fragrant and turning golden at the edges. Transfer the bacon mixture to the slow cooker; if you're in a hurry, the onions and garlic can also go directly into the cooker without pre-cooking.

3. Add the carrots, celery, chicken broth, 2½ cups water, barley, rosemary sprigs, salt, and pepper. Cover and cook for 6 to 7 hours on low or until the beans are tender.

4. Remove the rosemary stems. Add the chard leaves (discard stems) and chopped rosemary. Cover and cook about 45 minutes more or until the chard is tender.

Marlene Says: *This soup is an excellent source of fiber, Vitamin A and C, and potassium. It's as nutritious as it is delicious!*

NUTRITION INFORMATION PER SERVING (1 cup): Calories 110 | Carbohydrate 20g (Sugars 3g) | Total Fat 1g (Sat Fat .5g) | Protein 8g | Fiber 6g | Cholesterol 5mg | Sodium 320mg | Food Exchanges: 1 Starch, 1 Vegetable | Carbohydrate Choices: 1½ | Weight Watcher Plus Point Comparison: 2

Marlene's All-Purpose Marinara Sauce

ITALIAN FOOD LOVERS, REJOICE! When you convert to this amazing crockpot marinara, your days of being a stovetop sauce slave are over. This is another very versatile basic recipe (like my Chicken at the Ready, page 173). Use this in any dish calling for marinara sauce. The extended time in the slow cooker adds a richness and depth of flavor that rivals the sauce of any proud Italian grandmother. One batch makes the equivalent of two 26-ounce store-bought jars, but at a fraction of the price (and it freezes beautifully!).

MAKES **6** CUPS SAUCE

1 medium white onion, chopped, about 1¼ cup

1 tablespoon olive oil

3 cloves garlic, minced, about 1 tablespoon

1 (28-ounce) can crushed tomatoes

1 (8-ounce) can tomato sauce

1 (6-ounce) can tomato paste

½ cup dry red wine or reduced-sodium beef broth

1 cup water, plus additional, as required to thin

2 teaspoons sugar

1 tablespoon dried basil leaves

1 tablespoon dried oregano leaves

1. Place the onion and oil in a medium microwave-safe bowl and stir to combine. Cover and microwave on high power for 3 minutes; remove and stir. Microwave for another 2 minutes or until onions are softened and nearly translucent.

2. In a 4- to 6-quart slow cooker, place the onions and remaining ingredients (garlic through oregano leaves), stir to combine, and cover.

3. Cook on low for 6 to 8 hours or on high for 3 to 4 hours in any additional water and sugar to adjust thickness to your preference.

Marlene Says: *While convenient, jarred marinara varies in taste and nutritional content. A marinara that has less than 400 mg of sodium, 5 grams of sugar and 3 grams of fat is good-to-go.*

NUTRITION INFORMATION PER SERVING (½ cup): Calories 60 | Carbohydrate 11g (Sugars 4g) | Total Fat 1g (Sat Fat 0g) | Protein 2g | Fiber 2g | Cholesterol 0mg | Sodium 230mg | Food Exchanges: 1½ Vegetable | Carbohydrate Choices: ½ | Weight Watcher Plus Point Comparison: 1

Fast Fix Ratatouille

THIS CLASSIC FRENCH DISH is simple to make, great served hot or cold, and a tasty addition to any meal—indoors or out. Serve it as a side dish or double up the portion and top it with a tablespoon or two of reduced-fat feta for a farm fresh vegetarian entrée. Feel free to choose your favorite color peppers (though I do like to mix them up), and be careful not to overcook this dish. It's done when all the vegetables are cooked through, but still hold their shape. (Note: the vegetables really cook down. For a 4-quart slow cooker, halve the recipe.)

MAKES **8** SERVINGS

1 large eggplant cut into 1-inch cubes

3 medium zucchini (about 1 pound), cut into ½-inch rounds

2 medium yellow squash, cut into ½-inch rounds

1 large onion, cut in half lengthwise and then into ¼-inch slices

2 large peppers, cut into 1-inch pieces

3 cloves garlic, minced

2 tablespoons olive oil

3 sprigs fresh thyme or 1 teaspoon dried

½ cup chopped fresh flat leaf parsley

1 (14 ounce) can diced tomatoes (do not drain)

3 tablespoons tomato paste

¼ cup dry white wine or water

½ teaspoon salt

½ teaspoon black pepper

1. Combine all the ingredients in a 6-quart slow cooker and mix well.

2. Cook on high for 3½ to 4 hours. Stir carefully once every hour as vegetables start to give up some of their moisture.

3. Serve hot or cold, topped with optional fresh basil.

Marlene Says: *For ratatouille with an Italian twist, use only half the thyme and add 1 teaspoon of dried oregano to the ingredients before cooking. Serve sprinkled with grated Parmesan or Romano cheese.*

NUTRITION INFORMATION PER SERVING (generous ¾ cup): Calories 90 | Carbohydrate 16g (Sugars 8g) | Total Fat 3g (Sat Fat 0.5g) | Protein 3g | Fiber 5g | Cholesterol 0mg | Sodium 240mg | Food Exchanges: 2½ Vegetable | Carbohydrate Choices: 1 | Weight Watcher Plus Point Comparison: 2

Boston Baked Beans

WITH TWICE THE HOME-STYLE FLAVOR (and less than half the sugar) of canned baked beans, this highly nutritious side dish comes with two great options. Make it extra quick by starting with plain canned beans or more economical by starting with dry beans. Either way, these slow-cooked beans will have your partygoers clamoring for more.

MAKES **10** SERVINGS

4 (15-ounce) cans white beans, rinsed and drained, OR 1 bag of dry navy beans,

picked over and soaked overnight in cold water

1 large onion, chopped

½ cup tomato sauce

½ cup sugar-free maple syrup

⅔ cup granulated no-calorie sweetener

3 tablespoons molasses

2 tablespoons cider vinegar

2 teaspoons dry mustard

¾ teaspoon salt

½ teaspoon ginger

½ teaspoon liquid smoke

1. Place the rinsed, drained beans in a 4- to 6-quart slow cooker (if using dried beans, soak overnight, rinse and add to the slow cooker with 2 cups warm water). Add the remaining ingredients.

2. Stir and cook on low for 3 to 4 hours or on high for 1½ to 2 hours (stir halfway through and add more water, if needed, especially for dried beans). To thicken beans, remove lid for last 10 to 15 minutes of cooking time, stirring until desired consistency.

Marlene Says: *Organic canned beans are often lower in sodium, while all traditional brands now carry reduced-sodium beans. Draining and rinsing beans reduces the sodium another 40%. For Mixed-Up Boston Baked Beans, use 2 cans each white and black beans. To reduce the carbs, use 2 cans white beans and 2 cans black soybeans. Each serving will have 10 more calories, 12 grams fewer carbs, 5 grams more protein and 6 grams more fat.*

NUTRITION INFORMATION PER SERVING (½ cup): Calories 160 | Carbohydrate 30g (Sugars 5g) | Total Fat 1g (Sat Fat 0g) | Protein 9g | Fiber 9g | Cholesterol 0mg | Sodium 195mg | Food Exchanges: 1½ Starch | Carbohydrate Choices: 1½ | Weight Watcher Plus Point Comparison: 3

Creamy Slow Cooker Cheesecake Sundaes

GET ALL THE LUSCIOUSNESS OF CHEESECAKE without stressing about overcooking or cracks. Serve this fun dessert sundae-style with an ice cream scoop, topping it with fresh berries or sundae toppings. To add a "crust," garnish with graham crackers or reduced-fat vanilla wafers.

8 ounces low-fat cottage cheese

8 ounces light tub-style cream cheese, room temperature

8 ounces nonfat cream cheese, room temperature

2 tablespoons granulated sugar

1 cup granulated no-calorie sweetener (like Splenda)

1 tablespoon cornstarch

1¼ teaspoons vanilla extract

½ teaspoon almond extract

2 large eggs

2 large egg whites

½ cup light sour cream

2⅔ cups assorted fresh berries

1. Lightly spray a 4-cup heat-resistant bowl or baking dish (it should fit completely inside your slow cooker) with cooking spray.

2. With an immersion blender or food processor, puree the cottage cheese until completely smooth. Spoon into a bowl, add cream cheeses, and beat with an electric mixer until smooth. Add the sugar, sweetener, cornstarch and extracts. Beat again until smooth. On low speed, add the eggs, then the egg whites, beating briefly after each addition just to incorporate. Stir in the sour cream with a large spoon.

3. Pour the cheesecake mixture into the bowl and place inside the slow cooker. Add water to the cooker until it reaches about one-third the height of the bowl. Drape two folded paper towels under the lid to keep condensation from dripping onto the cheesecake (this is especially helpful when opening the lid). Cook on high for 1½ to 2 hours or until center of the cheesecake is just set (the edges should be firm, but the center still slightly soft. Check after 1½ hours).

4. Turn off the slow cooker, cock the lid halfway, and let the cheesecake cool in place for 15 minutes. Remove the cheesecake from the slow cooker and let cool completely. Place in the refrigerator to chill at least 4 hours more before serving. To serve, scoop ½ cup cheesecake into a small bowl and top with ⅓ cup fresh berries or set out the bowl and berries for a "sundae bar."

NUTRITION INFORMATION PER SERVING (1 sundae): Calories 150 | Carbohydrate 12g (Sugars 8g) | Total Fat 6g (Sat Fat 3g) | Protein 11g | Fiber 3g | Cholesterol 70mg | Sodium 280mg | Food Exchanges: 1 Lean Meat, 1 Carbohydrate, ½ Fat | Carbohydrate Choices: 1 | Weight Watcher Plus Point Comparison: 3

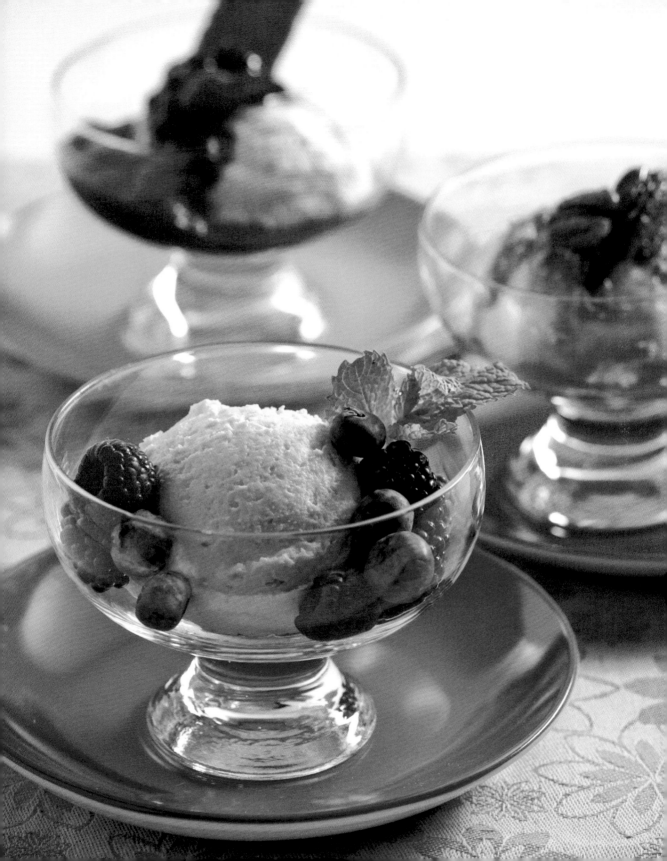

Slow Cooker Apples – Baked & Sauced

THE OLD-FASHIONED GOODNESS OF WARM BAKED APPLES returns with not one, but two, ways to enjoy them. Cook the apples until tender for delicious, warm, cinnamon-infused baked apples. They're great served plain or with a scoop of your favorite ice cream or frozen yogurt. Or continue cooking (as I accidentally did!) to make a comforting warm applesauce that leaves any jarred variety out in the cold.

MAKES **6** SERVINGS

6 medium Golden Delicious apples

3 tablespoons granulated no-calorie sweetener (or 4 packets)

1 tablespoon brown sugar

1 teaspoon cinnamon, divided

2 tablespoons sugar-free maple syrup

1 teaspoon vanilla

1 teaspoon butter

1. Wash the apples. Using a vegetable peeler, remove a ¾-inch strip from the top of each apple. Core the apples with an apple corer or a small paring knife, coring three-quarters of the way to the bottom of the apple.

2. In a small bowl, mix together the sweetener, brown sugar and ½ teaspoon cinnamon. Spoon 2 teaspoons of brown sugar mixture into each apple cavity.

3. Pour ⅓ cup water, syrup, ½ teaspoon cinnamon, and vanilla into the slow cooker. Place the apples into a 4 quart or larger slow cooker, cover, and cook on high for 2½ to 3½ hours.

4. For baked apples, carefully remove the apples from the slow cooker. Stir the butter into the cooking liquid and spoon the liquid over the apples.

Marlene Says: *For* **applesauce**, *continue to cook the apples for an additional hour. Remove the apples from the cooker with a large spoon and place in a large bowl. Mash the apples with a large fork or spoon, adding cooking liquid from the slow cooker until you reach the desired consistency.*

NUTRITION INFORMATION PER SERVING (1 apple or ½ cup applesauce): Calories 100 | Carbohydrate 24g (Sugars 19g) | Total Fat 1g (Sat Fat 0g) | Protein 0g | Fiber 4g | Cholesterol 0mg | Sodium 10mg | Food Exchanges: 1½ Fruit | Carbohydrate Choices: 1½ | Weight Watcher Plus Point Comparison: 3

pastas, pizzas, and more

Cajun Jambalaya Pasta

Sneaky Beef and Penne Skillet

Buffalo Chicken Pasta

Chicken Parmesan Pasta Toss

At-Home Pad Thai

Quick-Fix Turkey Chili Mac Skillet

Cheesy Seaside Shells

Chicken Fettuccine Alfredo

Creamy Pesto Penne – Two Ways

15-Minute Shrimp Fettuccine

Easy Eggplant Parmesan

Pizza Pasta Pie

Homemade Pizza Dough

Loaded Cheese and Pepperoni Pizza

Individual New York-Style Pizzas

I grew up eating spaghetti every week, so I simply can't imagine ever not eating pasta. That is why it gives me *great pleasure* to tell you that all of the incredibly *tempting* recipes in this chapter can be enjoyed by everyone—no matter what their diet.

Pasta takes center stage in this chapter with fourteen incredible new recipes. What's extra special is that every extraordinary dish is not only brimming with flavor, it's *perfectly proportioned* with just the right balance of pasta, satisfying protein, and colorful fresh vegetables—*to tickle your tastebuds*, yet keep your waistline and blood sugar in check. Contrary to popular belief, pasta need not be fattening or excessively raise blood sugar; it's a *good source* of protein, vitamins, and minerals and is actually moderate in calories and has a low glycemic index (the rate at which it raises blood sugar). Choosing whole grain or pastas *fortified* with protein or extra fiber is a healthy choice, while cooking your pasta al dente (slightly firm to the bite) reduces its impact on blood sugar. (Little known fact: larger, flatter pastas—*think fettuccini* instead of thin spaghetti—have the lowest glycemic impact.)

I'd love to be at your table when you dig into some of my newly beloved pasta dishes, such as my rendition of the #1 pasta dish at The Cheesecake Factory Restaurant—spicy Cajun Jambalaya Pasta—or *lusciously creamy* Cheesy Seaside Shells, or my *decadent*-tasting Chicken Fettuccine Alfredo, or my *kids' favorite*, Pizza Pasta Pie! These are dishes that make *everyone* smile. I'm also thrilled to bring you, after many requests, *better-for-you* pizza recipes. You won't need to go for takeout when you can serve up better-for-you Loaded Cheese and Pepperoni Pizza or ultra-thin-crust Individual New York Style *Pizzas right at home*. Pasta, pizza, and more…

CHEESE

Imagine not having pizza, macaroni and cheese, cheeseburgers, quesadillas, or cheesecake. A world without cheese is utterly unthinkable! Americans eat an average of more than 30 pounds of cheese per person each year. Admittedly, some types of cheese can be high in calories, sodium or fat, but there are also plenty of healthy reasons to love cheese!

Cheese is a great source of protein, calcium, Vitamin D, and phosphorus—and cheese can actually help boost your metabolism. A recent study found that increasing your consumption of dairy products, including cheese (while keeping calories in check), can help flatten your belly and lower your blood pressure. Here are some of my favorite healthy cheese-loving tips:

MARLENE'S SUPER CHEESY TIPS

1. Go bold with full-flavored cheese. Aged and strongly flavored cheeses offer loads of flavor with less quantity. Some examples are blue cheese, extra-sharp cheddar, and smoked gouda.

2. Sprinkle on Parm! Grated Parmesan cheese is high in calcium and modest in sodium. With just 23 calories per tablespoon it offers lots of bang for the cheese buck.

3. Opt for reduced-fat or reduced-sodium cheese. Light and reduced-fat versions work beautifully in a wide variety of dishes, from sandwiches and salads to pizzas and casseroles. Reduced-sodium cheeses (like those offered by Sargento brand) can be as delicious as they are nutritious.

4. Think outside the block. Low-fat cottage cheese delivers protein-rich cheesy goodness for a fraction of the fat and calories of cream cheese. A sneaky trick: puree it well and the curds disappear. Opt for part-skim or reduced-fat ricotta when cooking Italian specialties.

5. Keep your eye on the cheese. To keep quantity in check, use cheese to enhance, not overwhelm, your favorite dishes. Whenever possible, place cheese on top of the food, where you can see it and really taste it. Hidden cheese can mean hidden calories.

Cajun Jambalaya Pasta

THIS RECIPE WAS INSPIRED BY THE #1 PASTA DISH at Cheesecake Factory, Cajun Jambalaya Pasta. Their menu describes it as "shrimp and chicken sautéed with onion, tomatoes, and peppers in a very spicy Cajun sauce." What it doesn't say is that the dish is as rich in butter, oil and carbs as it is in Cajun flavor. This tasty makeover lets you enjoy the same crave-worthy ingredients and spicy flavor for a mere fraction of the fat and calories.

MAKES **4** SERVINGS

6 ounces linguine

8 ounces boneless, skinless chicken breast, cut into 1-inch pieces

5 teaspoons Cajun spice blend, divided

2 teaspoons olive oil

2 medium red or yellow bell peppers, sliced into strips

½ medium red onion, sliced into strips

8 ounces large raw shrimp, peeled and deveined

1 garlic clove, minced

¼ teaspoon ground black pepper

1 cup canned diced tomatoes, with juice

¼ cup reduced-sodium chicken broth

2 teaspoons butter

2 tablespoons fresh chopped parsley

1. Cook the pasta according to the package directions and set aside.

2. Place the chicken pieces into a medium bowl and toss with 3 teaspoons (or 1 tablespoon) Cajun spice.

3. Heat the oil in a large non-stick skillet over medium high heat. Add the chicken and sauté for 3 to 4 minutes or until cooked about halfway through. Add the peppers, onion and shrimp and sauté another 1 to 2 minutes or until the shrimp are pink.

4. Reduce the heat to medium. Add the garlic, black pepper, remaining 2 teaspoons Cajun spice, tomatoes, and chicken broth to the skillet and gently stir. Cook for 5 more minutes or until chicken is thoroughly cooked and vegetables tender. Swirl the butter into the sauce.

5. Place the pasta in a large bowl, toss with the sauce, and garnish with chopped parsley.

DARE TO COMPARE: An order of the Cajun Jambalaya Pasta at the Cheesecake Factory serves up 1,070 calories, over 50 grams of fat, and almost 100 grams of carbohydrate.

NUTRITION INFORMATION PER SERVING (1 ¾ cups): Calories 325 | Carbohydrate 38g (Sugars 0g) | Total Fat 6g (Sat Fat 1g) | Protein 30g | Fiber 6g | Cholesterol 115mg | Sodium 810mg | Food Exchanges: 3 Lean Meat, 2 Starch, 1 vegetable | Carbohydrate Choices: 2½ | Weight Watcher Plus Point Comparison: 8

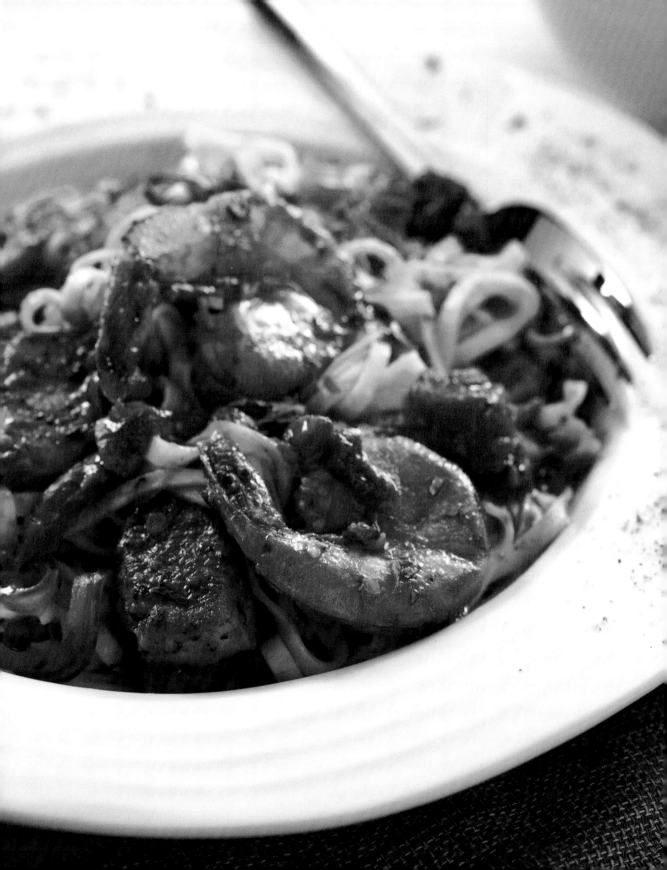

Sneaky Beef and Penne Skillet

LOOKING TO SNEAK MORE VEGETABLES into your family's diet? This ultra-easy one-pan no-chop skillet recipe will do the trick. It's packed with antioxidants and vitamin-rich bell peppers (but we'll just keep that ▓▓▓▓▓▓▓▓▓▓▓▓▓▓▓▓ makes them "disappear" into a beefy tomato sauce that's made cr▓▓▓▓▓▓▓▓▓▓▓▓▓▓▓umpkin. The result is a dish reminiscent of an Italian bolognese, co▓▓▓▓▓▓▓▓▓▓▓▓r that seals the sneaky deal.

MAKES **4** SERVINGS

1½ cups reduced-sodium V-8 juice

1¼ cups frozen bell pepper strips, thawed

12 ounces lean ground beef

½ cup frozen diced onion

1 tablespoon jarred minced garlic

1 (14-ounce) can no salt petite diced tomatoes

½ cup canned pumpkin

1 teaspoon dried basil

1 teaspoon brown sugar

½ teaspoon salt

½ teaspoon black pepper

1½ cups dry penne pasta

½ cup shredded low-fat Italian cheese blend

1. In a food processor, purée the V-8 and bell pepper strips and set aside.

2. Spray a large non-stick skillet with cooking spray and place over medium heat. Add the ground beef, onion, and garlic and cook for 8 to 10 minutes or until meat is browned.

3. Stir in the puréed mixture, tomatoes, pumpkin, basil, brown sugar, salt, and pepper and bring to a boil. Add the pasta, cover, reduce heat to low and cook for 23 to 25 minutes or until pasta is tender, stirring occasionally (add 1 to 2 tablespoons of water toward the end of cooking, if necessary).

4. Uncover the pan, sprinkle the cheese over pasta mixture and cover once again for 1 to 2 minutes or until cheese is melted.

Marlene Says: *Each serving of this cheesy, beefy dish delivers 3 servings of vegetables, 6 grams of fiber, and over 100% of the daily allowance for vitamins A and C. Use the leftover pumpkin to make the Spicy Sweet Potato Mash (page 230) or Cream Cheese Filled Pumpkin Muffins (page 57).*

NUTRITION INFORMATION PER SERVING (1¾ cups): Calories 330 | Carbohydrate 38g (Sugars 11g) | Total Fat 8g (Sat Fat 4g) | Protein 30g | Fiber 6g | Cholesterol 70mg | Sodium 480mg | Food Exchanges: 3½ Lean Meat, 3 Vegetable, 1 Starch | Carbohydrate Choices: 2 | Weight Watcher Plus Point Comparison: 8

Buffalo Chicken Pasta

IF YOU ARE A CHICKEN WINGS AFICIONADO, this is your pasta meal. Here is a dish layered with enticing texture and big flavors—a spicy pasta complemented with the same sides that are traditionally served with wings: crunchy celery, sweet carrot, and rich blue cheese. It's simple to make, but the final result is restaurant-worthy in taste and presentation.

MAKES **6** SERVINGS

8 ounces dry penne pasta

2 teaspoons canola oil

½ medium onion, diced

2 medium carrots, diced (½-inch)

3 ribs celery, diced (½-inch)

2 large garlic cloves, minced

1 pound skinless, boneless chicken breast

2 teaspoons paprika

2 teaspoons all-purpose flour

2 tablespoons hot sauce

1 (14.5-ounce) can diced tomatoes with juice

1 cup reduced-sodium chicken broth

2 teaspoons butter

½ cup crumbled blue cheese

¼ cup sliced green onions, including tops

1. While preparing the sauce, cook the pasta according to the package directions and set aside.

2. Heat the oil in a very large non-stick sauté pan over medium heat. Add the onion, carrots, and celery and sauté for 5 minutes, stirring occasionally. Add garlic and chicken and sauté for 4 to 5 more minutes or until chicken is almost cooked.

3. Sprinkle the paprika and flour over the mixture and stir to coat. Add hot sauce, tomatoes, and chicken broth, and simmer 2 to 3 minutes or until the sauce thickens and the chicken is cooked through. Swirl the butter into the sauce.

4. Place the pasta in a large serving dish. Pour sauce on top and toss gently to combine. Sprinkle the blue cheese and scallions over the pasta and serve.

Marlene Says: *Hot sauces vary in taste and sodium content. Try Frank's Red Hot Wings Sauce for an authentic buffalo wing flavor or Tabasco brand hot sauce if you want less sodium.*

NUTRITION INFORMATION PER SERVING (1½ cups): Calories 290 | Carbohydrate 35g (Sugars 7g) | Total Fat 7g (Sat Fat 3g) | Protein 25g | Fiber 6g | Cholesterol 10mg | Sodium 540g | Food Exchanges: 2 ½ Lean Meat, 2 Vegetable, 1 ½ Starch | Carbohydrate Choices: 2 | Weight Watcher Plus Point Comparison: 7

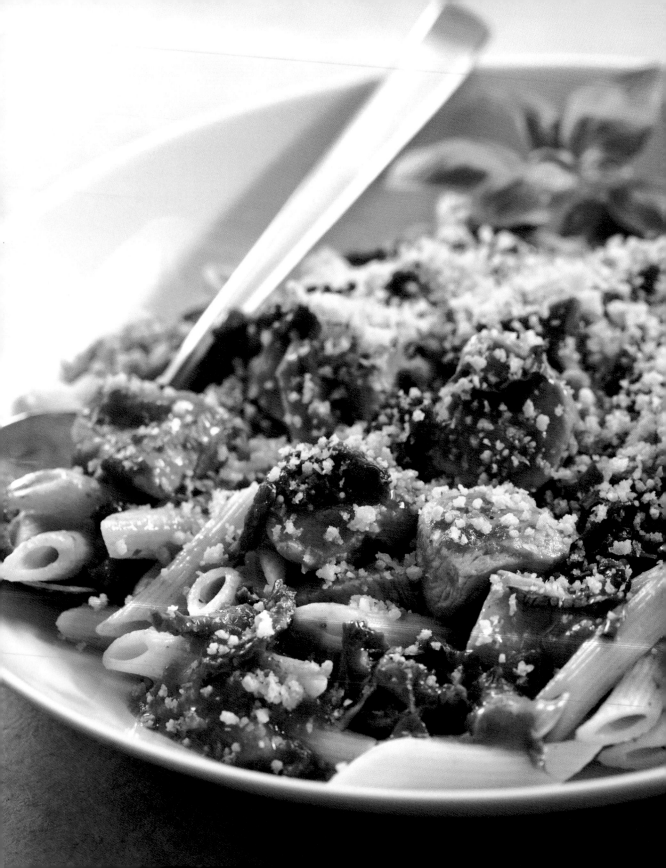

Chicken Parmesan Pasta Toss

CHICKEN PARM LOVERS, UNITE! Here are all the flavors and flair of traditional Chicken Parmesan served not on pasta, but in it. In addition to the main ingredients of chicken and fresh tomatoes, sun-dried tomatoes give this dish extra rich flavor and color (look for bagged soft, pliable sundried tomatoes). The crowning touch is a crunchy panko Parmesan topping, which layers on the great taste of crunchy, cheesy bread.

MAKES **4** SERVINGS

6 ounces (about 2 cups dry) penne pasta

2½ teaspoons olive oil, divided

½ cup grated Parmesan cheese, divided

⅓ cup panko breadcrumbs

12 ounces boneless, skinless chicken breast, cut into 1-inch pieces

3 garlic cloves, minced

1 teaspoon dried oregano

¼ teaspoon salt

¼ teaspoon black pepper

1 medium tomato, seeded and chopped (about 1 cup)

⅓ cup julienned sun-dried tomatoes

2 teaspoons cornstarch

1 cup reduced-sodium chicken broth

¼ cup fresh basil, finely chopped

1. While preparing the sauce, cook the pasta according to the package directions and set aside.

2. Heat 1 teaspoon oil in a large non-stick skillet over medium heat. Add the panko breadcrumbs and ¼ cup of the Parmesan. Stir well and toast until golden brown, about 1 to 2 minutes. Remove from pan and set aside.

3. Add remaining 1½ teaspoons oil and heat over medium heat. Add the chicken and garlic and sauté for 3 to 4 minutes or until the chicken is mostly cooked through. Sprinkle oregano, salt, and pepper over the chicken. Add both tomatoes and stir.

4. In a small bowl, whisk the cornstarch into the chicken broth and add to the pan. Cook for 1 to 2 minutes or until the sauce thickens and the chicken is cooked through. Add the fresh basil and sprinkle in remaining ¼ cup Parmesan.

5. Place the pasta in a large bowl, pour the sauce over and stir gently. Sprinkle the panko Parmesan crumbs over the pasta and serve.

NUTRITION INFORMATION PER SERVING: Calories 340 | Carbohydrate 41g (Sugars 4g) | Total Fat 9g (Sat Fat 2.5g) | Protein 29g | Fiber 5g | Cholesterol 60mg | Sodium 480mg | Food Exchanges: 3 Lean Meat, 2½ Starch, 1 Vegetable | Carbohydrate Choices: 2½ | Weight Watcher Plus Point Comparison: 9

At-Home Pad Thai

TRADITIONALLY SWIMMING IN OIL, sugar, and sodium, the beloved Thai noodle dish Pad Thai might more aptly be called "pad (your) thighs!" As it's one of my husband's favorite Thai dishes I yearned for a simple make-at-home version that would be easier on his wallet, my thighs, and of course, taste just as good as takeout. Now I have one. The choice of noodles is yours, but for real Thai flavor, the fish sauce is a must. Feel free to add additional garnishes. Our favorites are sliced limes and fresh cilantro.

MAKES **4** SERVINGS

5 ounces linguine pasta or rice noodles

2 tablespoons fresh lime juice

2 tablespoons reduced-sodium soy sauce

2 tablespoons granulated no-calorie sweetener (or 3 packets)

1½ tablespoons fish sauce

1 tablespoon ketchup

2 teaspoons minced garlic

2 teaspoons oil

8 ounces skinless boneless chicken breast, sliced

8 ounces large shrimp, peeled and deveined

1 large whole fresh egg, beaten

1 (8-ounce) package, or 2½ cups, mung bean sprouts

1¼ cups carrots, julienned or pre-shredded

3 tablespoons chopped peanuts

1. Cook pasta or soak rice noodles according to package instructions. In a small bowl, whisk together next 6 ingredients (lime juice through garlic). Set aside.

2. In a large wok or non-stick skillet, heat oil until hot. Add chicken and sauté for 3 to 4 minutes or until about half cooked. Add shrimp and cook just until pink. Push chicken and shrimp to one side of the pan, add the egg, stirring over heat until scrambled. Remove contents from pan, cover with foil, and set aside.

3. Return pan to heat. Add two tablespoons of water, 2 cups bean sprouts and ¾ cup carrots. Cover and cook for 2 to 3 minutes, stirring once, or until the vegetables are slightly softened. Remove the cover; add sauce, chicken mixture and noodles to the pan. With tongs toss everything together and cook for a minute or two to warm. Place in a large serving dish, top with peanuts and garnish with remaining sprouts and carrots.

DARE TO COMPARE: A restaurant order of Pad Thai can have as many as 1,400 calories and as much as 3,000 (yes, 3,000) mg of sodium. I think I prefer it At-Home!

NUTRITION INFORMATION PER SERVING (1½ cups): Calories 325 | Carbohydrate 36 (Sugars 4g) | Total Fat 8 g (Sat Fat 1g) | Protein 31g | Fiber 6g | Cholesterol 135mg | Sodium 660mg | Food Exchanges: 3 Lean Meat, 1½ Starch, 1½ Vegetable | Carbohydrate Choices: 2 | Weight Watcher Plus Point Comparison: 8

Quick-Fix Turkey Chili Mac Skillet

RING THE CHOW BELL for the easiest ever two-step stovetop dinner. This skillet meal is sure to please the hungriest of cowboys—and cowgirls. The wagon-wheel pasta not only makes this dish "campfire fun," it's also the perfect shape for holding the warm, hearty chili-style sauce. Mix it up by adding different-colored peppers or zucchini for extra color and fiber. Happy trails!

1 teaspoon canola oil

1 medium onion, diced

1 medium green bell pepper, diced

1 teaspoon minced garlic

1¼ pounds lean ground turkey

1 (14-ounce) can fire-roasted diced tomatoes

1 (6-ounce) can tomato paste

1 (4-ounce) can diced green chilies

1 tablespoon chili powder

1½ teaspoon ground cumin

¾ teaspoon dried oregano

6 ounces uncooked wagon wheels (about 2 cups dry)

1. Heat the oil in a large non-stick skillet over medium heat. Add the onion, peppers, and garlic, and sauté for 4 to 5 minutes or until the onion is transparent.

2. Add the turkey and cook, breaking up the meat for 4 to 5 minutes or until browned. Add the remaining ingredients and 1¾ cups water and stir well. Cover and cook 23 to 25 minutes or until the macaroni is tender. Adjust salt and pepper to taste. Dinner is served.

NUTRITION INFORMATION PER SERVING (1½ cups): Calories 370 | Carbohydrate 37g (Sugars 6g) | Total Fat 11g (Sat Fat 2.5g) | Protein 28g | Fiber 6g | Cholesterol 75mg | Sodium 320mg | Food Exchanges: 3½ Lean Meat, 1½ Starch, 1 Vegetable, 1 Fat | Carbohydrate Choices: 2 | Weight Watcher Plus Point Comparison: 9

Cheesy Seaside Shells

GET YOUR MAC 'N CHEESE FIX with this divine stove-to-table seafood skillet dish. Pink shrimp, sweet crabmeat and a touch of Old Bay seasoning blend beautifully into the velvety, creamy, cheesy sauce that coats the pasta shells. At only 320 calories per serving, you'll wonder how something so satisfying can keep (or get) you in ship-shape.

MAKES **6** SERVINGS

3 cups large shells, uncooked

1 cup low-fat milk

1 cup reduced-sodium chicken broth

1 tablespoon cornstarch

1 teaspoon olive oil

3 stalks celery, diced

2 cups sliced mushrooms

2 cloves garlic, minced

¾ cup shredded reduced-fat cheddar cheese

2 tablespoons light tub-style cream cheese

1½ teaspoons Old Bay seasoning

2 cups peas and carrots

12 ounces cooked salad or bay shrimp

8 ounces crab meat (chopped imitation crabmeat works well)

1. While preparing the sauce, cook the pasta according to package directions. Drain and place back in pot.

2. In a medium bowl, whisk together the milk, broth, and cornstarch until fully combined. Set aside.

3. Heat the oil in a large sauté pan over medium high heat. Add the celery, mushrooms (if desired), and garlic and sauté until the vegetables are soft, about 5 minutes. Add the peas and carrots and cook 2 minutes, or until moisture cooks off. Stir in the milk mixture until blended. Continue cooking, stirring constantly, for about 5 minutes or until thickened. Turn heat to low. Stir in the cheeses and Old Bay seasoning.

4. Add the pasta, shrimp, and crab. Stir and heat until seafood is warm, then add the cooked shells. Toss lightly and serve.

Marlene Says: *While this dish is nice and creamy as it is, swapping the low-fat milk for evaporated will add more creaminess along with an extra boost of calcium.*

NUTRITION INFORMATION PER SERVING (1½ cups): Calories 320 | Carbohydrate 39g (Sugars 5g) | Total Fat 5g (Sat Fat 3g) | Protein 28g | Fiber 3g | Cholesterol 120 mg | Sodium 620mg | Food Exchanges: 3 Lean Meat, 2 Starch, 1 Vegetable | Carbohydrate Choices: 2½ | Weight Watcher Plus Point Comparison: 8

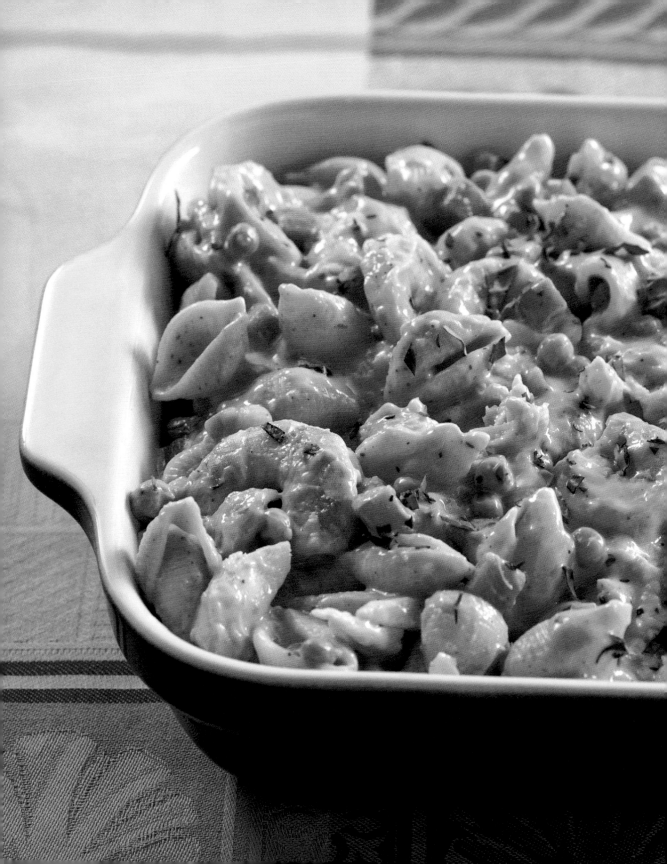

Chicken Fettuccine Alfredo

MMM, MORE LUSCIOUS ALFREDO! For this version I have added a new twist to my favorite Alfredo sauce—a bit of lovely rosemary. Add classic fettuccine noodles, tender mushrooms and flavorful zucchini and the result is a Chicken Alfredo more interesting, more flavorful, and far better for you than you will find in any restaurant.

MAKES **4** SERVINGS

6 ounces dry fettuccine pasta

2 small zucchini, cut in half lengthwise and sliced

1½ cups sliced mushrooms

Scant ¼ teaspoon garlic salt

⅔ cup low-fat milk

1 tablespoon plus 1 teaspoon cornstarch

⅔ cup reduced-sodium chicken broth

3 tablespoons light cream cheese

1 teaspoon minced garlic

½ teaspoon fresh rosemary, finely chopped

¼ teaspoon black pepper

6 tablespoons grated Parmesan cheese

Salt to taste

2 cups shredded cooked boneless, skinless chicken breast

1. While preparing the sauce, cook the pasta according to the package directions for al dente pasta. Drain the pasta, return to the pot, and cover.

2. Lay mushrooms on a plate covered with a paper towel. Lightly sprinkle with half the garlic salt and microwave for 30 seconds. Add zucchini to plate. Sprinkle zucchini with remaining garlic salt and microwave 30 more seconds. Set aside.

3. In a medium saucepan, whisk the milk and cornstarch until smooth. Whisk in the broth and place over low heat. Add the cream cheese, garlic, rosemary and pepper. Bring to a low simmer and cook until the sauce thickens, about 4 minutes. Whisk in the Parmesan and cook for 1 to 2 more minutes or until sauce is smooth. Add salt to taste.

4. Add the chicken to the pasta in pot and stir to warm. Add vegetables and sauce and toss to combine.

DARE TO COMPARE: A dinner entrée of Chicken Alfredo at the Olive Garden clocks in at 1,440 calories, close to 3 days' worth of saturated fat, over 100 grams of carb, and 2,000 mg of sodium. This dish is definitely better as a do-it-yourself-er!

NUTRITION INFORMATION PER SERVING: Calories 330 | Carbohydrate 40g (Sugars 5g) | Total Fat 7g (Sat Fat 3g) | Protein 29g | Fiber 6g | Cholesterol 60mg | Sodium 500mg | Food Exchanges: 4 Lean Meat, 2 Starch, 1 Vegetable, ½ Fat | Carbohydrate Choices: 2 | Weight Watcher Plus Point Comparison: 8

Creamy Pesto Penne – Two Ways

PRESTO! IT'S CREAMY PESTO, easy, economical and packed with flavor. For this slimmed down version I've added creamy goodness with a touch cottage cheese for a winning pasta dish that can be enjoyed two ways. Made with broccoli and beans, the recipe "as is" is a great vegetarian or Meatless Monday option. Swap out the beans for chicken and you've got a great Chicken and Broccoli Pesto Pasta that's always sure to please.

MAKES **4** SERVINGS

1 cup packed fresh basil leaves

1 tablespoon extra-virgin olive oil, divided

2 tablespoons chopped walnuts

2 tablespoons minced garlic

¼ teaspoon salt

¼ teaspoon black pepper

¼ cup low-fat cottage cheese

¼ cup shredded Parmesan cheese, divided

5 ounces dry penne pasta (about 1¾ cups)

¾ cup cannellini beans, rinsed and drained

4 cups broccoli florets

Freshly ground black pepper, optional

1. For the pesto, place the basil in a food processor (or use an immersion blender). Add 2 teaspoons of oil, 2 tablespoons of water, walnuts, garlic, salt and pepper, and pulse. Add cottage cheese and 2 tablespoons of Parmesan; process until smooth. Set aside.

2. Cook the pasta according to the package directions. Place the broccoli in a large microwave-safe dish, add 2 tablespoons of water, cover and microwave on high for 2 to 3 minutes or until the broccoli is crisp tender. Drain and set aside.

3. Drain the pasta, reserving 2 tablespoons of cooking water. Return pasta and water to the pot; add the beans, stir, and heat over low heat for 2 minutes. Turn off the heat. Pour the pesto over the penne and stir gently to combine. Add the broccoli and toss again.

4. Pour the pasta into a serving dish and sprinkle with remaining 2 tablespoons of Parmesan. Garnish with basil leaves and top with freshly ground black pepper, if desired.

Marlene Says: For **Chicken and Broccoli Pesto Pasta**, reduce broccoli florets to 3 cups, omit beans, and add 1½ cups cooked chicken to drained pasta. (Add 30 calories, 10 grams of protein, 2 grams fat; subtract 7 grams carbohydrate, 4 grams fiber.)

NUTRITION INFORMATION PER SERVING (1½ cups): Calories 300 | Carbohydrate 40g (Sugars 4g) | Total Fat 9g (Sat Fat 2g) | Protein 17g | Fiber 7g | Cholesterol 5mg | Sodium 430mg | Food Exchanges: 2½ Starch, 1 Lean Meat, 1 Vegetable, 1 Fat | Carbohydrate Choices: 2½ | Weight Watcher Plus Point Comparison: 8

15-Minute Shrimp Fettuccine

SO QUICK, SO EASY—in not much more time than it takes to cook and drain the pasta, dinner is served. Low-fat evaporated milk is the secret to this ultra-smooth, rich-tasting, restaurant-quality sauce that's created in just 15 minutes. You'll barely have time to set the table (or light the candles) before sitting down to this lovely meal.

MAKES **4** SERVINGS

6 ounces dry fettuccine

1 teaspoon olive oil

1 garlic clove, crushed

1 pound large raw shrimp, peeled and deveined

3 tablespoons sweet vermouth

1½ cups marinara (or one 14-ounce jar)

½ cup low-fat evaporated milk

½ teaspoon dried oregano

⅛ teaspoon black pepper

Pinch red pepper flakes

1. While preparing the sauce, cook the pasta according to the package directions, drain and set aside.

2. Heat the oil in a large non-stick saucepan over medium heat. Add the garlic, then the shrimp and cook until pink, about 1 to 2 minutes. Add the vermouth and sauté for one more minute. Remove the shrimp from the pan and cover to keep warm.

3. Add the spaghetti sauce, evaporated milk, oregano, black pepper, and red pepper flakes to the saucepan and whisk to combine. Bring the sauce to a simmer for 1 to 2 minutes or until heated through. Add the shrimp to the sauce and then toss with the pasta.

Marlene Says: *To quick-thaw shrimp, place frozen shrimp in a large bowl of cold water and continue to run cold water over them (letting excess water flow out of the bowl). Depending on the size of the shrimp, thawing should take between 10 to 15 minutes.*

NUTRITION INFORMATION PER SERVING (1½ cups): Calories 310 | Carbohydrate 40g (Sugars 12g) Total Fat 4g (Sat Fat .5g) | Protein 24g | Fiber 4g | Cholesterol 140mg | Sodium 420mg | Food Exchanges: 2½ Lean Meat, 2 Starch, 1 Vegetable | Carbohydrate Choices: 2½ | Weight Watcher Plus Point Comparison: 7

Easy Eggplant Parmesan

*IF YOU LOVE EGGPLANT, this is the dish for you. If you don't think you like eggplant, this is still a dish for you. My boys do **not** like eggplant—but they do like this dish. Why? Because it tastes nothing like eggplant (and of course, to them, that's a good thing). The trick here is to salt the slices of eggplant—drawing out any bitterness—before you start the dish. The result is a tender, mild Parmesan-style dish that everyone loves.*

MAKES **4** SERVINGS

1 medium globe eggplant (¾ to 1 pound)

½ teaspoon salt

⅓ cup flour

1 large egg

½ cup breadcrumbs

½ cup panko crumbs

1½ cups marinara sauce (or one 14-ounce jar)

¼ teaspoon red pepper flakes, optional

1 cup shredded part-skim mozzarella

2 tablespoons grated Parmesan cheese

2 tablespoons chopped fresh basil, optional

1. Preheat oven to 425°F. Generously spray a baking sheet with cooking spray.

2. Slice eggplant (with skin) into ¼-inch slices. Place eggplant in a bowl, toss with salt and let sit for 10 minutes. Lightly rinse eggplant and pat dry.

3. In a shallow bowl, mix together breadcrumbs and panko crumbs. In another shallow bowl, beat the egg until frothy. Place flour in a third bowl.

4. Dip eggplant in flour, then egg (letting excess egg drip off) and then into the breadcrumb mixture. Coat both sides and place eggplant slices on baking sheet. Bake for 20 minutes, flipping eggplant slices over after 10 minutes.

5. Add pepper flakes to marinara, if desired. Place ¾ cup marinara sauce in bottom of a 9 x 13-inch baking dish. Line baking dish with eggplant slices, slightly overlapping them, and top with remaining sauce. Sprinkle shredded cheeses on top. Bake for 15 minutes. Garnish with basil.

Marlene Says: *The Meatless Monday campaign from John Hopkins School of Public Health encourages us all to give up meat, if just for one day a week. Healthy meat-free meals are good for your body, the planet, and your wallet!*

NUTRITION INFORMATION PER SERVING: Calories 225 | Carbohydrate 23g (Sugars 5 g) | Total Fat 9g (Sat Fat 0g) | Protein14g | Fiber 3g | Cholesterol 45mg | Sodium 620mg | Food Exchanges: 2 Vegetable, 1 Starch, 1 Medium Fat Meat, 1 Fat | Carbohydrate Choices: 1 ½ | Weight Watcher Plus Point Comparison: 5

Pizza Pasta Pie

In the three weeks after I first made this recipe, I made it three more times! Fresh-cooked pasta forms the "crust" for this deep dish "pizza" layered with ricotta cheese, meaty marinara, and melted mozzarella cheese. This quick and easy dish is part pizza, part pasta, and part pie—and it delivers the flavor of lasagna. Could it get any better?

MAKES **6** SERVINGS

6 ounces dry spaghetti

1 large egg, lightly beaten

¼ cup, plus 2 tablespoons grated Parmesan cheese, divided

½ pound lean ground beef

2 cups sliced mushrooms, optional

1½ cups marinara sauce

½ teaspoon oregano

1 cup part-skim ricotta cheese

¾ cup shredded part-skim mozzarella cheese

1. Preheat the oven to 350°F. Lightly spray a 9-inch pie plate with cooking spray.

2. Cook the spaghetti according to the package directions, drain, rinse, and shake well to remove excess water. Place in a large bowl and toss with the egg and ¼ cup of the Parmesan cheese. Press the spaghetti on the bottom and up the sides of the prepared pie plate and set aside.

3. Spray a medium non-stick skillet with cooking spray and place over medium high heat. Add the beef and mushrooms, if desired, and cook for 5 to 7 minutes or until the beef is browned. Add the marinara sauce and oregano, stir to combine, and cook 3 to 4 minutes. Give the ricotta a stir and spoon onto the spaghetti crust, spreading evenly. Spoon the meat sauce on the ricotta layer. Sprinkle with the mozzarella and remaining Parmesan cheese.

5. Bake for 30 minutes or until fully heated through. Remove from oven and let stand 10 minutes before cutting into six wedges to serve.

Marlene Says: *To make a "deepdish" pie, use 8-ounces (or 4 cups cooked) spaghetti. (Adds 30 calories and 7 grams carbohydrate.)*

NUTRITION INFORMATION PER SERVING: Calories 290 | Carbohydrate 26g (Sugars 2g) | Total Fat 12g (Sat Fat 6g) | Protein 24g | Fiber 5g | Cholesterol 80mg | Sodium 410mg | Food Exchanges: 3 Lean Meat, 1 Starch, 1 Vegetable, 1 Fat | Carbohydrate Choices: 1½ | Weight Watcher Plus Point Comparison

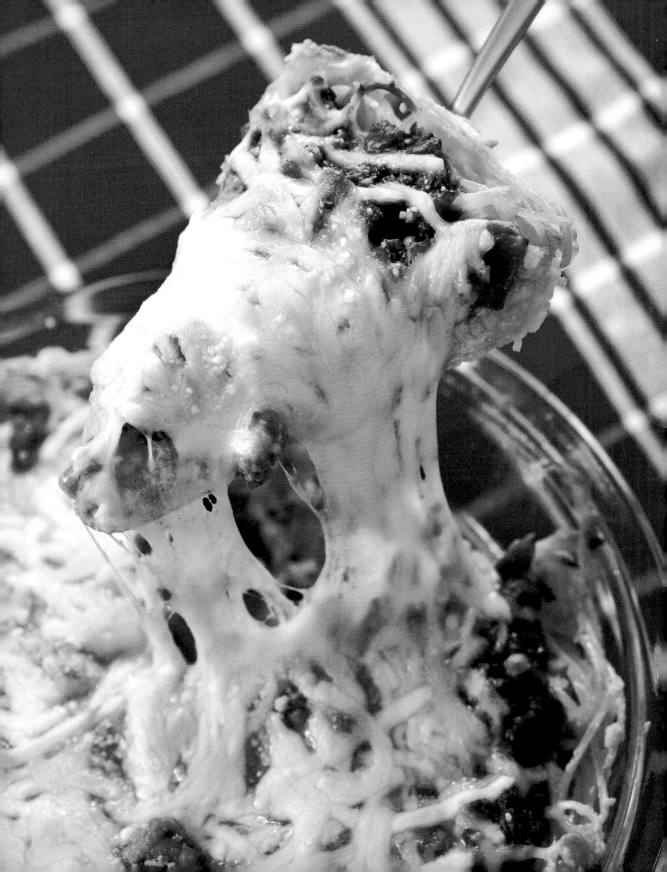

Homemade Pizza Dough

THE COMBINATION OF WHITE WHOLE-WHEAT and regular all-purpose flour makes this dough healthful and delicious, while the food processor makes it easy. Even if you have never made pizza dough before, I promise you, it's easier than you think. For a uniform and predictably crunchy crust, pre-bake the dough for 10 to 15 minutes at 425°F before adding the toppings. This dough can be used in any recipe that calls for pizza crust (it's equivalent to one 11-ounce refrigerated can of pizza crust).

MAKES **12** OUNCES PIZZA DOUGH

¾ cup white whole-wheat flour

¾ cup all-purpose flour

1 package instant yeast (2¼ teaspoons)

¼ teaspoon salt

¼ teaspoon sugar

½ cup warm water

2 teaspoons olive oil

1. Combine both flours, the yeast, salt, and sugar in a food processor and pulse to mix. Mix together the water and oil in a cup. With the food processor running, slowing pour in the water until a sticky dough begins to form. Continue to process until the dough becomes a ball and then process one more minute. (The dough should be nice and soft; if it's too dry to make a ball, add a touch more water. If it seems very sticky, add 1 more tablespoon of flour).

2. Spray a large bowl with cooking spray. Place the dough in the bowl, turning to coat. Cover the bowl with plastic wrap or a damp towel and let rise about an hour or until doubled in size. Punch down and let the dough rest for about 10 minutes before rolling it out.

Marlene Says: *After punching down the dough, it can be placed in a bowl and covered, or wrapped in plastic and placed in the refrigerator for later use. Keeps well up to two days.*

NUTRITION INFORMATION PER SERVING (one-sixth crust): Calories 130 | Carbohydrate 24g (Sugars 1g) | Total Fat 2g (Sat Fat 0g) | Protein 4g | Fiber 3g | Cholesterol 0mg | Sodium 200mg | Food Exchanges: 1½ Starch | Carbohydrate Choices: 1½ | Weight Watcher Plus Point Comparison: 3

Loaded Cheese and Pepperoni Pizza

YES, YOU CAN HAVE PEPPERONI ON YOUR PIZZA AND EAT IT TOO! I've had many requests for a better-for-you pizza recipe, so this was no place to get skimpy. The great news is that when it comes to tasty veggie toppings, the more you load on, the healthier the pizza gets. A loaded slice of this pizza has just over 200 calories, and when paired with a salad it's a fulfilling, yet nutritious, meal. Day or night, now you can always say yes to pizza!

MAKES **6** SERVINGS

2 cups sliced mushrooms

1 medium green bell pepper, sliced crosswise into ¼-inch rings

1 thin prepared pizza crust, like Boboli

6 tablespoons pizza sauce

½ cup roasted red peppers, chopped

¾ cup shredded reduced fat Italian blend cheese, like Sargento

12 slices (about ¾ ounce) turkey pepperoni slices, cut in halves

½ cup slivered red onion

2 tablespoons grated Parmesan cheese

1. Preheat the oven to 450°F and position a rack in the middle of the oven.

2. Place a paper towel on a microwave-safe plate, spread the mushrooms and bell pepper on the paper towel, and microwave for 1 minute.

3. Place the crust on a baking sheet and spread the pizza sauce over the crust. Top evenly with the red peppers and Italian cheese. Layer the pizza with the green bell pepper, pepperoni halves, and red onion.

4. Sprinkle the Parmesan on top and bake in the middle of the oven for 15 minutes or until the cheese is melted and the crust is browned. Cut into six pieces.

Marlene Says: *The trick to piling on the veggies without piling on excess moisture is to cook the vegetables slightly first. I've found that one quick minute in the microwave on a paper towel liner does a great job of getting the veggies pizza-ready.*

NUTRITION INFORMATION PER SERVING (one slice): Calories 220 | Carbohydrate 31 (Sugars 3g) | Total Fat 7 g (Sat Fat 2g) | Protein 13g | Fiber 3g | Cholesterol 15mg | Sodium 680mg | Food Exchanges: 1½ Starch, 1½ Vegetable, 1 Lean Meat | Carbohydrate Choices: 2 | Weight Watcher Plus Point Comparison: 6

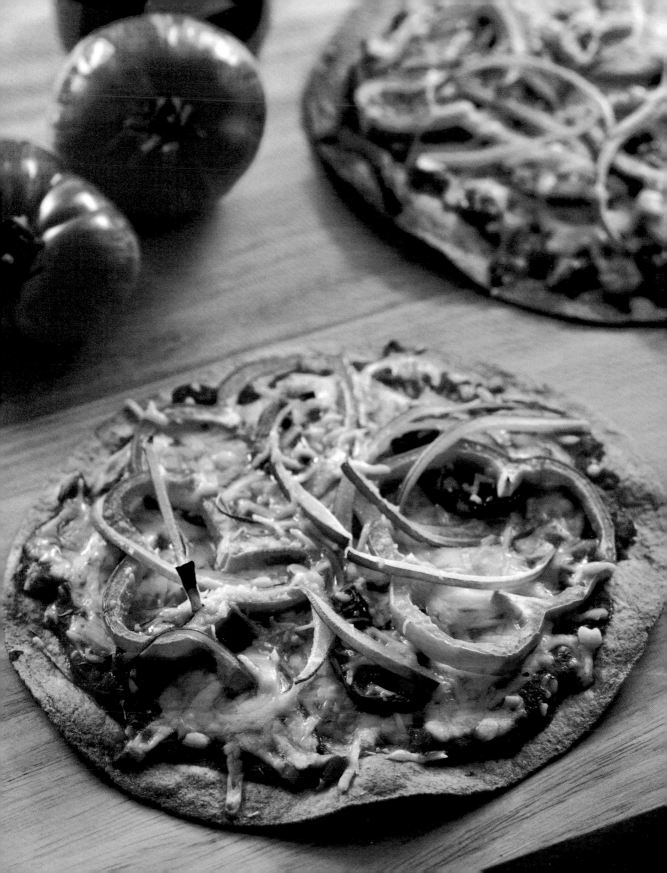

Individual New York-Style Pizzas

WITH THE PERFECT TRIO OF TOPPERS—mushrooms, onions, and bell pepper—this pizza tastes like a classic pizza should. The surprise is the thin crispy crust fashioned with a carb-conscious high-fiber tortilla. And what a surprise it is—not one of the crispy-pizza-crust-loving men in my family could tell that the crust (which reminded my son Stephen of a pizza he ate in Italy) was actually a tortilla. If you like an even crisper crust, move the pizza directly onto the oven rack for the last minute of baking.

MAKES **1** SERVING

1 high fiber tortilla (like Mission Carb Balance)

2 tablespoons pizza sauce

3 tablespoons reduced-fat Italian cheese

1 cup sliced mushrooms

3 sliced green pepper rings (or ⅓ cup chopped)

¼ cup slivered red onion

½ teaspoon oregano

1 teaspoon Parmesan cheese

1. Preheat oven to 425°F.

2. Place the tortilla on baking pan and spray lightly with cooking spray. Bake for 4 minutes or until lightly crisped. While tortilla is baking, place a paper towel on a microwave-safe plate, spread the mushrooms and bell pepper on the paper towel, and microwave for 1 minute.

3. Remove tortilla from oven; top with sauce and cheese, then mushrooms, pepper and onion. Crush oregano over pizza and sprinkle with Parmesan. Bake for 4 minutes or until cheese is melted and crust is crisped to your liking.

Marlene Says: *I used Mission Carb Balance 8-inch tortillas to test this pizza and loved the results. Regular flour tortillas will give you similar results—but not the whopping 11 grams of fiber!*

NUTRITION INFORMATION PER SERVING (entire pizza): Calories 220 | Carbohydrate 26g (Sugars 4g) | Total Fat 8g (Sat Fat 4g) | Protein 13g | Fiber 13g | Cholesterol 0mg | Sodium 590 mg | Food Exchanges: 2 Vegetables, 1 Medium Fat Meat, 1 Starch, 1 Fat | Carbohydrate Choices: 1½ | Weight Watcher Plus Point Comparison: 5

sides that make the meal

Classic Creamed Spinach

Lemony Buttery Green Beans

Fresh Orange-Glazed Carrots

Oven-Fried Broccoli Bites

Smoky Garlicky Greens

Inside-Out Stuffed Mushrooms

Sauteed Cabbage, Onions, and Apples

Roasted Onions with Sweet Balsamic Glaze

Fresh Asparagus with Hollandaise Sauce

Easy Everyday Vegetable Latkes

Light-as-a-Feather Zucchini Casserole

Creamy Golden Mashed Potatoes

Sour Cream and Onion Smashed Potatoes

Fiesta Lime Rice

Spicy Sweet Potato Mash

10-Minute Broccoli, Cheese, and Rice Skillet

Quick-Fix Macaroni and Cheese Muffins

Cheesy Skillet Cornbread

Everyday Garlic Toast

Just once wouldn't it be nice to hear about something incredibly *delicious* that you should be eating *more* of instead of less? Well, there is such a thing—*tasty, nutritious vegetables*. Chockfull of vitamins, minerals, antioxidants and powerful phytochemicals, vegetables are Mother Nature's way of keeping us *healthy, happy,* and *beautiful*. Because vegetables are also low in calories, high in fiber, and virtually fat- and sodium-free, the USDA suggests that almost one-third of a healthy plate be filled with non-starchy vegetables. Another one-fourth should be filled with *wholesome* grains or starches (like bread, potatoes, pasta or rice). If you combine the amounts for *vegetables and grains*, this means that more than half of every healthy meal should be composed of "sides"!

But we don't eat for health, we eat for taste—and when it comes to *great taste*, vegetables rarely make the cut. I would like to change that, and I think my Oven-Fried Broccoli Bites are a *great start*. When drenched in *creamy* Ranch-style dressing, *coated* in seasoned breadcrumbs and oven-fried, good ol' broccoli becomes a side that can make the meal, just like my Classic Creamed Spinach. It took eight tries to create a healthy yet truly *decadent-tasting* creamed spinach recipe, but one bite and I think you'll agree: it was worth the effort! When this stellar side is front and center, it elevates any meal. Smoky Garlicky Greens are *the perfect complement* for Chicken Chicken Fried Steak; Sautéed Onions and Apples lend a tasty hand to Crispy Pork Scaloppini; and Lemony Buttery Green Beans and Creamy Golden Mashed Potatoes are *just the ticket* for Sunday dinner with a Fast Fabulous Roast Chicken. If you're a potato lover, be sure to check out the healthy reasons I still root for America's favorite vegetable, *the almighty spud.*

POTATOES

We love our potatoes. On Thanksgiving Day alone, Americans eat over 100 *million pounds* of them. But, unfortunately, when potatoes and health are mentioned in the same sentence, what we often think of are high carbs and empty calories. The real truth, however, is that when prepared in the right way (and eaten in the proper portion size) potatoes can fit easily, deliciously—and nutritiously—in any diet. Familiar, economical, healthy, and highly satisfying, America's favorite vegetable is something to root for. Here are seven reasons why:

SEVEN SPUD-TACULAR POTATO FACTS:

1. Potatoes are diet-friendly. Fat-free, gluten-free, and low in sodium, a medium (5.3-ounce) potato has just 110 calories. It's the rich preparations and tempting toppings that sabotage nature's naturally skinny spuds.

2. Potatoes satisfy. Calorie for calorie, boiled potatoes lead all foods when ranked according to their satiety value (the ability to make you feel full). Ranking *below* potatoes are fish, apples and oats!

3. Potatoes can help reduce blood pressure. Potatoes lead all produce picks in potassium content. Studies show a diet high in potassium can reduce the effects of sodium on blood pressure.

4. Potatoes are packed with nutrients. Potatoes contain all 22 amino acids (the building blocks of protein) and are an excellent source of vitamin C. Colorful red, yellow, orange, and purple potatoes rival vegetable superstars broccoli and Brussels sprouts when it comes to antioxidants.

5. Potato salads are extra blood-sugar friendly. Cooked and cooled potatoes are high in resistant starch, a type of starch that is "resistant" to digestion which acts like fiber to slow the rise of blood sugar.

6. Potatoes are super when sweet! A single sweet potato or yam packs over 200% of the daily requirement for Vitamin A, as well as 5 healthy grams of fiber.

7. Potatoes are ultra-easy to prepare. For a marvelous microwave "baked" potato, cut and remove a thin wedge, about ¼-inch wide, 1 inch deep and 3 inches long, from a clean baking spud. Microwave on high for 10 to 12 minutes or until soft. The steam from the potato will escape, creating a dry, fluffy oven baked-style interior.

Classic Creamed Spinach

ONCE RESERVED FOR ONLY THE MOST SPECIAL OCCASIONS, creamed spinach moved to everyday-dish status when it became a customer favorite at Boston Market restaurants. The problem with creamed spinach is that it's usually made with cream and butter—or loads of bacon—making it an everyday diet killer. I am proud to share this recipe, as it significantly lightens the load, but not the decadent quality, of silky creamed spinach.

MAKES **6** SERVINGS

2 (10-ounce) packages frozen chopped spinach

2 teaspoons butter

½ cup finely chopped shallots or onions

2 cloves garlic, minced

2 teaspoons cornstarch

1½ cups low-fat milk

½ teaspoon liquid smoke

3 tablespoons light cream cheese

¾ teaspoon seasoned salt (I use Lawry's 25% less sodium)

¼ teaspoon fresh ground pepper

2 tablespoons grated Parmesan cheese

1. Place the spinach in a large microwave-safe bowl, add ½ cup of water, cover, and microwave on high for 9 minutes. Move the spinach to a colander and use a small pot lid or plate to press down firmly, squeezing out the cooking liquid until the spinach is dry.

2. In a large non-stick skillet over medium heat, melt the butter. Add the shallots and cook until soft and translucent, about 3 minutes. Add the garlic and sauté for 1 minute.

3. Stir the cornstarch into the milk along with the liquid smoke. Add the mixture to the pan, bring to a simmer, and simmer for 2 minutes or until slightly thickened. Reduce heat to low and stir in the cream cheese, seasoned salt and pepper. Cook until smooth.

4. Stir in spinach and increase the heat to medium. Turn the spinach in the sauce and cook for 2 to 3 minutes or until thoroughly coated (if adding spinach creates excess water, continue cooking until thick again). Stir in Parmesan cheese and serve.

DARE TO COMPARE: The average restaurant side order of creamed spinach serves up 280 calories, over 20 grams of fat (most of it saturated), and a hefty 600 mg of sodium. This decadent-tasting side impressively serves up a full day's worth of vitamin A, 25% of the daily requirement for calcium and vitamin C, and a good dose of both iron and fiber.

NUTRITION INFORMATION PER SERVING (½ cup): Calories 100 | Carbohydrate 10 (Sugars 6g) | Total Fat 3g (Sat Fat 1.5g) | Protein 8g | Fiber 3g | Cholesterol 10mg | Sodium 290 mg | Food Exchanges: 1 Vegetable, ½ Low-Fat Milk, ½ Fat | Carbohydrate Choices: ½ | Weight Watcher Plus Point Comparison: 2

Lemony Buttery Green Beans

I FIRST ENCOUNTERED A VERSION OF THIS DELIGHTFUL SIDE DISH at Buca di Beppo, the Italian restaurant chain known for delicious food and hefty family-style portions. I was so impressed by the simply adorned yet flavorful beans that I immediately headed to my kitchen to duplicate them. Don't let the simple ingredients fool you—this dish is a great addition for everyday meals and special occasions.

MAKES **6** SERVINGS

1 pound fresh green beans, trimmed

2 tablespoons butter

Juice of one large lemon (about 3 tablespoons)

⅛ teaspoon salt

⅛ teaspoon freshly ground black pepper or to taste

1. Fill a large saucepan with water and bring to a boil. When the water comes to a boil, add beans and bring back to a boil. Reduce the heat to medium high and boil for 2 to 3 minutes or until the beans are crisp tender or to your liking. Drain immediately and set aside (Step 1 can be done in advance).

2. In a large non-stick sauté pan, melt the butter over low heat. Whisk in the lemon juice, increase the heat to medium, and continue to whisk to form a sauce. Do not let brown.

3. Add the cooked green beans to the sauté pan, toss in the sauce to coat, and season with salt and pepper. Serve immediately.

Marlene Says: *There aren't many vegetable dishes more versatile than perfectly cooked green beans. They complement everything from Good 'n Easy Garlic Chicken (page 238), and Nut-Crusted Fish Fillets (page 276) to Mile High Meatloaf (page 260).*

NUTRITION INFORMATION PER SERVING (½ cup)**:** Calories 60 | Carbohydrate 5g (Sugars 2g) | Total Fat 4g (Sat Fat 2.5g) | Protein 1g | Fiber 2g | Cholesterol 10mg | Sodium 90mg | Food Exchanges: 1 Vegetable, 1 Fat | Carbohydrate Choices: 1 | Weight Watcher Plus Point Comparison: 2

Fresh Orange-Glazed Carrots

THIS DISH TAKES ORANGE-GLAZED CARROTS to new flavor heights with everyone's favorite holiday spices. It's a delicious side for the buffet table, an Easter ham, or Thanksgiving turkey, as well as an everyday grilled pork chop or salmon fillet.

MAKES **6** SERVINGS

1 pound fresh baby carrots

1 medium orange, juiced and finely zested

⅛ teaspoon cornstarch

⅜ teaspoon ground cinnamon

⅛ teaspoon ground ginger

Pinch ground cloves

Pinch salt

1½ teaspoons brown sugar

1 tablespoon butter

1. Bring ½ cup of water and carrots to a boil in a medium sauté pan over medium high heat. Cover, reduce the heat to medium low, and cook for 8 to 10 minutes or until the carrots are crisp tender.

2. While carrots are cooking, whisk together the orange juice (you may need to add water to make a full ⅓ cup), cornstarch and spices. Uncover the pan, add the orange juice mixture, brown sugar, and butter, and stir to evenly distribute. Bring to a simmer for 2 to 3 more minutes or until the juice forms a glaze and the carrots are tender.

3. Stir in the orange zest and serve.

Marlene Says: *How much is a "pinch"? Some guidelines say one-eighth of a teaspoon, but after conducting my own "pinch test," measuring the amount of spice pinched between my forefinger and thumb, I found the measure to be closer to one-sixteenth of a teaspoon.*

NUTRITION INFORMATION PER SERVING (½ cup each): Calories 60 | Carbohydrate 10g (Sugars 6g) | Total Fat 2g (Sat Fat 1g) | Protein 1g | Fiber 2g | Cholesterol 5mg | Sodium 140mg | Food Exchanges: 1 Vegetable, ½ Fat | Carbohydrate Choices: 1 | Weight Watcher Plus Point Comparison: 2

Oven-Fried Broccoli Bites

WHILE MANY COOKING GUIDES use a one size fits all approach to oven frying, I disagree. The initial preparation, the dipping and crumb mixtures, and even the oven temperature for a food like broccoli are very different than what works for, say, zucchini. For this recipe I discovered that dipping the broccoli in a creamy Ranch-flavored dip before coating it with breadcrumbs turned out to be the special step that had everyone clamoring for more.

MAKES **4** SERVINGS

4 cups bite-sized broccoli florets, with stems

¼ cup low-fat buttermilk

2 tablespoons light mayonnaise

¼ teaspoon garlic powder

¼ teaspoon onion powder

⅛ teaspoon black pepper

½ cup panko breadcrumbs

3 tablespoons breadcrumbs

⅛ teaspoon salt

1 teaspoon vegetable oil

1. Preheat the oven to 400°F. Place the broccoli and 1 tablespoon of water in a medium microwave-safe bowl. Cover and microwave on high for 90 seconds. Carefully uncover the bowl and place the broccoli on a paper-towel-lined plate to cool. Set aside.

2. In a small bowl, whisk together the next 5 ingredients (buttermilk through pepper). In a separate shallow bowl or pie plate, combine both types of breadcrumbs and the salt. Drizzle the oil over the crumbs and toss to mix lightly.

3. Holding a broccoli floret by the stem, dip and twist the floret top through the buttermilk mixture to coat, then roll in the crumbs. Place the coated floret onto a baking sheet and repeat until all florets are coated. Spray lightly with cooking spray.

4. Bake the florets for 12 minutes. (If you would like your Bites extra crispy or more browned, place them under the broiler for 1 minute before serving.)

DARE TO COMPARE: With over 6 grams of fat per "bite," just three cheesy Broccoli Bites at Bennigan's restaurant will set you back 286 calories. That's a whole lotta calories for a little bite of broccoli!

NUTRITION INFORMATION PER SERVING (¾ cup): Calories 100 | Carbohydrate 15g (Sugars 3g) | Total Fat 3.5g (Sat Fat 0.5g) | Protein 4g | Fiber 2g | Cholesterol 5mg | Sodium 330mg | Food Exchanges: 1 Vegetable, ½ Starch, 1 Fat | Carbohydrate Choices: 1 | Weight Watcher Plus Point Comparison: 2

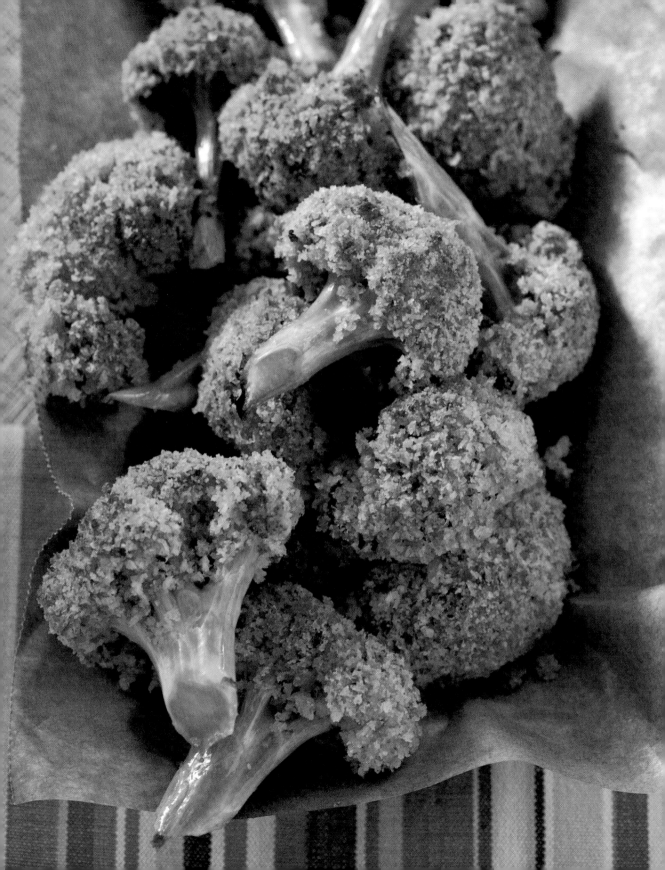

Smoky Garlicky Greens

IF YOU HAVE EVER BEEN CURIOUS ABOUT HOW TO COOK GREENS, this quick-fix version of the Southern specialty is the way to go. I start with mild-tasting, fast-cooking Swiss chard and cook it with a Southern flair, taking care to reduce the usual fat and sodium while allowing the garlicky, smoky, spicy flavors to shine. If desired, you can substitute another Southern favorite—collard greens. Start with 1 pound and use only the leaves. When cooking, add an additional 5 minutes to the simmer time.

MAKES 2 SERVINGS

1 slice center cut bacon, cut in half

½ cup chopped onion

1½ teaspoons minced garlic

½ cup reduced-sodium chicken broth, divided

¼ teaspoon black pepper

¼ teaspoon liquid smoke

1 bunch chard, about ¾ pound, coarsely chopped

1 teaspoon cider vinegar

⅛ teaspoon crushed red pepper flakes or ¼ teaspoon hot sauce, optional

1. In a large non-stick skillet, cook the bacon over medium heat, turning until crisp. Remove bacon, crumble, and set aside.

2. Add the onion to any drippings, stir and cook for 3 to 4 minutes or until translucent. Stir in the garlic, and cook for 30 seconds.

3. Stir in ¼ cup broth, pepper, and liquid smoke. Using tongs, add half the greens, turning to coat. Let cook down for 2 to 3 minutes, then stir in the remaining greens, toss briefly, reduce heat to medium low, and cover the skillet. Let simmer for 5 minutes. Uncover and stir in the remaining ¼ cup of broth. Cook, stirring occasionally, for an additional five minutes or until the greens are tender and stems are crisp tender.

4. Stir in the vinegar and, if desired, crushed red pepper or hot sauce. Place the greens in a serving dish and top with the crumbled bacon.

Marlene says: *Greens are jam-packed with vitamins, minerals, and disease-fighting antioxidants. Multiple studies have also shown Swiss chard can help blood sugar regulation—maybe that's one reason it has been named one of the world's healthiest vegetables.*

NUTRITION INFORMATION PER SERVING (about ¾ cup): Calories 80 | Carbohydrate 12g (Sugars 5g) | Total Fat 2g (Sat Fat 1g) | Protein 6g | Fiber 4g | Cholesterol 5mg | Sodium 390mg | Food Exchanges: 2 Vegetable | Carbohydrate Choices: ½ | Weight Watcher Plus Point Comparison: 1

Inside-Out Stuffed Mushrooms

HERE'S AN EASY WAY TO BRING A PARTY FEEL to your dinner table. While I love stuffed mushrooms, just hearing the term conjures up work as much as it does satisfaction. Not anymore. This clever dish brings together the great flavor of stuffed mushrooms in a dish that takes just minutes to prepare. Unique and versatile, these mushrooms are a great accompaniment to beef, chicken or fish dishes.

MAKES **4** SERVINGS

1 pound medium whole mushrooms

2 teaspoons sherry

1 small clove garlic, pressed

2 teaspoons olive oil, divided

3 tablespoons Italian breadcrumbs

3 tablespoons grated Parmesan cheese

⅛ teaspoon dried thyme, crushed

⅛ teaspoon salt

⅛ teaspoon pepper

1. Preheat the oven to 350°F. Clean, trim stems, and quarter mushrooms. Place the mushrooms in a large microwave-safe bowl. Microwave on high power for 2 to 2½ minutes, stirring after 1 minute, or until the mushrooms begin to soften. Remove and drain the mushrooms, discarding the liquid.

2. Place the mushrooms in a 1½-quart baking dish. Add the sherry, garlic, 1 teaspoon of olive oil, and stir to combine. In a small bowl, combine the breadcrumbs, Parmesan, thyme, salt, and pepper. Stir 2 tablespoons of the crumb mixture into the mushrooms and mix well to coat. Let sit for 5 minutes.

3. Mix the remaining 1 teaspoon of olive oil into the remaining crumbs. Sprinkle over the mushrooms and bake for 15 minutes or until the crumbs are golden brown.

Marlene Says: *Mushrooms are magical when it comes to your health, leading all other vegetables in cancer-fighting selenium and bone-enhancing vitamin D. They're also high in heart-healthy fiber and blood pressure-reducing potassium.*

NUTRITION INFORMATION PER SERVING (½ cup): Calories 90 | Carbohydrate 8g (Sugars 3g) | Total Fat 3g (Sat Fat 1g) | Protein 6g | Fiber 2g | Cholesterol 5mg | Sodium 300mg | Food Exchanges: 1 Vegetable, ½ Lean Meat, ½ Fat | Carbohydrate Choices: ½ | Weight Watcher Plus Point Comparison: 2

Sautéed Cabbage, Onions, and Apples

THIS FLAVORFUL GERMAN-STYLE CABBAGE dish is big on taste yet modest in sodium content, making it not only a wonderful side dish, but a wonderful replacement for sodium-saturated sauerkraut. Lightly sweet, tangy, sour and peppery, cabbage never had it so good. Serve as a side for any pork dish or use it as a topping for burgers and brats.

MAKES **8** SERVINGS

1 teaspoon canola oil

½ small head cabbage, cored and thinly sliced

1 small sweet onion, thinly sliced, about 1 cup

1 medium apple, peeled, quartered, cored and sliced

1 tablespoon cider vinegar

½ teaspoon caraway seeds

¾ cup reduced-sodium chicken broth

1 teaspoon brown sugar

¼ teaspoon salt

⅛ teaspoon pepper

1 tablespoon butter

1. Heat the oil in a large skillet over medium high heat. Add the cabbage and onion and sauté for 5 to 6 minutes, stirring occasionally, until the cabbage is lightly browned and starts to wilt. Add the apple and sauté for 1 minute.

2. Add the vinegar, caraway seeds, broth, brown sugar, salt, and pepper. Stir to combine. Cover and cook on medium heat for 5 minutes. Remove the lid and cook another 3 to 5 minutes to allow liquid to reduce slightly.

3. Stir in the butter, remove from heat, cover and let stand for 5 to 10 minutes. Serve warm or at room temperature.

DARE TO COMPARE: A ½ cup serving of canned or bottled sauerkraut can have as much as 700 mg of sodium. This superior "sauerkraut substitute" keeps fresh for 3 to 4 days when stored covered in the refrigerator.

NUTRITION INFORMATION PER SERVING (½ cup): Calories 45 | Carbohydrate 7g (Sugars 2g) | Total Fat 2.5 g (Sat Fat 1g) | Protein 1g | Fiber 2g | Cholesterol 5mg | Sodium 90mg | Food Exchanges: 1 Vegetable | Carbohydrate Choices: ½ | Weight Watcher Plus Point Comparison: 1

Roasted Onions with Sweet Balsamic Glaze

TEMPTED BY A WONDERFUL SALE on Vidalia onions last year, I stocked up, only to realize I was running out of ways to prepare them. I turned to my good friend Diane Welland, author of The Complete Idiot's Guide to Eating Clean, and asked if she had any good onion recipes. This simple irresistible dish is the result of our conversation. Delicious with everything from burgers and chicken to roasted pork and beef tenderloin, these onions make me look forward to buying them at any price.

MAKES **8** SERVINGS

2 large red onions (about 1¼ pounds)

2 teaspoons olive oil

¼ teaspoon salt

¼ cup balsamic vinegar

1 tablespoon brown sugar

1. Preheat the oven to 425°F. Peel onions, cut in quarters, and place in a flat microwave-safe baking dish, with one of the cut edges down. Cover the dish and microwave on high for 5 minutes or until the onion layers start to soften and separate. Uncover the onions and move them to the oven. Cook for 20 minutes or until the onions are well-browned on the outside and tender on the inside (tips or spots may blacken and that's fine).

2. About 10 minutes before the onions finish cooking, stir the vinegar and brown sugar together in a small pot and simmer over medium high heat for 8 to 10 minutes or until syrupy and reduced by one-half (watch carefully near the end of cooking— once reduced, the glaze can quickly burn). Set aside.

3. Remove the onions from the oven, turn cavity side up and immediately drizzle or brush onions with balsamic glaze.

Marlene Says: *A few tips for this recipe. 1) For easier clean-up, transfer the microwaved onions to a foil-lined dish. 2) Red onions are sweeter than yellow and look terrific glazed with the balsamic syrup, but any large onion will do. 3) A small sprig of fresh rosemary placed in the covered onion dish lends the wonderful essence of rosemary to the onions.*

NUTRITION INFORMATION PER SERVING (one onion wedge): Calories 30 | Carbohydrate 5g (Sugars 4g) | Total Fat 1g (Sat Fat 0g) | Protein 0g | Fiber 0g | Cholesterol 0mg | Sodium 110mg | Food Exchanges: 1 Vegetable | Carbohydrate Choices: 0 | Weight Watcher Plus Point Comparison: 1

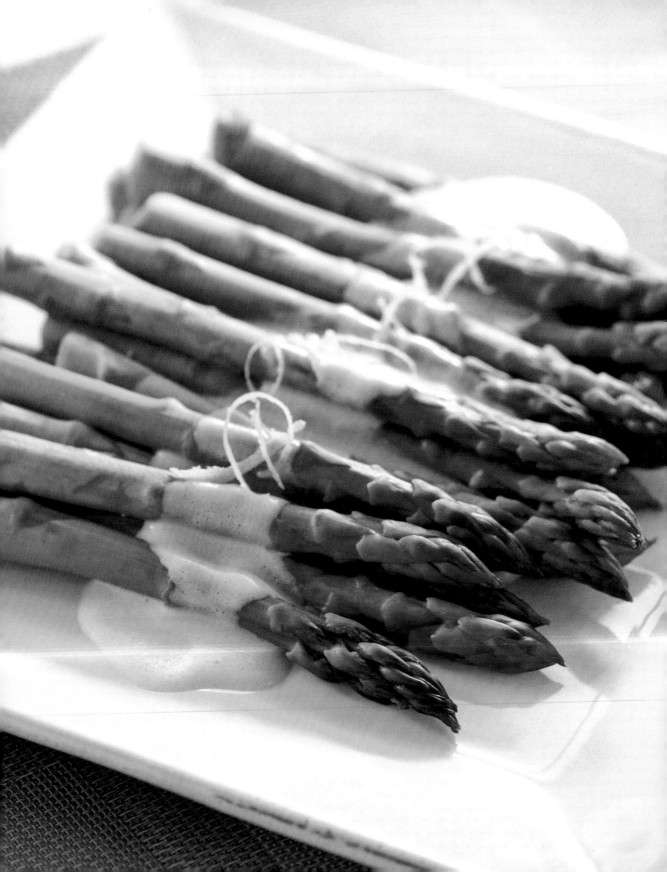

Fresh Asparagus with Hollandaise Sauce

DINING OUT WHILE WATCHING YOUR WAISTLINE (and your health) can be difficult. This steakhouse favorite side is one of the reasons why. While exceedingly delicious, hollandaise sauce is also notoriously high in fat and calories. Essentially made from butter and egg yolks, it's hard to imagine the words "healthy" and "hollandaise" could ever fit together. But here it is, healthy hollandaise, still rich, but now only in taste. Enjoy it here with fresh steamed asparagus and again in the Eggs Benedict on page 86.

MAKES **6** SERVINGS

Hollandaise Sauce

1 large egg

¼ cup liquid egg substitute

1½ tablespoons lemon juice

2 tablespoons water

¼ teaspoon Dijon mustard

⅛ teaspoon salt

2 tablespoons butter, melted

Cayenne pepper to taste

Asparagus

1½ pounds medium asparagus spears, washed and ends trimmed

⅛ teaspoon black pepper or to taste

1. For the hollandaise sauce, fill a medium saucepan or bottom part of a double boiler halfway with water. Place over medium heat and bring to simmer.

2. In a small metal bowl or the top part of a double boiler, add the first 6 ingredients (egg through salt) and whisk together until very foamy, about 1 minute. Place bowl over the simmering water (do not let it touch the water) and whisk constantly until sauce thickens and increases in volume. As soon as the eggs begin to cook around the edges, remove the bowl and set on a dish towel. The sauce should be thick enough to coat a spoon.

3. Continue to whisk the sauce for another 30 seconds. Slowly drizzle in the melted butter and cayenne pepper, whisking until well incorporated. Set aside.

4. Place the asparagus in a large microwave-safe baking dish. Add ¼ cup water, cover, and microwave on high power for 3 to 4 minutes or until spears are tender; Serve with Hollandaise.

DARE TO COMPARE: A side of asparagus with hollandaise averages 200 calories. The difference when compared to this recipe: an additional 120 calories and 13 grams of fat!

NUTRITION INFORMATION PER SERVING (4 to 5 asparagus spears, 2 tablespoons sauce): Calories 80 | Carbohydrate 6g (Sugars 3g) | Total Fat 5g (Sat Fat 3g) | Protein 5g | Fiber 2g | Cholesterol 45mg | Sodium 90mg | Food Exchanges: 1 Vegetable, 1 Fat | Carbohydrate Choices: ½ | Weight Watcher Plus Point Comparison: 2

Easy Everyday Vegetable Latkes

*MOVE OVER POTATOES, HERE COMES SQUASH! These marvelous mini pancakes, tradition-ally made from potatoes, come together in only minutes. Zucchini, squash, and carrot lend a healthy boost to these tasty latkes, which also double nicely as a light meal. Most importantly, this is **the** recipe that will get kids (and adults) to eat their veggies. Need a bit more help? Try topping the cooked latkes with a dusting of grated Parmesan.*

MAKES **4** TO **6** SERVINGS

1 medium zucchini, trimmed (about 8 ounces)

1 medium yellow squash, trimmed (about 8 ounces)

¼ teaspoon salt

1 large egg

1 large egg white

1 small carrot, peeled and grated

¼ cup grated onion

½ teaspoon black pepper

¼ cup all-purpose flour

2 tablespoons cornmeal

¾ teaspoon baking powder

1. Using the medium grate on a food processor or grater, grate the zucchini and squash. Place in a colander, sprinkle with salt, and set in the sink for 5 minutes.

2. Whisk the egg and egg white together in a large bowl. Add the remaining ingredients and stir to combine. Using a small plate or pan lid, press firmly on the squash until you have squeezed out all of the excess liquid. Add the squash to the egg and carrot mixture and stir to combine.

3. Spray a large non-stick skillet with cooking spray and place over medium heat. Pour a scant ¼ cup of batter into the skillet and spread in a 3½-inch circle. Cook for 1 to 2 minutes on the first side or until golden on the bottom. Flip and cook another 1 to 2 minutes. Repeat for a total cooking time of about 5 to 6 minutes or until latkes are nicely browned on both sides and slightly crisp.

MARLENE SAYS: *This recipe is very versatile. For more latke fun, try adding ⅓ cup corn for a pleasingly sweet flavor, 2 to 3 tablespoons of grated Parmesan cheese for cheesy goodness, or 2 to 3 tablespoons finely diced red bell pepper for more color.*

NUTRITION INFORMATION PER SERVING (2 latkes): Calories 60 | Carbohydrate 10g (Sugars 2g) | Total Fat 1g (Sat Fat 0g) | Protein 3g | Fiber 2g | Cholesterol 30mg | Sodium 150mg | Food Exchanges: 1 Vegetable, ¼ Starch | Carbohydrate Choices: 1 | Weight Watcher Plus Point Comparison: 1

Light-as-a-Feather Zucchini Casserole

DURING THOSE HOT SUMMER DAYS when the zucchini won't stop producing, this delightful and tasty casserole will make you grateful for the abundant crop. While conventional veggie bakes can weigh you down, here whipped egg whites give a lovely light texture to this casserole, making it silky and airy yet satisfying enough to serve on its own as a light summertime lunch.

MAKES **8** SERVINGS

4 teaspoons margarine or butter, divided

6 cups coarsely grated zucchini (about 1½ pounds)

1 cup finely chopped onion

½ cup finely chopped red bell pepper

1 tablespoon all-purpose flour

1 cup low-fat evaporated milk

1 teaspoon Dijon mustard

½ teaspoon garlic salt

⅛ teaspoon fresh ground pepper

¾ cup shredded reduced-fat sharp cheddar cheese

2 large egg whites

¼ cup panko breadcrumbs

1. Preheat the oven to 400°F. Lightly spray a 9 x 9 x 2-inch glass or ceramic baking dish with cooking spray.

2. In a large non-stick skillet, heat 1 teaspoon of margarine over medium heat. Add the zucchini, onion, and bell pepper and cook for 10 to 15 minutes or until the liquids have evaporated. Transfer to a bowl and set aside.

3. Add 2 teaspoons of margarine to the pan over medium heat. Add flour and cook for 1 minute, stirring constantly. Add the milk, Dijon, garlic salt, and pepper and whisk until mixture thickens, about 4 to 5 minutes. Remove from heat and stir in the cheese until blended. Pour over the zucchini mixture, stir, and let cool while you prepare the egg whites.

4. In a small bowl, beat the egg whites until soft peaks form. Gently fold the egg whites into zucchini mixture. Pour the mixture into the prepared baking dish. Melt the remaining teaspoon of margarine, combine it with the breadcrumbs, and sprinkle on top.

5. Bake for 35 to 40 minutes or until heated through.

NUTRITION INFORMATION PER SERVING (generous ½ cup): Calories 90 | Carbohydrate 10g (Sugars 6g) | Total Fat 3g (Sat Fat 2g) | Protein 7g | Fiber 2g | Cholesterol 10mg | Sodium 250mg | Food Exchanges: 1 Vegetable, 1 Lean Meat | Carbohydrate Choices: 1 | Weight Watcher Plus Point Comparison: 2

Creamy Golden Mashed Potatoes

ONE OF MY FUN TRICKS is to add a sweet potato or two to my mashed white potatoes. I recently received a copy of a wonderful book called No More Whine with Dinner *by my colleagues, the Meal Makeover Moms, and was delighted to see a similar mix. Moms Janice Bissex and Liz Weiss did me one better and upped the ante by lacing their luscious slightly sweet spuds with a bit of cream cheese. Yum! Please do try these. It was very nice of the Moms to allow me to pass on this ever-so-slightly adapted version of their fabulous recipe.*

MAKES **8** SERVINGS

2 pounds Yukon Gold potatoes, peeled and cut into 1-inch cubes, about 4 cups

1 pound sweet potatoes, peeled and cut into 1-inch cubes, about 2½ cups

¼ cup low-fat milk

¼ cup light cream cheese

¾ teaspoon salt

⅛ teaspoon black pepper

1 tablespoon butter

1. Place the potatoes and sweet potatoes in a large saucepan and add enough cold water to cover. Cover and bring to a boil. Reduce the heat and cook, covered at a low boil, until very tender, about 12 minutes.

2. Drain the potatoes well and return them to the pot. Place over low heat and add 2 tablespoons of the milk, cream cheese, salt, and pepper. Use an electric hand mixer or immersion blender to blend lightly until smooth. Add additional milk, if necessary, transfer the potatoes to a serving dish and swirl in the butter before serving.

NUTRITION INFORMATION PER SERVING (½ cup): Calories 140 | Carbohydrate 26g (Sugars 8g) | Total Fat 2.5g (Sat Fat 1.5g) | Protein 2g | Fiber 3g | Cholesterol 5mg | Sodium 410mg | Food Exchanges: 1½ Starch, ½ Fat | Carbohydrate Choices: 1½ | Weight Watcher Plus Point Comparison: 3

Sour Cream and Onion Smashed Potatoes

I GET A BIT SNEAKY with these smashed potatoes, but I have science on my side. A recent nutrition study showed that adding pureed veggies, such as cauliflower, to otherwise calorically more dense dishes resulted in participants eating fewer calories and feeling just as satisfied. For mashed potatoes I find that the perfect sneaky cauliflower/potato ratio is 50/50. The cauliflower literally disappears, leaving only the potato taste, and in the case of this recipe, the taste of yummy sour cream and fragrant green onions.

MAKES **6** SERVINGS

1 pound unpeeled Yukon Gold potatoes, cubed, about 3 cups

1 pound cauliflower, cut into florets, or 3 cups florets

½ cup diced green onion

1 teaspoon vegetable oil

½ teaspoon onion powder

⅓ cup light sour cream

¼ teaspoon salt or to taste

¼ teaspoon black pepper

1. Place the potatoes in a large pot of water, bring to a boil, and cook for 5 minutes.

2. Add the cauliflower and reduce the heat to medium low. Cook an additional 15 minutes or until the potatoes and cauliflower are tender.

3. While the potato/cauliflower mix is cooking, stir together the green onion and oil in a small microwave-safe bowl, cover, and microwave for 1 minute.

4. Drain the potato mixture in a colander. Remove excess water by pressing down on the mixture twice with the lid of a pot or a small plate. Transfer the potato mixture back to the pot and add the remaining ingredients. Using a hand masher or electric mixer, process until smooth (do not overmix).

Marlene Says: *If you wish to omit the cauliflower and make a potatoes-only side dish, use 1½ pounds of potatoes and add 3 to 4 tablespoons milk along with the sour cream. It will make 6 one-half cup servings with 120 calories and 23 grams of carb per serving.*

NUTRITION INFORMATION PER SERVING (⅓ cup): Calories 100 | Carbohydrate 18g (Sugars 3g) | Total Fat 2g (Sat Fat 1g) | Protein 4g | Fiber 3.5g | Cholesterol 5mg | Sodium 135mg | Food Exchanges: 1 Starch, 1 Vegetable | Carbohydrate Choices: 1 | Weight Watcher Plus Point Comparison: 3

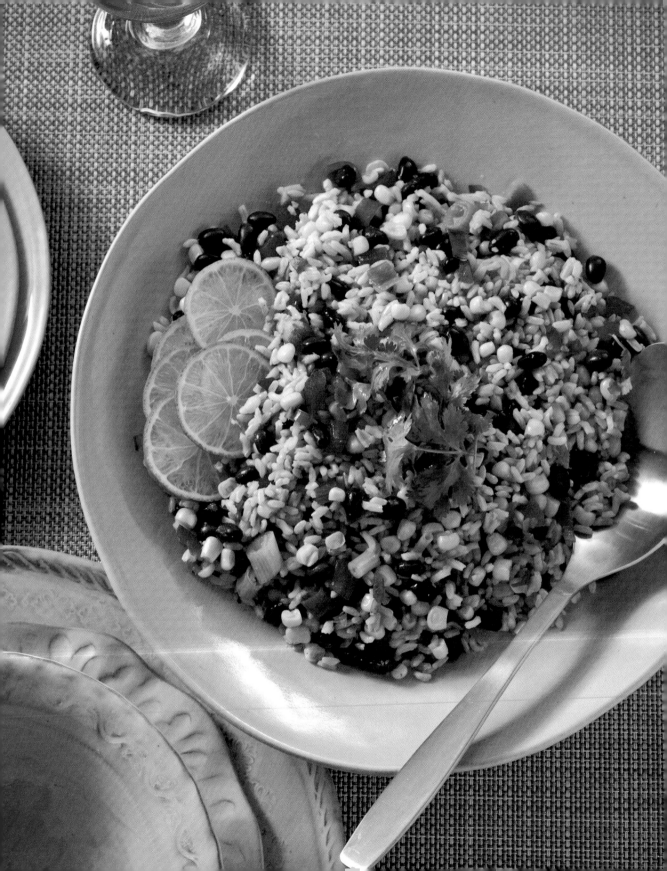

Fiesta Lime Rice

MY BOYS RECENTLY TOLD ME Chipotle Mexican Grill has the **best** Mexican rice. I am excited to say that this recipe has all the components of the rice they love—and more! Like Chipotle's beloved rice, it has the tasty combination of lime juice, chopped cilantro and a pinch of salt, but I've kicked it up a notch by adding a smattering of fiber-rich black beans, colorful red pepper, and sweet corn for a party-worthy rice that's easy enough to prepare every day. I think there is a new best rice in town.

MAKES **4** SERVINGS

⅔ cup instant brown rice (like Uncle Ben's Fast and Natural)

¾ cup canned black beans, rinsed and drained

¼ cup frozen corn, thawed

⅓ cup diced red pepper

1 medium green onion, white and green parts, finely diced

1 medium lime

2 tablespoons chopped cilantro

¼ teaspoon salt

1. Place the rice and 1¼ cups water in a medium saucepan and bring to a boil. Reduce heat to medium low, cover, and cook for 10 minutes. Remove the pan from heat and fluff the rice with a fork.

2. Immediately add the beans, corn, red pepper, green onion, and lime juice to the rice, toss gently to combine, and cover. Let sit for 3 to 4 minutes to warm added ingredients. Remove cover, stir in cilantro and salt to taste. Serve.

DARE TO COMPARE: This versatile rice side has one-third fewer calories and carbohydrates and four times the fiber as the same serving size of plain white or Chipotle Mexican Grill Cilantro Lime Rice. Note: While instant brown rice offers the health benefits of regular brown rice, it has a light texture and is closer in color to white rice.

NUTRITION INFORMATION PER SERVING (¾ cup): Calories 120 | Carbohydrate 23g (Sugars 2g) | Total Fat 1 g (Sat Fat 0g) | Protein 4g | Fiber 4g | Cholesterol 0mg | Sodium 250 mg | Food Exchanges: 1½ Starch, ½ Vegetable | Carbohydrate Choices: 1½ | Weight Watcher Plus Point Comparison: 3

Spicy Sweet Potato Mash

SPICY, SWEET, AND SAVORY, this sweet potato dish has it all! Using my pureed veggie trick once again, canned pumpkin lightens the load and ups the nutrition while taking care to preserve the traditional sweet potato flavor we all love. With just a pat of butter and a spoonful of sugar-free syrup, you can "splurge" with these sweet potatoes all year round.

MAKES **6** SERVINGS

1½ pounds dark sweet potatoes (or yams)

1 tablespoon butter or margarine

½ teaspoon dried thyme

1 cup canned pumpkin

1½ tablespoons sugar-free maple flavored syrup

¾ teaspoon seasoned or table salt

½ teaspoon black pepper

⅛ teaspoon cayenne pepper or to taste

1. To prepare the sweet potatoes, wash and pierce each potato with a fork and place in the microwave. Cook on high for 10 minutes or until sweet potatoes are soft.

2. Slice the potatoes in half lengthwise and scoop the flesh into a large, microwave-safe bowl. Add the butter and mix until well incorporated.

3. Crush the thyme in with your fingers and add the pumpkin, syrup, salt, pepper, and cayenne pepper. Using a potato masher or a large fork, mash the potatoes until smooth. Place the potato mash back into the microwave and heat for 1 minute or until hot.

Marlene Says: *Pumpkin is an excellent source of Vitamin A and fiber. One-half cup of creamy canned pumpkin has only 40 calories and 5 fabulous grams of fiber.*

NUTRITION INFORMATION PER SERVING (½ cup)**:** Calories 150 | Carbohydrate 31g (Sugars 14g) | Total Fat 2.5g (Sat Fat 1g) | Protein 4g | Fiber 5g | Cholesterol 0mg | Sodium 250 mg | Food Exchanges: 2 Starch | Carbohydrate Choices: 2 | Weight Watcher Plus Point Comparison: 4

10-Minute Broccoli, Cheese, and Rice Skillet

FRESH, YET CONVENIENT, this home-style side is sure to become a new family favorite. Chockfull of nutty brown rice, tender broccoli and cheesy sauce, it comes together in just 10 minutes and beats the packaged variety in every way.

1 cup quick-cooking brown rice (like Uncle Ben's Fast and Natural)

1 (15 ounce) can reduced sodium chicken broth (or 2 cups)

3 cups broccoli florets, cut into bite-sized pieces, about 6 ounces

¼ teaspoon garlic powder, optional

1 can condensed cheddar cheese soup (like Campbells)

¼ teaspoon black pepper or more to taste

1. In a medium saucepan, combine the brown rice and broth over medium high heat and bring to a boil. Reduce the heat to medium low, cover and simmer for 3 minutes.

2. Add the broccoli and garlic powder, (if desired), cover and cook for 4 minutes.

3. Stir in the soup and pepper and cook 2-3 minutes or until heated through.

DARE TO COMPARE: A one-half cup portion of packaged "Cheddar Broccoli Rice Sides," prepared as suggested, has 280 calories, 650 mg of sodium, and 0 grams fresh broccoli.

NUTRITION INFORMATION PER SERVING (²/3 cup)**:** Calories 125 | Carbohydrate 25g (Sugars 1g) | Total Fat 2g (Sat Fat 1g) | Protein 5g | Fiber 2g | Cholesterol 10mg | Sodium 300mg | Food Exchanges: 1½ Starch, ½ Vegetable | Carbohydrate Choices: 1½ | Weight Watcher Plus Point Comparison: 3

Quick-Fix Macaroni and Cheese Muffins

I LOVE TO USE CUPCAKE AND MUFFIN TINS as intended—for cupcakes and muffins (both savory and sweet)—but I also love to use them for pies, meatloaf, and now, macaroni and cheese. Yes, macaroni and cheese! You simply mix cooked macaroni with a few ingredients, scoop it into muffin tins, and presto: healthy, portion-controlled, marvelous macaroni and cheese that you can eat out of hand. Perfect for a light lunch, a picnic, or your next tailgate adventure, these really are fun.

MAKES **12** SERVINGS

8 ounces small elbow macaroni (about 2½ cups)

2 cups reduced-fat sharp cheddar cheese

2 teaspoons cornstarch

1 cup low-fat milk

1 large egg

½ teaspoon garlic salt

½ cup panko breadcrumbs

2 teaspoons melted butter

1. Preheat the oven to 400°F. Place paper or foil liners in a 12-cup muffin tin and spray lightly with non-stick baking spray

2. Cook the macaroni according to the package directions. Drain and immediately return to the pot. Add the cheese and stir until it is nearly melted.

3. In a medium bowl, whisk together the cornstarch and milk. Add the egg and whisk until smooth. Pour the milk mixture over the macaroni and mix well.

4. In a small bowl combine the butter and the breadcrumbs. Scoop the macaroni mixture evenly into the prepared muffin tins (it will be wet and milky, but don't worry, it will bake up fine). Sprinkle 2 teaspoons crumbs on each and bake for 20 minutes.

Marlene Says: *While any elbow macaroni will do, I used Ronzoni Smart Taste pasta, a white pasta that's fortified with fiber, calcium and vitamins for these delicious, nutritious, calcium-rich "muffins."*

NUTRITION INFORMATION PER SERVING (1 muffin): Calories 130 | Carbohydrate 18g (Sugars 2g) | Total Fat 3g (Sat Fat 1g) | Protein 9g | Fiber 3g | Cholesterol 20mg | Sodium 210mg | Food Exchanges: 1 Starch, 1 Lean Meat | Carbohydrate Choices: 1 | Weight Watcher Plus Point Comparison: 3

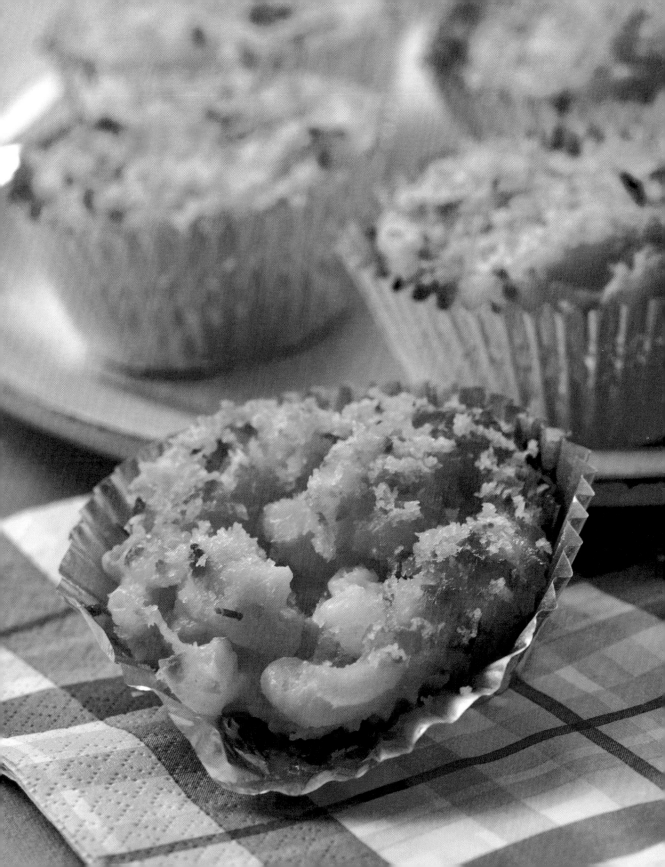

Cheesy Skillet Cornbread

THIS SUPER MOIST YET "LIGHT" RENDITION of Southern style cornbread may be lighter, but it keeps the true corn flavor and cake-like texture intact. To add extra Southern flair I've even added cottage cheese and cooked it up in a skillet. Pair it with my Smoky Garlicky Greens (page 218) and Grilled Pork with Memphis-Style Barbecue Sauce (page 269) to the delight of any fit and food-loving Southern belle or gentleman.

MAKES **10** SERVINGS

1 cup cornmeal

1 cup white whole-wheat flour

1 tablespoon baking powder

½ teaspoon baking soda

¼ cup granulated no-calorie sweetener (or 6 packets)

⅛ teaspoon salt

⅛ teaspoon pepper

½ cup diced onion

1 cup buttermilk

½ cup low-fat cottage cheese

2 large eggs, beaten

3 tablespoons butter or margarine, melted

1 teaspoon canola oil

1. Preheat the oven to 425°F. Place a 10-inch cast iron skillet in the oven to heat it.

2. In a large bowl, whisk together the first seven ingredients (cornmeal through pepper) until well combined.

3. Place the onion in a medium microwave-safe bowl and microwave on high for 30 seconds. Add the buttermilk, cottage cheese, eggs, and melted butter to the bowl and stir well to combine. Make a well in the center of the dry ingredients and pour in the buttermilk mixture. Mix with a spoon until all ingredients are combined.

4. Carefully remove the hot skillet from the oven, spray with the oil, and pour the batter into the skillet, spreading evenly. Bake for 20 to 25 minutes or until cornbread springs back when touched lightly in center.

Marlene Says: *No skillet? Bake the cornbread in an 8-inch square baking pan or make muffins. Spray the baking pan or 12 muffin cups with non-stick cooking spray. Bake at 375°F for 20 to 22 minutes, or 13 to 15 minutes, respectively.*

NUTRITION INFORMATION PER SERVING (1 slice): Calories 160 | Carbohydrate 21g (Sugars 2g) | Total Fat 5g (Sat Fat 1.5g) | Protein 6g | Fiber 2g | Cholesterol 40mg | Sodium 290mg | Food Exchanges: 1½ Starch, ½ Lean Meat | Carbohydrate Choices: 1½ | Weight Watcher Plus Point Comparison: 4

Everyday Garlic Toast

THIS ELEVENTH-HOUR RECIPE ADDITION may become one of your standbys—as it is mine. I am not exactly sure why I hesitated so long before adding it (perhaps because it has become second nature to me), but after two readers in one week shared their desperate need to find a healthier option to the buttery pre-made loaves of garlic bread their families craved, the time had come. With the delicious taste of butter, the goodness of olive oil, and the yum of garlic and cheese, the only thing missing from this garlic toast is half the fat and 45% of the refined carbs (to slash the fat and carbs even further see my Super Skinny Garlic Bread variation below).

MAKES **4** SERVINGS

4 slices sourdough bread (like Francisco's)

1 clove garlic

2 teaspoons butter

2 teaspoons olive oil

¼ teaspoon garlic salt

4 teaspoons grated Parmesan cheese

1. Preheat the oven to 400°F. Place oven rack in top position.

2. Mince garlic (I use a garlic press) into a small microwave-safe cup or bowl. Add the butter and olive oil. Microwave on high heat for 45 seconds or until butter is melted.

3. Brush bread slices with garlic mixture, sprinkle lightly with garlic salt, and dust with Parmesan cheese (I simply grate a dusting of Parmesan directly onto the bread—it measures out to about 1 teaspoon for each piece).

4. Place the baking sheet on top oven rack and bake garlic bread slices for 7 to 8 minutes or until tops are golden brown.

Marlene Says: *For **Super Skinny Garlic Bread**, substitute light white bread for sourdough. Spray bread lightly with cooking spray and bake for 5 minutes or until tops are firm but not golden brown. Cut garlic clove in half and rub bread slices with exposed garlic. Sprinkle bread with garlic salt and Parmesan, return to oven, and bake until golden brown (50 calories, 1 gram of fat, 9 carbs, 2 grams fiber, and 1 point each per slice).*

NUTRITION INFORMATION PER SERVING: Calories 100 | Carbohydrate 11g (Sugars 0g) | Total Fat 4g (Sat Fat 2g) | Protein 3g | Fiber 0g | Cholesterol 40mg | Sodium 280mg | Food Exchanges: 1Starch, 1 Fat | Carbohydrate Choices: 1 | Weight Watcher Plus Point Comparison: 2

fast and fit
chicken dishes

Good 'n Easy Garlic Chicken

Fast and Fabulous Roast Chicken

Chicken Chicken Fried Steak with Cream Gravy

Chicken Cordon Bleu

Sticky Lemon Chicken

Triscuit "Fried" Chicken Fingers

Cheesecake Factory-Style Chicken Madeira

1-2-3 Basic Balsamic Chicken

Super Simple Chicken Pizzaiolo

General Tso's Chicken

Curried Cashew Chicken Stir-Fry

Chicken Enchilada Bake

One Pan Creamy Turkey and Rice Skillet

Turkey Kabobs with Greek Cucumber Yogurt Dip

The slogan may state that beef is "what's for dinner," but the truth is that it's chicken, not beef, that graces our dinner tables most often. Inexpensive and *versatile*, chicken is the ultimate weeknight wonder ingredient when it comes to preparing quick and easy *protein packed meals*.

There are no other entrée recipes that get more raves than the ones I create with chicken. High in protein and low in fat and calories, chicken and turkey breast meat have long been a dieter's best friend, but let's face it, plain 'ol chicken doesn't hold a candle to the *seductive* taste of chicken that's been *fried, stuffed,* or blanketed in a sweet or creamy sauce. In this chapter you will find recipes for the creamy, "fried," stuffed, *and sauced chicken* entrees that make chicken entrees #1. These recipes are, quite honestly, some of the ones my *own family loves* most. The first time my son, James, tasted the Triscuit-"Fried" Chicken Tenders, his only comment was to request that I "make more." My discerning husband, Chuck, said that the Sticky Lemon Chicken tasted like it came from a *wonderful* Chinese restaurant, and my son, Stephen (who was being extra careful about eating healthy at the time), questioned me not once but three times about whether the *Super Simple* Chicken Pizzaiolo he was eating was really healthy. Such comments give me the confidence to say, without hesitation, that the recipes in this chapter are not only good for you; they all hit the *great–taste* mark. Last, I knew traditional Southern *comfort food* had finally met *its* match when after reworking the Chicken Chicken Fried Steak with Cream Gravy recipe for *days*, the first bite made me feel like I'd been transported to a Southern diner. Chicken, in all its *beloved* glory, it's what for dinner now.

Good 'n Easy Garlic Chicken

THIS IS THE PERFECT WEEKNIGHT STAPLE—quick, easy, healthy, and good! A quick flattening of the chicken breasts ensures they cook up fast and tender, while pantry staples add great flavor. Pair this recipe with my 10-Minute Broccoli, Cheese and Rice Skillet (page 231) for a family-friendly meal that can be prepared in no time flat.

MAKES **2** SERVINGS

1 teaspoon garlic powder

½ teaspoon onion powder

½ teaspoon reduced-sodium or regular seasoned salt

2 boneless, skinless chicken breasts (about ⅔ pound)

1 teaspoon oil

¼ cup reduced-sodium chicken broth

2 teaspoons butter

1. In a small bowl, stir together the garlic powder, onion powder, and seasoned salt. Set aside.

2. Wrap the chicken breasts in plastic wrap, gently pound to ¼- to ½-inch thickness, and coat them with the seasoning mix.

3. Heat the oil in a medium non-stick skillet over medium high heat. Add the chicken and cook for 2 minutes on each side, until well browned and barely cooked through.

4. Pour the chicken broth into the skillet, tilting to evenly distribute the broth. Cover, reduce heat to medium low, and cook chicken for an additional 3 minutes or until cooked through. Transfer the chicken to plates or a single serving plate.

5. Swirl the butter into the broth and reduce the mixture slightly. Pour the sauce over the chicken and serve.

Marlene Says: *This recipe can easily be doubled. When doubling the broth, add ¼ cup as directed in Step 4 and the additional ¼ cup with the butter in Step 5.*

NUTRITION INFORMATION PER SERVING: Calories 220 | Carbohydrate 2g (Sugars 0g) | Total Fat 8g (Sat Fat 2.5g) | Protein 34g | Fiber 0g | Cholesterol 100mg | Sodium 220mg | Food Exchanges: 4½ Lean Meat, 1 Fat | Carbohydrate Choices: 0 | Weight Watcher Plus Point Comparison: 5

Fast Fabulous Roast Chicken

SUNDAY NIGHT CHICKEN GETS A MONDAY NIGHT MAKEOVER. This is my go-to recipe for fabulous roast chicken—made in under an hour! The trick to reducing the normal roasting time is to butterfly the chicken, spread it open, place it in a roasting pan and bake it in a very hot oven. In 45 minutes you have a chicken with beautiful crispy skin and juicy tender meat. Feel free to swap in your own favorite roast chicken seasonings.

MAKES **4** SERVINGS

1 tablespoon olive oil

1 roasting chicken, about 4 pounds

¾ teaspoon seasoned salt

½ teaspoon garlic powder

½ teaspoon fresh rosemary, finely minced

¼ freshly ground black pepper or to taste

1. Preheat the oven to 450°F. Spray the bottom of a roasting pan with cooking spray.

2. Remove giblets, rinse chicken inside and out, and pat dry. Place chicken breast side down on a cutting board, and using a sharp knife or sturdy kitchen shears, cut along both sides of the backbone to remove it. Turn the chicken over, opening the back, and press firmly on the breast with the heel of your hand to flatten the chicken. Rub the chicken with the oil, and sprinkle with seasoned salt, garlic powder, rosemary, and pepper. (Feel free to rub some of the seasonings under the skin as well.)

3. Place the chicken in the roasting pan breast side up and put it in the oven. After 30 minutes, check the chicken and cover the breast with foil if the skin is already well browned. Bake 15 more minutes or until juices run clear when pierced and thigh meat registers 175 to 180 degrees on a meat thermometer.

Marlene Says: *The nutritional content for this dish varies depending on the chicken part. Three and one-half ounces of cooked breast meat (about one-half of one of the breasts) without the skin has 140 calories and 3 grams fat; one skinless thigh averages 120 calories and 5 grams fat; a leg has 100 calories and 3 grams fat; and a wing (with skin) averages 100 calories with 6 grams fat.*

NUTRITION INFORMATION PER SERVING (3.5 ounces—average of light and dark meat): Calories 175 | Carbohydrate 0g (Sugars 0g) | Total Fat 6g (Sat Fat .5 g) | Protein 28g | Fiber 0g | Cholesterol 30mg | Sodium 25mg | Food Exchanges: 3½ Lean Meat | Carbohydrate Choices: 0 | Weight Watcher Plus Point Comparison: 4

Chicken Chicken Fried Steak with Cream Gravy

GOODBYE BEEF, HELLO CHICKEN! This is good, really good [...] *ee days of cooking flour- and crumb-coated chicken breasts in every conceivable (healthy) f* [...] *ctured myself sitting in a greasy-spoon diner as I sampled the delightful results of the final tast* [...] *s recipe. Perfectly coated and loaded with flavor, the only thing missing is 75% of the fat and s* [...] *more than half the usual carbs and calories. While devouring a serving of this dish, my son Ste* [...] *d me not once, but twice, "Are you sure this is healthy?"*

MAKES **4** SERVINGS

Chicken Chicken Fried Steak

4 boneless, skinless chicken breasts, about 1 pound

6 tablespoons all-purpose flour, divided

1 egg white

½ cup buttermilk

1 teaspoon baking soda

2 cups cornflake cereal, finely crushed

½ teaspoon onion powder

½ teaspoon garlic powder

⅛ teaspoon salt

⅜ teaspoon black pepper

¼ teaspoon dried thyme

1 tablespoon canola oil

Cream Gravy

1. Preheat the oven to 350°F. Cover the chicken breasts in plastic wrap and gently pound to ½-inch thickness. Set aside.

2. Place 2 tablespoons of flour in a shallow bowl. In another shallow bowl, whisk together the egg white, buttermilk and baking soda. In a third shallow bowl, mix the cornflake crumbs with 4 tablespoons flour, onion powder, garlic powder, salt, pepper, and thyme.

3. Coat each chicken breast with flour, dip into egg mixture, allowing excess egg to drip off, and roll in crumbs. Heat the oil in a large non-stick skillet over medium high heat. Add the chicken and cook until undersides are golden brown. Spray top with cooking spray and turn. Cook two minutes and transfer pan to oven for 5 to 6 minutes or until cooked through.

4. While chicken is baking prepare Cream Gravy (page 242). To serve, place each chicken steak on a plate and top with ¼ cup gravy.

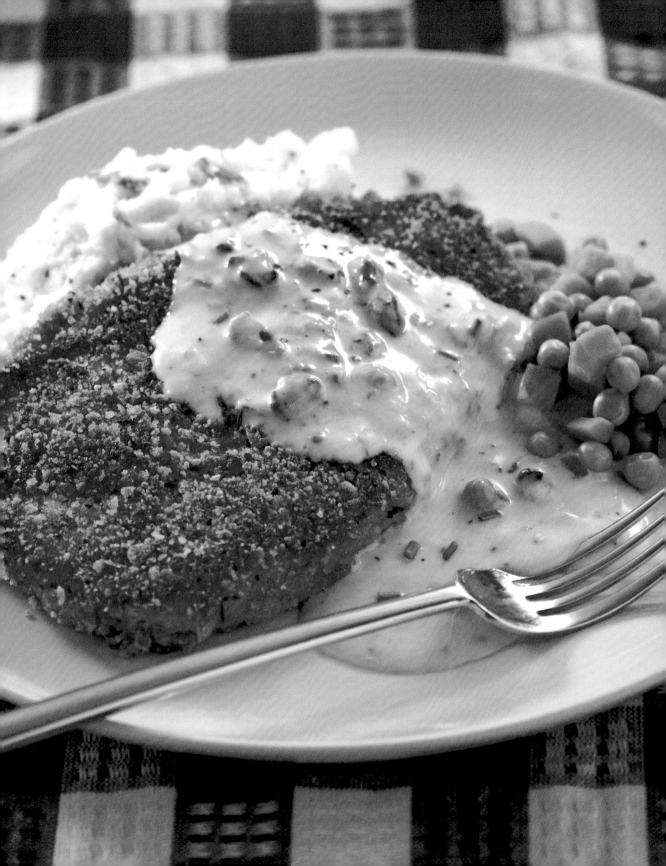

Cream Gravy

1 slice center-cut bacon, cut in half

2 tablespoons all-purpose flour

1 cup reduced-sodium chicken broth

⅛ teaspoon black pepper

Pinch of thyme

3 tablespoons nonfat half-and-half

Pinch of salt, optional

1. In a small saucepan cook the bacon over moderate heat, turning until crisp. Remove the bacon, mince, and set aside.

2. Add flour to the pan and slowly whisk in ½ cup of broth, stirring until smooth. Add the remaining broth and ⅛ teaspoon pepper. Finely crush thyme into the gravy with your fingers. Bring to a boil, reduce heat, and simmer for 3 to 4 minutes, whisking occasionally until gravy thickens.

3. Whisk in the nonfat half-and-half and the minced cooked bacon and simmer 1 more minute. Adjust salt to taste and serve ¼ cup over each "steak."

DARE TO COMPARE: A traditional Southern recipe for Chicken Fried Steak with Cream Gravy averages 600 calories and 25 grams of fat. When served with a side of grits the plate total jumps to 1,000 calories and 50 grams of fat. When paired with a side of Sour Cream and Onion Smashed Potatoes (page 227), the grand total for my Southern Chicken Chicken Fried Steak "fix" is just 380 calories and 10 grams of fat!

NUTRITION INFORMATION PER SERVING: Calories 280 | Carbohydrate 22g (Sugars 3g) | Total Fat 8g (Sat Fat 1g) | Protein 29g Fiber 1g Cholesterol 75mg | Sodium 600mg | Food Exchanges: 3½ Lean Meat, 1½ Starch | Carbohydrate Choices: 1½ | Weight Watcher Plus Point Comparison: 7

Chicken Cordon Bleu

MY GOOD FRIEND AND COLLEAGUE, chef Michelle Dudash, collaborated with me to create this elegant, yet simple rendition of the classic French chicken dish. My two teenage boys then used this recipe to prepare me a lovely Mother's Day dinner. They said that it was easy. I say, "Success!" Note: You can forgo the sauce, but I don't recommend it. It's a delicious addition that will make you look like a culinary star.

MAKES 4 SERVINGS

3 tablespoons
all-purpose flour

1 teaspoon onion powder

¼ teaspoon salt

¼ teaspoon freshly
ground black pepper

¾ cup panko breadcrumbs

½ teaspoon paprika

1 tablespoon olive oil

1 large egg

4 boneless, skinless
chicken breasts (about 1
pound)

2 teaspoons Dijon mustard

2 (1-ounce) slices Swiss or
Gruyere cheese, cut into
quarters

4 thin (½-ounce) slices
natural deli ham

⅓ cup nonfat half-and-half

1 teaspoon Dijon mustard

½ teaspoon of chicken
bouillon cube

1. Preheat the oven to 375°F. Combine the flour, onion powder, salt, and pepper in a shallow dish. Place breadcrumbs and paprika into another shallow dish. Drizzle in the oil and stir well. In a third medium bowl, whisk together the egg with 2 teaspoons water.

2. With a very sharp knife, slice a pocket about halfway into the thick "hump" side of each chicken breast, taking care not to cut all the way through. With a mallet, lightly pound the "hump" to flatten the breast.

3. Spread ½ teaspoon of Dijon inside each pocket. Wrap each slice of ham around two stacked cheese pieces and place one deeply in each breast. Firmly press the edges to close.

4. Coat chicken breasts with flour and dip into the egg. Roll breasts in crumb mixture and place on a baking sheet. Bake for 18 minutes or until centers are cooked through.

5. For the sauce, in a small saucepan, whisk together the remaining ingredients. Heat gently (do not boil) over medium low for 3 to 4 minutes or until thickened, whisking occasionally. Pour one tablespoon of sauce over each breast and serve.

NUTRITION INFORMATION PER SERVING: Calories 250 | Carbohydrate 9g (Sugars 1g) | Total Fat 10g (Sat Fat 3g) | Protein 34g | Fiber 0g | Cholesterol 70mg | Sodium 460mg | Food Exchanges: 4½ Lean Meat, ½ Starch | Carbohydrate Choices: ½ Weight Watcher Plus Point Comparison: 7

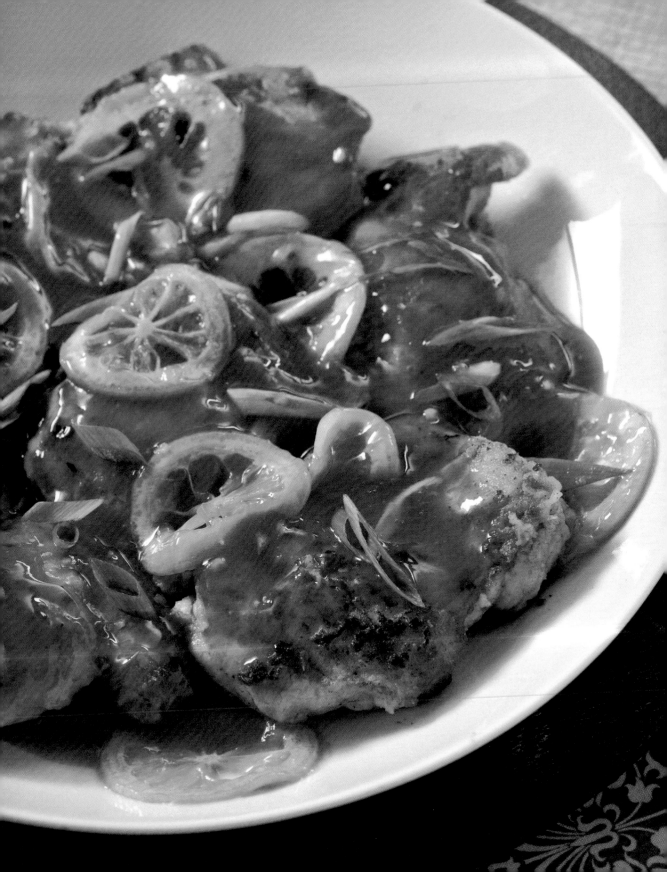

Sticky Lemon Chicken

LIKE MY QUICKER-THAN-TAKEOUT ORANGE CHICKEN from Eat What You Love, *this make-over will inspire you to cook Chinese food at home more often. Made with fresh lemon, fragrant ginger, and sticky honey, this one-pan dish is quick to put together but will have you lingering at the dining table. Sweet, tart, and oh-so-lemony, the scrumptious sauce that coats the tender chicken thighs will make you forget about going out.*

MAKES **4** SERVINGS

⅓ cup fresh lemon juice

⅓ cup granulated no-calorie sweetener (or 8 packets)

1 tablespoon honey

¼ cup reduced sodium chicken broth

1½ tablespoon reduced sodium soy sauce

½ teaspoon grated ginger

1 tablespoon cornstarch

8 boneless, skinless chicken thighs, well-trimmed

2 tablespoons all-purpose flour

2 teaspoons canola oil

½ lemon, thinly sliced

3 sliced green onions, white parts and green tops, divided

1. To make the sauce, whisk together the first 7 ingredients (lemon juice through cornstarch) in a small saucepan. Place the pan over low heat and simmer until clear and slightly thickened. Remove and set aside.

2. Roll the chicken in the flour, shaking to remove excess.

3. Heat the oil in a large non-stick skillet over medium high heat. Add the chicken and cook until well browned on both sides, about 4 to 5 minutes per side.

4. Reduce the heat to medium low. Sprinkle all of the white part and half of the green tops of the onions over the chicken. Add the sauce and simmer for 3 to 4 minutes or until the chicken is just about cooked through and the sauce has thickened. Add the lemon slices to the sauce and cook for 2 more minutes. Sprinkle with remaining green onion tops and garnish with additional fresh lemon slices, if desired.

DARE TO COMPARE: The average restaurant order of Lemon Chicken serves up as much as 1,400 calories, over 150 grams of carbohydrate (the equivalent of 10 servings of bread), and the amount of sugar in 32 ounces of regular Coca-Cola—all in one meal!

NUTRITION INFORMATION PER SERVING (2 thighs): Calories 235 | Carbohydrate 11g (Sugars 5g) | Total Fat 7g (Sat Fat 2g) | Protein 28g | Fiber 0g | Cholesterol 125 mg | Sodium 420mg | Food Exchanges: 4 Lean Meat, 1 Carbohydrate | Carbohydrate Choices: 1 | Weight Watcher Plus Point Comparison: 5

Triscuit® "Fried" Chicken Tenders

TURNS OUT THE BELOVED TRISCUIT® CRACKER makes for one fine "fried" chicken. The texture of the crushed crackers is terrific and when combined with just the right spices you get fantastic fried chicken flavor and the perfect crunch in every delicious bite. If your market doesn't carry Dijonnaise, substitute 3 tablespoons of Dijon mustard blended with 1 tablespoon of light mayo (this combo also tastes great on sandwiches).

MAKES **4** SERVINGS

18 original Triscuit® crackers*

½ teaspoon garlic powder

½ teaspoon onion powder

½ teaspoon black pepper

¼ teaspoon dried thyme, crushed

¼ cup Dijonnaise

1 pound chicken breast tenders, cut into eight 2-ounce strips

1. Set cooking rack in the lower third of the oven and preheat to 425°F. Spray a large baking pan well with cooking spray.

2. Place the crackers in a resealable plastic bag and finely crush them with a rolling pin or mallet. Transfer the crumbs to a shallow flat bowl and add the garlic powder, onion powder, pepper, and thyme.

3. Coat the chicken with the Dijonnaise. Roll the chicken in the crumb mixture until evenly coated. Place crumb-coated chicken on the baking sheet and bake for 7 minutes. Lightly spray chicken strips with cooking spray, turn, and bake for 7 more minutes or until golden brown.

VARIATION: *To make* **Cheesy Crunchy Chicken Tenders***, replace the Triscuit® crumb mixture with 1½ cups crushed reduced-fat cheddar cheese crackers mixed with ¼ teaspoon black pepper. Bake as directed.*

* *Note: Reduced-fat Triscuits are not recommended for this recipe.*

NUTRITION INFORMATION PER SERVING (2 strips): Calories 230 | Carbohydrate 15g (Sugars 0g) | Total Fat 7g (Sat Fat 0.5g) | Protein 27g | Fiber 2g | Cholesterol 70mg | Sodium 435 mg | Food Exchanges: 3½ Lean Meat, 1 Starch | Carbohydrate Choices: 1 | Weight Watcher Plus Point Comparison: 6

Cheesecake Factory®-Style Chicken Madeira

FASHIONED AFTER THE #1 CHICKEN DISH at the ever-popular Cheesecake Factory, my version still gives you the fabulous layers of flavor, but without the crazy calories and fat. I like to pair this with a side of steamed asparagus, but feel free to place a few cooked spears between the chicken and cheese (in Step 4), if you want to serve it the way the restaurant does.

MAKES **4** SERVINGS

4 boneless, skinless chicken breasts (about 1 pound)

¼ teaspoon plus ⅛ teaspoon salt, divided

½ teaspoon black pepper, divided

1 tablespoon canola oil, divided

1 (8-ounce) package sliced mushrooms

½ cup red onion, finely diced

1 cup Madeira wine

¾ cup reduced sodium beef broth, divided

2 teaspoons cornstarch

2 teaspoons honey (or brown sugar)

1 teaspoon dried Italian seasoning

1 teaspoon butter

2 slices part-skim mozzarella cheese, cut in half

1. Cover the chicken breasts in plastic wrap and gently pound flat to ½-inch thickness. Season chicken with ¼ teaspoon each of salt and pepper.

2. Heat 2 teaspoons oil in a large non-stick skillet over medium high heat. Add the chicken and cook for 4 to 5 minutes or until well browned. Turn the chicken and cook for 3 more minutes or until barely cooked through. Transfer to a plate and keep warm.

3. Reduce the heat to medium. Add the remaining teaspoon of oil and mushrooms and cook for 2 minutes. Add the onions and cook for 3 more minutes or until softened. Add the wine and ½ cup broth and simmer until three-quarters of the liquid evaporates.

4. In a small bowl, whisk together the cornstarch and remaining ¼ cup broth and add to the skillet with the honey, Italian seasoning, remaining ⅛ teaspoon salt and ¼ teaspoon pepper. Simmer for 1 minute or until thickened. Swirl in the butter, add the chicken back to the pan and top each breast with cheese. Turn to heat low and cover skillet for 2 to 3 minutes to melt cheese. Place chicken on plates and top with sauce.

DARE TO COMPARE: The "Factory" entrée is served with mashed potatoes, but with 1,420 calories and 44 grams of saturated fat you would think it was served on cheesecake!

NUTRITION INFORMATION PER SERVING: Calories 330 | Carbohydrate 16g (Sugars 13g) | Total Fat 10g (Sat Fat 2.5g) | Protein 28g | Fiber 1g | Cholesterol 85mg | Sodium 550mg | Food Exchanges: 4 Lean Meat, 1 Vegetable, ½ Carbohydrate | Carbohydrate Choices: 1 | Weight Watcher Plus Point Comparison: 7

1-2-3 Basic Balsamic Chicken

WHILE IT'S FUN TO TRY A NEW RECIPE that's novel or has a lot going on, let's face it, the more basic a recipe, the more likely you are to make it again. That's why I had to include this ultra-easy recipe. Taking advantage of one of today's best pantry staples, sweet-tart balsamic vinegar, I've created a healthy family-pleasing dish with minimal effort. For me, that's basic at its very best.

MAKES **4** SERVINGS

⅓ cup balsamic vinegar

⅓ cup chicken broth

⅛ teaspoon dried thyme

2 teaspoons sugar or honey

1 teaspoon butter

2 teaspoons olive oil

4 boneless, skinless chicken breasts (about 1 pound)

1 tablespoon all-purpose flour

Salt to taste

Pepper to taste

1. In a very small saucepan, stir together the vinegar, broth, thyme, and sugar, and simmer over medium heat, stirring occasionally, until it reduces by half and is syrupy, about 8 to 10 minutes. Stir in butter, remove from heat and keep warm.

2. While sauce cooks, cover the chicken breasts in plastic wrap and gently pound to ½-inch thickness. Lightly coat each chicken breast with flour and season with salt and pepper to taste.

3. Heat the oil in a medium non-stick skillet over medium high heat. Add the chicken and cook for 3 to 4 minutes on the first side or until very well browned. Reduce heat to medium, turn the chicken, and cook for 2 minutes. Add 1 tablespoon water to the pan, cover, and cook two more minutes or until chicken is cooked through. Place the chicken on plates and drizzle 1½ tablespoons balsamic glaze over each breast.

NUTRITION INFORMATION PER SERVING: Calories 220 | Carbohydrate 7 g (Sugars 1g) | Total Fat 7g (Sat Fat 4g) | Protein 31g | Fiber 0g | Cholesterol 90mg | Sodium 220mg | Food Exchanges: 4½ Lean Meat, ½ Carbohydrate | Carbohydrate Choices: ½ | Weight Watcher Plus Point Comparison: 6

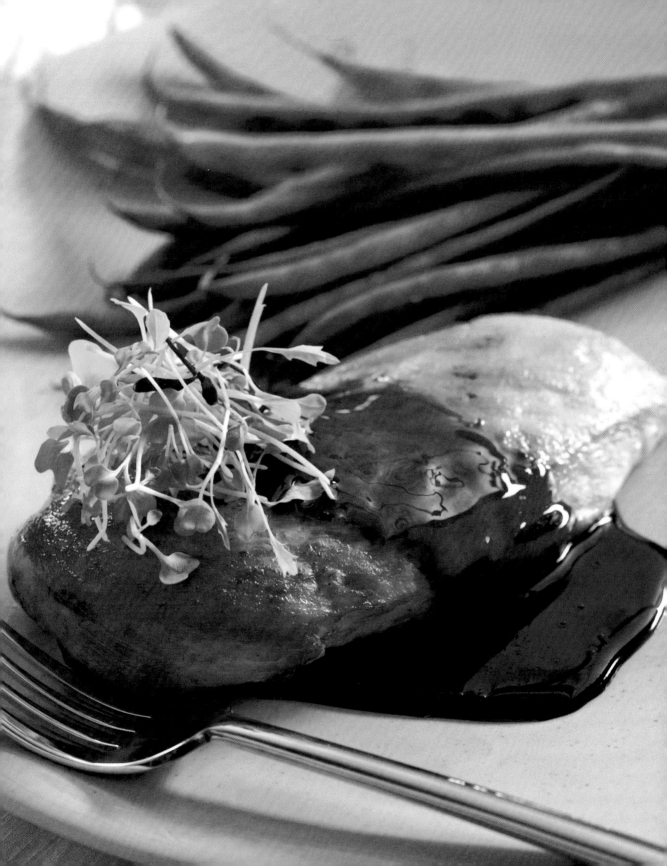

Super Simple Chicken Pizzaiolo

THIS PIZZA-INSPIRED DISH is not only super simple, but also just plain super. With just a handful of ingredients and in less than 30 minutes you can have a dinner on the table that the whole family will love. (In fact, the first time I made this my hungry husband and teenage sons loved it so much, they barely left me a bite.) A nice way to round out the meal is to serve it with whole-grain blend pasta and a fresh green salad.

MAKES **4** SERVINGS

1 (14-ounce) jar marinara sauce (or 1½ cups)

4 boneless, skinless chicken breasts (about 1 pound)

½ teaspoon black pepper

½ cup grated Parmesan cheese

½ cup shredded reduced-fat Italian blend cheese

16 slices turkey pepperoni

½ teaspoon dried oregano

1. Preheat the oven to 450°F. Spread the marinara sauce in a 10-inch pie plate or 9 x 9-inch ceramic or glass baking dish. Crumble the dried oregano and sprinkle it over the sauce.

2. Cover the chicken breasts in plastic wrap and gently pound to ½-inch thickness. Sprinkle the chicken breasts with the black pepper.

3. Spread the Parmesan in a shallow dish. Roll the chicken in the Parmesan and lay the breasts on top of the marinara. Bake for 13 minutes.

4. Remove the chicken from the oven, sprinkle with the Italian blend cheese and oregano, top with pepperoni slices and bake another 5 to 7 minutes or until the chicken is cooked through.

Marlene Says: *You can reduce the sodium in this dish by purchasing a low-sodium marina sauce or using Marlene's All-Purpose Marinara (page 181). Swapping out the pepperoni for 1 cup of sliced mushrooms will slash another 130 mg of sodium.*

NUTRITION INFORMATION PER SERVING: Calories 275 | Carbohydrate 8g (Sugars 1g) | Total Fat 11g (Sat Fat 4g) | Protein 35g | Fiber 0g | Cholesterol 90mg | Sodium 810mg | Food Exchanges: 5 Lean Meat, 1 Vegetable, ½ Fat | Carbohydrate Choices: ½ | Weight Watcher Plus Point Comparison: 7

General Tso's Chicken

UPON HEARING I WAS LIGHTENING UP this much-loved dish, a reader—and avid General Tso's Chicken fan—volunteered to be the first to try it out. Linda's verdict? Two chopsticks up! While the ingredient list may look long, the time commitment is short and well worth it for yummy, take-out quality General Tso's chicken, now with only 300 calories per serving.

MAKES **4** SERVINGS

1 cup reduced-sodium chicken broth

2 tablespoons low-sodium soy sauce

1 tablespoon rice vinegar

4 teaspoons cornstarch

3 tablespoons granulated no-calorie sweetener (or 4 packets)

1 tablespoon brown sugar

1 tablespoon minced garlic

1 teaspoon ketchup

¼ teaspoon red pepper flakes

½ cup sliced onion

3 cups broccoli small florets

¼ cup all-purpose flour

¼ teaspoon black pepper

1 pound boneless, skinless chicken breast, cut into 1-inch pieces

1 egg, beaten

2 tablespoons canola oil

1. To make the sauce, in a medium-sized bowl thoroughly whisk together the first nine ingredients (chicken broth through red pepper flakes). Add onion and set aside.

2. Place the broccoli in a microwave-safe bowl. Add 2 tablespoons of water, cover, and microwave for 2 minutes. Set aside.

3. In a small bowl, mix flour and black pepper. Roll chicken into beaten egg, letting excess egg drip off, and coat the chicken with the seasoned flour.

4. Heat 1 tablespoon of the oil in a large non-stick wok or skillet over medium high heat. Add half of the chicken and cook 4 to 5 minutes or until well browned and cooked through. Transfer chicken to a bowl and cover. Heat remaining oil and repeat.

5. Whisk the sauce, pour it into the wok, and stir until it thickens and clears. Add the chicken and broccoli, toss well, and cook 1 to 2 minutes or until heated through.

DARE TO COMPARE: An order of General Tso's chicken packs a wallop with the average restaurant order loaded with as many as 1,200 calories and over 3,000 mg of sodium!

NUTRITION INFORMATION PER SERVING (1½ cups): Calories 300 | Carbohydrate 19g (Sugars 6g) | Total Fat 12g (Sat Fat 1g) | Protein 29g | Fiber 3g | Cholesterol 125mg | Sodium 510mg | Food Exchanges: 3½ Lean Meat, 1 Vegetable, 1 Starch, ½ Fat | Carbohydrate Choices: 1 Weight Watcher Plus Point Comparison: 8

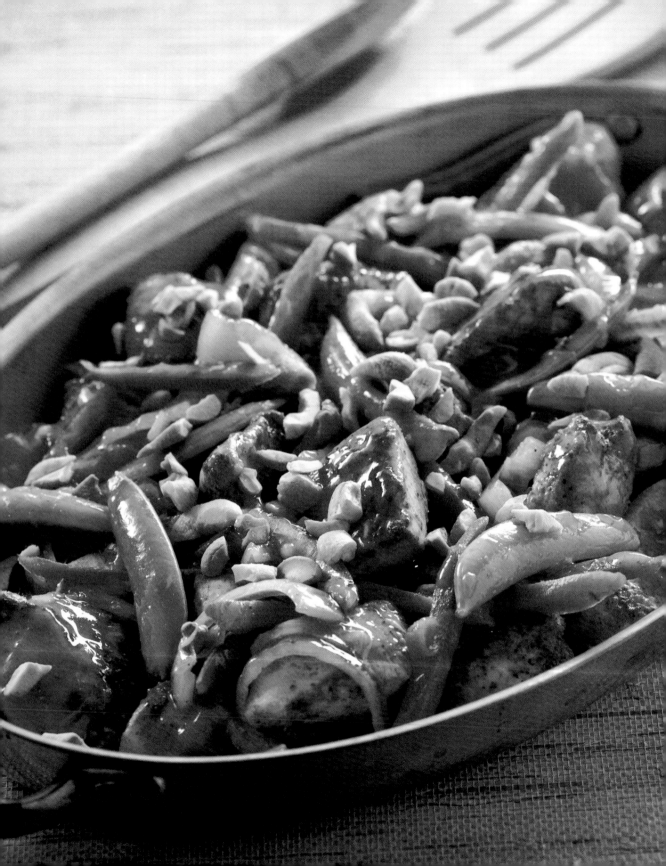

Curried Cashew Chicken Stir-Fry

KISSED WITH CURRY, this Asian chicken stir-fry is bursting with colorful veggies, crunchy cashews, and a sweet, yet savory, sauce. When it's this fresh, fast, and oh so easy, who needs Chinese delivery?

1 pound boneless, skinless chicken breasts, cubed

2 teaspoons curry powder, divided

¼ teaspoon salt, divided

1 tablespoon lemon juice

6 tablespoons low-sugar apricot preserves

3 teaspoons canola oil, divided

1 clove garlic, minced

1 (15-ounce) bag fresh sugar snap peas (or 4 cups)

2 medium carrots, peeled and cut into strips

½ medium red onion, cut into strips

¼ cup chopped cashews

1. Coat the chicken with 1 teaspoon curry powder and ⅛ teaspoon salt. Set aside.

2. Mix together the remaining 1 teaspoon curry powder, ⅛ teaspoon salt, lemon juice, preserves, and ¾ cup water in a small bowl and set aside.

3. Add 2 teaspoons oil to a large non-stick skillet and place over medium high heat. Add the chicken and cook 4 to 5 minutes or until browned and almost cooked through. Remove the chicken, cover and set aside.

4. Add the remaining teaspoon of oil and the garlic to the skillet. Add the snap peas, carrots, and red onions, and stir fry for one minute. Add ¼ cup of water, cover, and steam for 3 minutes. Return the chicken and sauce to the skillet, stir, and heat briefly while tossing the chicken and vegetables with the sauce. Transfer the curried chicken to a serving dish, sprinkle with cashews, and serve.

Marlene Says: *Feel free to toss a few more cashews into this dish if your calorie budget permits. Even though they're high in calories, studies show that people who eat nuts at least twice a week are less likely to be overweight. The key to enjoying nuts is healthy moderation, which means 1 ounce (or about ¼ cup) as a snack serving.*

NUTRITION INFORMATION PER SERVING (1½ cups): Calories 310 | Carbohydrate 25 g (Sugars 15g) | Total Fat 11g (Sat Fat 1g) | Protein 29g | Fiber 5g | Cholesterol 70mg | Sodium 360mg | Food Exchanges: 4 Lean Meat, 3 Vegetable, ½ Carbohydrate, ½ Fat | Carbohydrate Choices: 1½ | Weight Watcher Plus Point Comparison: 8

Chicken Enchilada Bake

IF YOU ARE A TEX-MEX FAN, this is your chicken casserole. Studded with fiber-rich black beans and brimming with spicy enchilada sauce, this baked dish is soft and saucy just like a good enchilada should be. While I find it difficult, I suggest you resist the temptation to dig in straight from the oven. Waiting 10 minutes sets the casserole for cutting and serving.

MAKES 6 SERVINGS

½ cup chopped onion

¾ cup reduced-sodium chicken broth

2 cloves minced garlic

¼ teaspoon black pepper

¾ cup light sour cream

2 tablespoons all-purpose flour

2 cups shredded cooked chicken breast

4 (6-inch) reduced-carb high-fiber flour tortillas

1 (10-ounce) can red enchilada sauce

¾ cup rinsed, drained, canned black beans

1 (4-ounce) can chopped green chilies, drained

1 cup shredded reduced-fat Mexican Blend cheese

½ cup minced fresh cilantro

1. Preheat the oven to 350°F.

2. In a medium pot over medium heat, combine the onion, chicken broth, garlic, and pepper and bring to a boil. Reduce to a simmer, cover, and cook for about 3 minutes or until onions are tender.

3. In a small bowl, mix the sour cream and flour until smooth. Add to the pot and cook, stirring occasionally, until thickened (about 5 minutes). Remove from the heat and stir in the shredded chicken. Set aside.

4. Spray a 2-quart casserole dish with non-stick cooking spray. Cut tortillas into 1-inch-long strips and line the bottom of the dish with them. Top with a layer of the chicken filling, then the black beans, then the green chilies, and end with the enchilada sauce.

5. Bake for 25 minutes. Top with the cheese and bake for another 5 minutes or until the cheese has melted. Let it sit for 10 minutes before cutting. Top with fresh cilantro.

Marlene Says: *For a firmer bake, add another layer of tortilla strips by cutting three additional tortillas into strips and laying them over the green chilies before adding the enchilada sauce (adds 40 calories and 1 point more per serving).*

NUTRITION INFORMATION PER SERVING (one-sixth recipe): Calories 250 | Carbohydrate 25g (Sugars 4g) | Total Fat 7g (Sat Fat 2.5g) | Protein 22g | Fiber 8g | Cholesterol 60mg | Sodium 570 mg | Food Exchanges: 2½ Lean Meat, 1½ Starch | Carbohydrate Choices: 1½ Weight Watcher Plus Point Comparison: 6

One Pan Creamy Turkey and Rice Skillet

CANNED SOUP RECIPES ARE USUALLY a lot more about convenience than taste, but this recipe puts great taste and convenience on equal footing. The crunch of water chestnuts, the tang of soy sauce, and the fresh mushrooms perk up the other ingredients to make this stick-to-the-ribs dish a true one-pan wonder. (Please feel free to substitute chicken for the turkey.)

MAKES **5** SERVINGS

2 teaspoons canola oil

1¼ pound skinless, boneless turkey breast cutlets, cut into 1-inch cubes

1½ cups sliced mushrooms

1 teaspoon minced garlic, about 1 clove

2 tablespoons sherry

1 can (10.75 ounces) reduced-fat cream of chicken soup

½ cup low-fat evaporated milk

2 tablespoons reduced sodium soy sauce

1½ cups quick-cooking brown rice (uncooked)

1 (5-ounce) can sliced water chestnuts, drained

2½ cups frozen French cut green beans, defrosted

Salt and pepper to taste

1. Heat the oil in a large non-stick skillet over medium high heat. Add the turkey and cook for 3 minutes. Add the mushrooms and garlic and cook for 2 more minutes or until mushrooms are softened.

2. Deglaze the pan with the sherry, stirring it into the meat and mushrooms. Add the soup, evaporated milk, soy sauce and 1 cup water to the skillet. Stir to blend. Stir in the rice and water chestnuts and bring to a boil. Cover, reduce heat to medium low, and cook for 5 minutes.

3. Uncover, add the green beans, and continue to simmer for 12 to 15 minutes or until the rice is tender.

NUTRITION INFORMATION PER SERVING (1 ½ cups): Calories 395 | Carbohydrate 47g (Sugars 8g) | Total Fat 5g (Sat Fat 1g) | Protein 40g | Fiber 6g | Cholesterol 90mg | Sodium 590mg | Food Exchanges: 4 Lean Meat, 3 Starch, 1 Vegetable | Carbohydrate Choices: 3 | Weight Watcher Plus Point Comparison: 10

Turkey Kabobs with Greek Cucumber Yogurt Dip

I'M NOT SURE WHAT I LIKE BEST about this recipe—the aromatic Greek flavors or its variety of options. Switch it up and use chicken breast, lamb loin or lean beef for the kabobs. Skewer different vegetables like zucchini chunks ⬚⬚⬚⬚⬚⬚⬚⬚ Or make extra dip for a raw veggie tray. Whatever you do, you'll have a delicious, h⬚⬚⬚⬚⬚⬚⬚⬚⬚⬚⬚ean in every bite.

MAKES **4** SERVINGS

1 small cucumber, peeled and seeded

¾ cup low-fat or nonfat plain Greek-style yogurt

¼ cup light sour cream

3 garlic cloves, minced, about 1½ teaspoons, divided

3 teaspoons olive oil, divided

2 teaspoons lemon juice

⅛ teaspoon salt

½ teaspoon Dijon mustard

1 tablespoon red wine vinegar

1 teaspoon dried oregano

¼ teaspoon black pepper

pinch of salt

20 ounces turkey tenderloin, cut into 24 1½-inch pieces

24 cherry tomatoes

1 small red onion, cut into 1½-inch squares

1. In a small bowl, combine the cucumber, yogurt, sour cream, 1 teaspoon garlic, 1 teaspoon oil, lemon juice, and salt. Cover and refrigerate.

2. In a medium bowl, combine the Dijon, vinegar, remaining garlic, 2 teaspoons oil, oregano, pepper, and salt. Add the turkey, toss well, and let marinate for 15 minutes.

3. Preheat the grill on medium high. Alternate turkey, tomatoes, and onion squares on each skewer. Place skewers on the grill and cook for 6 to 7 minutes, turning once or until well browned and cooked through. Serve with cucumber sauce.

Marlene Says: *The cucumber dip, also known as tzatziki, makes a delicious, light dip for crudité and a sauce for pita sandwiches. If you make it ahead, reduce the garlic to two cloves, as its flavor intensifies over time.*

NUTRITION INFORMATION PER SERVING: Calories 250 | Carbohydrate 10g (Sugars 7g) | Total Fat 7g (Sat Fat 2g) | Protein 36g | Fiber 2g | Cholesterol 95mg | Sodium 260mg | Food Exchanges: 4½ Lean Meat, ½ Low-Fat Milk, ½ Vegetable | Carbohydrate Choices: ½ | Weight Watcher Plus Point Comparison: 6

lean beef, pork, and fish

Mile High Meatloaf (Times Two!)

East Meets West Salisbury Steak

Steak Diane

Biscuit and Burger Pie

Crispy Pork Scaloppini

P.F. Chang's-Style Mongolian Beef

15-Minute Maple Glazed Pork Chops

Sassy Grilled Pork with Memphis-Style BBQ Sauce

Skillet Pork and Peppers

Plum Good Pork

Shrimp Scampi

Simply Southwestern Tilapia

Nut-Crusted Fish Fillets

Honey Walnut Shrimp

Grilled Salmon with Raspberry Chipotle Sauce

Easy 20-Minute Fish Stew

The MyPlate healthy eating guide for Americans recommends one-fourth of our lunch and dinner plates be filled with lean protein to help *strengthen* our muscles, *fortify* our health, and even *trim our waistlines*. For starters, if your idea of protein means beef, I've got you covered. With the help of my healthy beef chart (page 259), flavorful lean beef choices such as beef tenderloin, top sirloin and 93% lean ground beef—and *delicious* recipes for comfort foods like Mile High Meatloaf (Times Two!) and Biscuit and Burger Pie—it's *easy to enjoy* the great taste of *lean beef* while keeping good health in mind.

In the US, beef is a *popular* choice for dinner, but it's pork that wins the prize as the most widely eaten meat worldwide. The *good news* for those who love pork is that today's pork is leaner than ever before. Pork tenderloin and lean center-cut loin pork chops are my go-to picks in this chapter for flavorful *"love 'em" lean pork dishes* like Grilled Pork with Memphis-Style BBQ Sauce and Crispy Pork Scaloppini. Italian food lovers are sure to love the Skillet Pork and Peppers in which spice rubbed pork tenderloin gives fatty sausage a run for its money.

And last, when it comes to *fish and seafood*, the message from health authorities and the dietary guidelines for Americans are clear: *eat more!* Specifically, aim to eat fish at least *twice a week* to protect your heart and reduce your risk of stroke. Personally, I love fish and seafood and am confident that the ease of preparation and scrumptious taste of dishes like sweet Honey Walnut Shrimp, *crunchy* Southwestern-Style Tilapia, *buttery* Shrimp Scampi, and the sophisticated Grilled Salmon with Raspberry Chipotle Sauce will have you clamoring to fill your plate with the *treasures of the sea*.

BEEF

Nothing says all-American like a thick burger or a juicy steak. The good news for beef lovers is that beef can be as nutritious as it is delicious—provided it's lean and eaten in moderation. Packed with high-quality, satisfying protein and ten essential nutrients, lean beef can keep your waistline trim and your body strong.

One of the keys to enjoying better-for-you beef is knowing what constitutes "lean." The tricky part in getting this equation right is that the lean and fat percentages listed on beef labels are based on weight—not calories. That means that for a package of 80% lean ground beef, 80% of the *weight* of the ground beef is lean and 20% is fat. Unfortunately, due to water weight, that 20% fat contributes a whopping 61% of the total *calories*. (Yes, over one-half of the calories in ground beef labeled 20% fat are from fat.) This comparison chart, which includes % fat calories, can help you understand what's *really* lean when it comes to beef. (The USDA defines lean meat as having no more than 10 grams of fat per 3-ounce cooked serving.)

Average 3-ounce cooked serving:	Calories:	Total Fat:	Sat Fat:%	Fat Calories:	Cholesterol:
93% Lean Ground	160	7g	3g	39%	70mg
90% Lean Ground	180	10g	5g	50%	70mg
85% (85/15) Ground	215	13g	6g	56%	75mg
80% (80/20) Ground	235	16g	7g	61%	75mg
Top Sirloin Steak	160	5g	2g	29%	75mg
Beef Tenderloin	175	8g	3g	41%	70mg
Ribeye	250	18g	8g	64%	85mg
Eye of Round	145	4g	1.5g	25%	53mg
Lean Stew Meat	160	6g	3g	34%	75mg
Brisket	165	5g	2g	27%	50mg
All Beef Hotdog	240	23g	9g	86%	45mg

TIP: *Rinsing cooked ground beef can significantly reduce the fat content. To rinse ground beef, brown meat, drain excess fat, blot meat with paper towels, and then rinse meat with hot water. The beefy flavor will remain, but up to 50% of the fat will be removed. I recommend this technique for 80% ground beef only and for use in recipes where the meat is browned, alone or with onions, before other ingredients are added, such as chilies and casseroles.*

Mile High Meatloaf (Times Two!)

IN MY SEARCH FOR A NEW MEATLOAF RECIPE, my makeover of the Cheesecake Factory's Mile High Meatloaf unanimously took the taste prize. But when it came to baking time and convenience, it lost out to recipes for smaller loaves. My simple solution—create two meals for the price of one! Cook two loaves at the same time, or, bake one and refrigerate the remaining mix for 2 days or freeze it for up to two weeks. It's great taste—times two! (If your idea of meatloaf means ketchup on top, mix 3 tablespoons ketchup with 1 teaspoon molasses and ½ teaspoon liquid smoke and slather on before baking. Adds 10 calories and 2 grams carb.)

MAKES **10** SERVINGS

1 small onion, diced (about 1 cup)

1¼ pounds 93% lean ground turkey

¾ pound lean ground beef

½ cup low-fat cottage cheese

2 large eggs

½ medium green bell pepper, diced

¾ cup dry breadcrumbs

¼ cup ketchup

¼ cup red wine (or beef broth)

2 teaspoons Dijon mustard

½ teaspoon black pepper

½ teaspoon salt

½ cup reduced-fat shredded sharp cheddar cheese

1. Preheat oven to 350°F.

2. In a small microwave-safe bowl, cover and cook onions on high heat for 1 minute. Scoop onions into a large bowl and add remaining ingredients. Knead mixture with a spoon or by hand until just uniform. Divide meatloaf mixture in half. Form into 2 loaves about 8 inches long and 4 inches wide (or create one loaf and wrap and refrigerate or freeze the other half of mixture). Place loaves onto a foil-lined sheet pan.

3. Cover loosely with foil and bake for 20 minutes. Remove foil and bake for an additional 25 to 30 minutes or until well browned and meat thermometer registers at least 165°F. Let stand for 10 minutes before serving.

Marlene Says: *To cook refrigerated meatloaf mix, form loaf and let sit at room temperature for 20 minutes before baking (may take up to 15 minutes longer to cook). For frozen meatloaf mix, thaw mixture overnight in the refrigerator before cooking.*

NUTRITION INFORMATION PER SERVING (one-fifth of one loaf): Calories 195 | Carbohydrate 9g (Sugars 2g) | Total Fat 8g (Sat Fat 2g) | Protein 23g | Fiber 1g | Cholesterol 30mg | Sodium 340mg | Food Exchange: 3 Lean Meat, ½ Starch | Carbohydrate Choices: ½ | Weight Watcher Plus Point Comparison: 4

East Meets West Salisbury Steak

EAST MEETS WEST WITH MY NEW SPIN on Salisbury steak. Crunchy water chestnuts, flavorful green onions, and sweet red peppers give this "steak" a delightful flavor with a subtle crunch, but it's the extraordinary pan sauce that will have you touting your good fortune. Quick cooking, tastes-like-white, instant brown rice is the perfect complement.

MAKES **4** SERVINGS

1 pound lean ground beef

½ cup chopped water chestnuts

½ cup chopped green onion, divided

¼ cup finely diced red bell pepper

2½ tablespoons hoisin sauce, divided

3 teaspoons minced ginger, divided (fresh or jarred, not dried)

⅛ teaspoon black pepper

½ cup reduced-sodium beef broth

1 tablespoon rice vinegar

1 teaspoon brown sugar

1. In a medium bowl, lightly mix the beef, water chestnuts, ¼ cup green onions, bell pepper, 1½ tablespoons hoisin sauce, 2 teaspoons ginger, and pepper. Shape into four 3½-inch patties.

2. Spray a large non-stick skillet with cooking spray and place over medium heat. Add the patties and cook for 4 minutes on each side until cooked through. Remove the cooked "steaks," cover, and set aside.

3. With the skillet still over medium heat, add the beef broth, 1 tablespoon hoisin sauce, vinegar, 1 teaspoon ginger, brown sugar, and ¼ cup green onions to the pan. Cook for 1 to 2 minutes or until the sauce is slightly thickened. Return the steaks to the skillet and cook for 1 to 2 minutes, until thoroughly heated through. Serve topped with hoisin pan sauce.

Marlene Says: *If you're watching carbs or calories, serve the Salisbury steaks over a bed of finely sliced Napa cabbage or spinach instead of rice.*

NUTRITION INFORMATION PER SERVING (1 steak with sauce): Calories 225 | Carbohydrate 13g (Sugars 7g) | Total Fat 9g (Sat Fat 4g) | Protein 27g | Fiber 1g | Cholesterol 40mg | Sodium 350mg | Food Exchanges: 3½ Lean Meat, 1 Starch, 1 Fat | Carbohydrate Choices: 1 | Weight Watcher Plus Point Comparison: 6

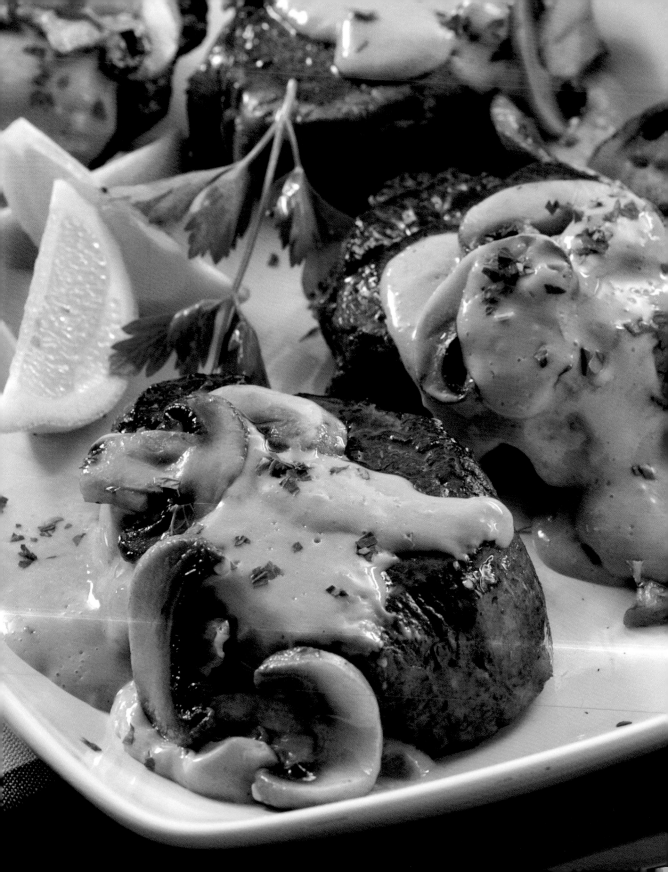

Steak Diane

SAUTÉING STEAKS, rather than grilling or broiling them, works beautifully with very tender cuts, such as filet mignon, and also allows you to create wonderful pan sauces. Fine restaurants take advantage of this with tableside preparation of the show-stopping entree known as Steak Diane. With its rich-tasting sauce, this translation is perfect for special occasions, yet lean and simple enough for every day.

MAKES **4** SERVINGS

⅓ cup nonfat half-and-half

1½ teaspoons cornstarch

4 (5-ounce) filets mignon, 1-inch thick

Salt and pepper to taste

2 teaspoons butter, divided

1 cup sliced mushrooms

1 tablespoon finely chopped shallots

⅓ cup reduced-sodium beef broth

1 tablespoon brandy or dry sherry

½ teaspoon Dijon mustard

2 teaspoons Worcestershire sauce

1 lemon, cut into 4 wedges, optional

Finely chopped fresh parsley

1. In a small bowl whisk together half-and-half and cornstarch. Set aside.

2. Pat the filets dry and season with the salt and pepper. Add 1 teaspoon of butter to a non-stick skillet and place over medium high heat. Add the steaks to the pan and cook each side for 5 minutes for medium rare (or to 145° F) or 1 to 2 minutes more per side (to 155° F) for medium. Remove from pan, cover, and set aside.

3. Add the remaining teaspoon of butter, then the mushrooms and shallots. Cook for 3 minutes or until slightly softened. Pour in the beef broth and brandy and stir, scraping the brown bits from the bottom. Stir in the half-and-half and cornstarch mixture and cook for 3 to 4 minutes or until thickened. Remove saucepan from heat and stir in mustard and Worcestershire sauce.

4. To serve, squeeze a wedge of lemon over the steak, if desired, and top with ¼ cup sauce. Sprinkle with chopped parsley.

DARE TO COMPARE: Order a small filet topped with creamy béarnaise at a steakhouse and you're looking at 680 calories and 14 grams of artery-clogging saturated fat.

NUTRITION INFORMATION PER SERVING (1 steak with sauce): Calories 265 | Carbohydrate 6g | (Sugars 2g) | Total Fat 12g (Sat Fat 4.5g) | Protein 30g | Fiber 1g | Cholesterol 90mg | Sodium 260mg | Food Exchanges: 4 Lean Meat, 1 Fat | Carbohydrate Choices: ½ | Weight Watcher Plus Point Comparison: 7

Biscuit and Burger Pie

WITH ITS BBQ-TINGED BEEF tucked under a warm biscuit topping, this casserole is hearty home-style comfort food at its best. Always a hit with kids (both young and old), it's a shoo-in for your next family-favorite meal. If you love the flavor of baked beans (and could use some extra fiber), try tossing ¾ cup of pinto or kidney beans into the meat mixture. Serve it with a salad and dinner is complete.

MAKES **6** SERVINGS

1 cup sugar-free root beer

1 (6-ounce) can tomato paste

¼ cup ketchup

2 tablespoons Worcestershire sauce

1 tablespoon liquid smoke

½ teaspoon garlic powder

½ teaspoon onion powder

¼ teaspoon black pepper

½ cup chopped celery

1 pound lean ground beef

1½ cups chopped red bell pepper

1½ cups reduced-fat baking mix (like Bisquick Heart Smart)

½ cup low-fat milk

4 tablespoons shredded reduced-fat cheddar cheese

2 tablespoons finely chopped green onion

1. Preheat oven to 400°F.

2. In a medium saucepan, whisk together the first 8 ingredients (root beer through black pepper). Place over medium low heat and cook for 10 minutes, stirring occasionally.

3. Spray a large non-stick skillet with non-stick cooking spray and place over medium high heat. Add celery and sauté for one minute. Add beef and bell pepper and cook for 5 minutes or until the beef is cooked and celery tender. Drain any excess liquid and add sauce. Mix well and transfer to an 8 x 8-inch baking dish. Set aside.

4. In a medium bowl, mix together the remaining ingredients until a soft dough forms. Spoon tablespoons of the dough onto the casserole. Spread the dough with a spoon or your fingers, leaving a 1-inch border on all sides.

5. Bake for 10 to 12 minutes or until top is golden brown.

NUTRITION INFORMATION PER SERVING (one-sixth recipe): Calories 295 | Carbohydrate 35g (Sugars 4g) | Total Fat 8g (Sat Fat 3g) | Protein 23g | Fiber 3g | Cholesterol 50mg | Sodium 490mg | Food Exchange: 2½ Lean Meat, 1½ Starch, 2 Vegetable | Carbohydrate Choices: 2 | Weight Watcher Plus Point Comparison: 8

Crispy Pork Scaloppini

RECENTLY, MY FAMILY TOOK A TRIP to Germany to visit relatives. While there, my two teenage boys quickly figured what to do when faced with a restaurant menu that wasn't in English—look for pork "schnitzel" (thinly pounded boneless pork, which is breaded and then fried). After a week of watching them eat the fatty fare, I remember thinking that I could do better—and now I have. Still crisp, but with more flavor and less fat, this pork dish is one my boys now enjoy healthfully at home.

MAKES **4** SERVINGS

1 pound pork tenderloin or thin center cut boneless pork loin chops

¼ cup all-purpose flour

1 large egg

½ cup plain breadcrumbs

¼ cup freshly grated Parmesan cheese

¼ teaspoon salt or more to taste

⅛ teaspoon ground black pepper

½ teaspoon dried parsley

1 tablespoon canola oil

1 lemon, zested and cut in wedges, optional

1. Cut the tenderloin into eight ¾- to 1-inch thick slices and pound to ¼-inch thickness (if using chops, pound if necessary).

2. Place the flour in a shallow bowl. Place the egg in the second bowl and whisk lightly. Place the breadcrumbs, cheese, salt, pepper and parsley in a third bowl and toss to mix well.

3. Gently coat the pork slices with flour. Dip each cutlet into the egg, shaking lightly to remove excess, and coat with crumbs. Repeat until all the pork is coated.

4. Heat 1½ teaspoons of the oil in a large non-stick skillet over medium high heat. Add half of the pork cutlets, reduce heat to medium, and cook for 2 to 3 minutes or until underside is well browned. Spray the pork lightly with non-stick cooking spray, turn, and cook for 2 to 4 minutes on second side or until done. Repeat with remaining cutlets.

5. Serve immediately, topped with a squeeze of fresh lemon and a sprinkling of lemon zest, if desired.

Marlene Says: *Complete your German-style meal with Sour Cream and Onion Smashed Potatoes (page 227) and Sautéed Cabbage, Onions, and Apples (page 220).*

NUTRITION INFORMATION PER SERVING (2 cutlets): Calories 290 | Carbohydrate 15g (Sugars 1g) | Total Fat 11g (Sat Fat 4g) | Protein 30g | Fiber 1g | Cholesterol 130mg | Sodium 450mg | Food Exchanges: 4 Lean Meat, 1 Starch, ½ Fat | Carbohydrate Choices: 1 | Weight Watcher Plus Point Comparison: 7

P.F. Chang's®-Style Mongolian Beef

THE FIRST TIME MY BOYS tasted Mongolian Beef was at a P.F. Chang's and it set the bar for them for what Mongolian Beef should taste like—most notably, they adored the sweet and savory sauce that coats the meat. I knew I hit it right with my version when after just one bite my son Stephen ran off with the entire plateful! (This sauce is sinfully sweet, just like P.F. Chang's; if you prefer it less sweet, simply use less sweetener.)

MAKES **4** SERVINGS

3 tablespoons reduced-sodium soy sauce

1 tablespoon dry sherry

¼ cup granulated no-calorie sweetener (or 6 packets)

1 tablespoon molasses

2 teaspoons cornstarch

1 tablespoon minced garlic

½ teaspoon minced ginger

1 pound lean boneless sirloin

1 tablespoon cornstarch

2 teaspoons canola oil

2 medium carrots, cut into matchsticks

1 small red bell pepper, cut into ¼-inch strips

4 stalks green onion, green and white parts, sliced ¼-inch thick on the diagonal

2 teaspoons sesame oil

1. In a small saucepan, combine the first 7 ingredients (soy sauce through ginger). Add ⅓ cup water and heat for 1 to 2 minutes. Remove from heat and set aside.

2. Slice the meat across the grain into very thin slices, ⅛-inch thick. Lightly toss the beef with 1 tablespoon cornstarch. Heat the oil in a non-stick wok or large sauté pan over medium high heat. Add the beef and cook for 30 to 60 seconds or until no longer pink, stirring frequently. Remove the beef from pan and set aside.

3. Add the carrots and bell peppers to the pan and stir-fry for 2 minutes. Add the sauce mixture and green onions, cover, and cook for 2 minutes. Uncover and simmer for 1 minute longer or until the sauce thickens slightly. Add the meat back to the pan with the sesame oil and toss until coated.

DARE TO COMPARE: An order of Mongolian Beef at P.F. Chang's China Bistro has 1,011 calories and 45 grams of fat, but the real killer is the sodium—4,020 mg worth!

NUTRITION INFORMATION PER SERVING (1 generous cup): Calories 300 | Carbohydrate 15g (Sugars 6g) | Total Fat 13g (Sat Fat 4.5g) | Protein 32g | Fiber 2g | Cholesterol 90mg | Sodium 490mg | Food Exchanges: 4 Lean Meat, 1 Vegetable, ½ Carbohydrate, ½ Fat | Carbohydrate Choices: 1 | Weight Watcher Plus Point Comparison: 7

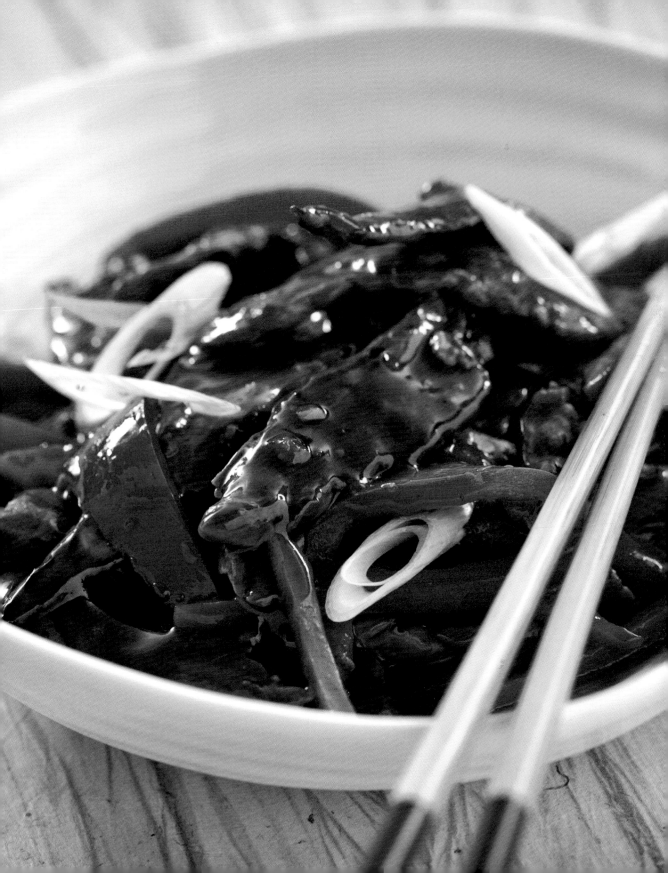

15-Minute Maple Glazed Pork Chops

A PACKAGE OF LEAN PORK CHOPS and a few short minutes are all you need to get dinner on the table with this fast-fix recipe. My very favorite way to serve them is with the Spicy Sweet Potato Mash (page 230). The flavors complement each other perfectly.

MAKES **4** SERVINGS

4 (5-ounce) thin-cut boneless center cut pork chops

Salt and pepper to taste (about ¼ teaspoon each)

2 slices center cut bacon

1 large shallot, minced

Pinch of dried thyme

⅓ cup sugar-free maple syrup

3 tablespoons cider vinegar

1 teaspoon brown sugar

¾ teaspoon whole grain or Dijon mustard

1. Pat the pork chops dry and sprinkle them with the salt and pepper. Place a large nonstick skillet over high heat and add the bacon to the pan. Cook for 3 to 4 minutes or until bacon is cooked. Remove, crumble or chop, and set aside. Remove extra fat if more than one tablespoon.

2. Place the chops into the pan and cook for 2 minutes or until nicely browned. Turn the pork chops and cook other side, about 3 to 4 more minutes for thin chops. Remove chops from pan, place on plate, cover and set aside.

3. Add the shallot and thyme to the pan. Cook over medium-high heat until the shallot is softening and beginning to brown, about 2 minutes. Add syrup, vinegar, brown sugar, and mustard and stir. Simmer sauce for 2 minutes or until mixture starts to bubble. (Add back some of the juices from the plate pork is on if needed to thin). Adjust salt and pepper to taste.

4. Pour sauce over pork chops and garnish with chopped bacon.

NUTRITION INFORMATION PER SERVING: Calories 210 | Carbohydrate 3g (Sugars 1g) | Total Fat 10g (Sat Fat 2g) | Protein 33g | Fiber 0g | Cholesterol 90mg | Sodium 260mg | Food Exchange: 4 Lean Meat | Carbohydrate Choices: 0 | Weight Watcher Plus Point Comparison: 6

Sassy Grilled Pork with Memphis-Style BBQ Sauce

INSPIRED BY THE FOOD NETWORK'S Tennessee barbecue masters, the Neelys, this recipe brings Memphis style to the table. Seasoned with paprika, mustard and molasses, the sweet & spicy tomato-y BBQ sauce kicks some serious sass when spooned over ultra- tender lean grilled pork tenderloin. I can't wait to get back "In the Kitchen" to share this with QVC host and Southern boy David Venable, aka Mr. Foodie—he's going to love this!

MAKES **4** SERVINGS

¼ cup reduced-sugar ketchup

2 tablespoons granulated no-calorie sweetener (or 3 packets)

1 tablespoon cider vinegar

1 teaspoon molasses

1 teaspoon Worcestershire sauce

¾ teaspoon paprika

½ teaspoon onion powder

¼ teaspoon mustard powder

⅛ teaspoon liquid smoke

⅛ teaspoon black pepper

1¼ pounds pork tenderloin, well trimmed

1. To make the sauce, whisk together the first 10 ingredients (ketchup through black pepper), along with 2 tablespoons of water, in a very small saucepan. Bring to a simmer and cook for 4 to 5 minutes or until reduced slightly. Set aside.

2. Preheat the grill on medium high or place a non-stick grill pan over medium high heat. When heated, place the tenderloin on the grill or grill pan, and cook for 4 to 5 minutes, turning several times to brown on all sides.

3. Reduce heat to medium and brush the sauce on all sides of the tenderloin. Cook the tenderloin another 8 to 12 minutes or until a meat thermometer reads 145°F, brushing on more sauce while the tenderloin cooks.

4. Remove tenderloin from the grill or grill pan and let it rest for 5 minutes. To serve, slice the meat and spoon the remaining sauce over the top.

DARE TO COMPARE: All pork is not created equal! While the fattiest cuts, such as pork butt and ribs, have as much as 20 grams of fat in a 4-ounce portion, lean pork tenderloin has a mere 3 grams of fat in a 3-ounce cooked serving.

NUTRITION INFORMATION PER SERVING: Calories 190 | Carbohydrate 3g (Sugars 2g) | Total Fat 5g (Sat Fat 2.5g) | Protein 30g | Fiber 0g | Cholesterol 85mg | Sodium 280mg | Food Exchanges: 4 Lean Meat | Carbohydrate Choices: 0 | Weight Watcher Plus Point Comparison: 4

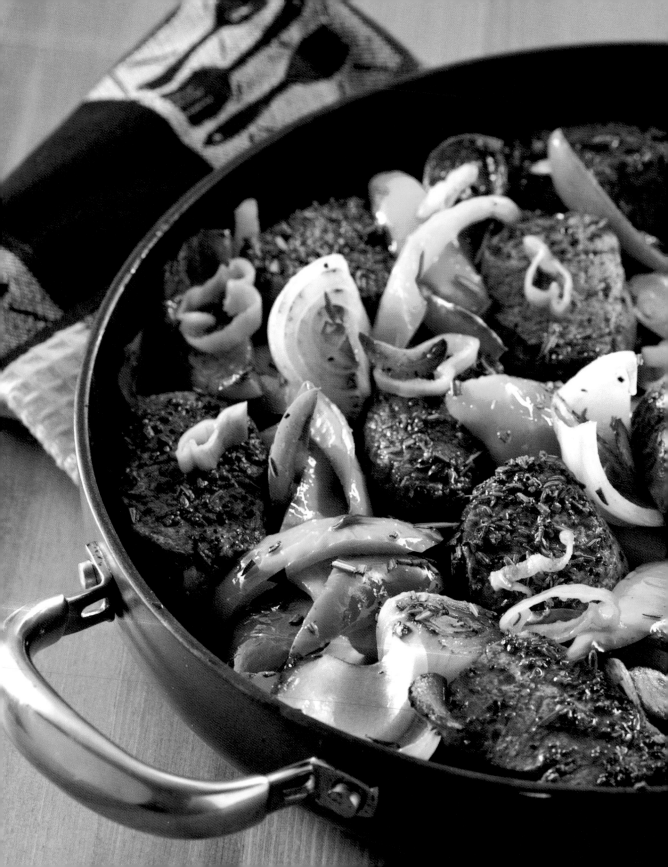

Skillet Pork and Peppers

IF YOU LIKE TRADITIONAL ITALIAN-STYLE SAUSAGE AND PEPPERS, you will love this dish. Pork tenderloin is coated with a sausage rub and then seared to perfection with sweet onions and a rainbow of bell peppers. Bottled pepperoncini finishes the dish, adding a tangy, pickle-like flavor that complements the Italian seasonings and sautéed vegetables to a tee.

MAKES 4 SERVINGS

½ teaspoon salt

¾ teaspoon black pepper

2 teaspoons fennel seeds, crushed

2 teaspoons oregano

1 teaspoon garlic powder

1 teaspoon paprika

1 pound pork tenderloin

1 tablespoon olive oil, divided

2 cups yellow onion (about 1 large), cut into ¼-inch slices

3 garlic cloves, minced

2 medium green bell peppers, cut into ½-inch slices

1 medium red or yellow bell pepper, cut into ½-inch slices

1 teaspoon fresh rosemary, chopped

2 tablespoons sweet vermouth or water

¼ cup pickled pepperoncini, cut into thin slices

1. Mix the first 6 ingredients (salt through paprika) in a small bowl. Cut the pork into 12 equal slices (about ½- to ¾-inch wide each). Coat the pork thoroughly with the spice rub.

2. Heat 2 teaspoons of the oil in a large sauté pan over medium high heat. Add the pork to the skillet and sear for 2 minutes on each side or until browned (the middle will be pink). Transfer the slices to a plate and set aside.

3. Add the remaining teaspoon of olive oil to the pan, reduce heat to medium, and add the onion and garlic. Sauté for 3 minutes or until browned and slightly softened. Add the bell peppers, rosemary and vermouth, and cook for 7 to 8 minutes, turning the peppers until they are crisp tender. Add the pepperoncini and cook for 1 minute.

4. Return the pork to the pan, reduce heat to low, cover and cook for 5 minutes or until peppers are tender and pork is thoroughly cooked.

NUTRITION INFORMATION PER SERVING (3 pieces of pork plus peppers): Calories 250 | Carbohydrate 13g (Sugars 7g) | Total Fat 10g (Sat Fat 2.5g) | Protein 25g | Fiber 3g | Cholesterol 75mg | Sodium 380mg | Food Exchanges: 3 ½ Lean Meat, 2 Vegetables | Carbohydrate Choices: 1 | Weight Watchers Point Comparison: 6

Plum Good Pork

FASHIONED AFTER MY POPULAR PORK TENDERLOIN with Cranberry Pan Sauce, this dish pairs dried plums (formerly known as prunes), with tender sliced pork. It's quick, easy, delicious, impressive, and elegant enough to be served on the best occasions. Please don't be deterred by the plums (or the prune juice)—it's truly plum good!

MAKES **4** SERVINGS

1¼ pounds pork tenderloin

1 teaspoon olive or canola oil

1 small shallot, minced

¼ cup chicken stock

¼ cup prune juice

¼ ruby port wine

⅓ cup chopped dried plums

1 teaspoon Dijon mustard

1 heaping tablespoon no-sugar-added boysenberry preserves

1 tablespoon butter

¼ teaspoon salt

¼ teaspoon black pepper

1. Preheat the oven to 400°F. Lightly season pork with salt and pepper to taste.

2. Heat the oil in a large non-stick skillet over medium high heat. Add the tenderloins and brown well on all sides. Remove the meat and transfer to a baking sheet. Roast in the oven for 20 minutes or until a meat thermometer reads 145°F. Remove from the oven, cover and let rest 5 to 10 minutes.

3. While the meat roasts, make the pan sauce. Add the shallot to the skillet and sauté for 2 minutes. Add the stock, prune juice and port and cook over low heat for 5 to 8 minutes until the mixture reduces slightly. Stir in the plums, Dijon, and preserves, and continue to cook for 3 to 5 minutes or until the sauce becomes syrupy. Remove from heat and swirl in the butter. Season with the salt and pepper (or more to taste).

4. To serve, slice the meat and lay it onto plates. Spoon the sauce over each serving.

Marlene Says: *Prune juice brings richness to the sauce but its flavor is not distinct. Most stores carry individual cans in six-packs and I simply purchase one can. If you like, you can replace it with more port. Alternatives for the port wine are prune or cranberry juice.*

NUTRITION INFORMATION PER SERVING (4 ounces meat and sauce): Calories 290 | Carbohydrate 11g (Sugars 5g) | Total Fat 9g (Sat Fat 3g) | Protein 32g | Fiber 1g | Cholesterol 120mg | Sodium 290mg | Food Exchanges: 4 Lean Meat, 1 Fruit | Carbohydrate Choices: 1 | Weight Watcher Plus Point Comparison: 7

Shrimp Scampi

SWEET PLUMP SHRIMP DOUSED in butter, white wine, lemon and garlic—what could be better? This recipe will satisfy every shrimp fan. You get all the real ingredients and traditional scampi flavor, with only 240 calories per serving. Be sure to have a chunk of crusty bread to mop up every bit of the leftover sauce. Enjoy.

MAKES **4** SERVINGS

2 green onions, white and green parts, thinly sliced

1 tablespoon minced garlic, about 4 cloves

½ cup dry white wine

Juice of one lemon, about 3 tablespoons

2 tablespoons butter

⅛ teaspoon each salt and pepper or to taste

Pinch of red pepper flakes or to taste

1¼ pound medium shrimp, peeled and deveined

1. Spray a large non-stick skillet with non-stick cooking spray and place over medium heat. Add the green onion and sauté for 2 minutes. Add the garlic and sauté for 1 minute.

2. Add the wine, lemon juice, butter, salt, pepper, and red pepper flakes, bring to a simmer, and reduce by half.

3. Add the shrimp to the pan and cook for 1 to 2 minutes per side, turning when the shrimp is pink. Cook down sauce to incorporate shrimp juices. Season with additional black pepper to taste and serve.

Marlene Says: *Love shrimp, but not the cholesterol? Good news: while shrimp is high in cholesterol, studies show that it's not cholesterol, but saturated fat that appears to increase the risk of heart disease. With just 2 tablespoons of butter for four servings instead of the whole sticks commonly used at restaurants, this dish fits in any healthy diet.*

NUTRITION INFORMATION PER SERVING: Calories 240 | Carbohydrate 5g (Sugars 1g) | Total Fat 8g (Sat Fat 4g) | Protein 29g | Fiber 1g | Cholesterol 230mg | Sodium 290mg | Food Exchanges: 4 Lean Meat, 1 Fat | Carbohydrate Choices: 0 | Weight Watcher Plus Point Comparison: 5

Simple Southwestern Tilapia

A PINCH OF TACO SEASONING, a dash of lime, and a smidgen of cayenne add a kick of the Southwest to moist-on-the-inside, crunchy-on-the-outside tilapia filets. For a quick 30-minute dinner, just add Fiesta Lime Rice (page 229) and salsa.

MAKES **4** SERVINGS

1 lime, juice and zest

2 tablespoons light mayonnaise

1 pound tilapia filets

1¼ cups reduced-fat cheese crackers

1 tablespoon taco seasoning (40% less sodium)

2 tablespoons cornmeal

Pinch cayenne pepper

1. Preheat the oven to 450°F. Spray a baking sheet with cooking spray.

2. Zest and juice the lime and place in a shallow flat bowl. Whisk in the mayonnaise, add the fish filets and marinate for 5 minutes.

3. Place the crackers in a plastic bag, crush with a rolling pin, and place crumbs on a plate. Add the taco seasoning and cornmeal and mix well.

4. Coat the filets with the cracker mixture and place on the prepared baking sheet. Bake for 5 minutes, turn the filets over, and bake for 5 to 7 minutes or until the fish flakes with a fork. Serve with optional salsa.

NUTRITION INFORMATION PER SERVING (1 filet)**:** Calories 250 | Carbohydrate 18g (Sugars 1g) | Total Fat 9g (Sat Fat 3.5g) | Protein 26g | Fiber 1g | Cholesterol 30mg | Sodium 295mg | Food Exchanges: 3½ Lean Meat, 1 Starch | Carbohydrate Choices: 1 | Weight Watcher Plus Point Comparison: 7

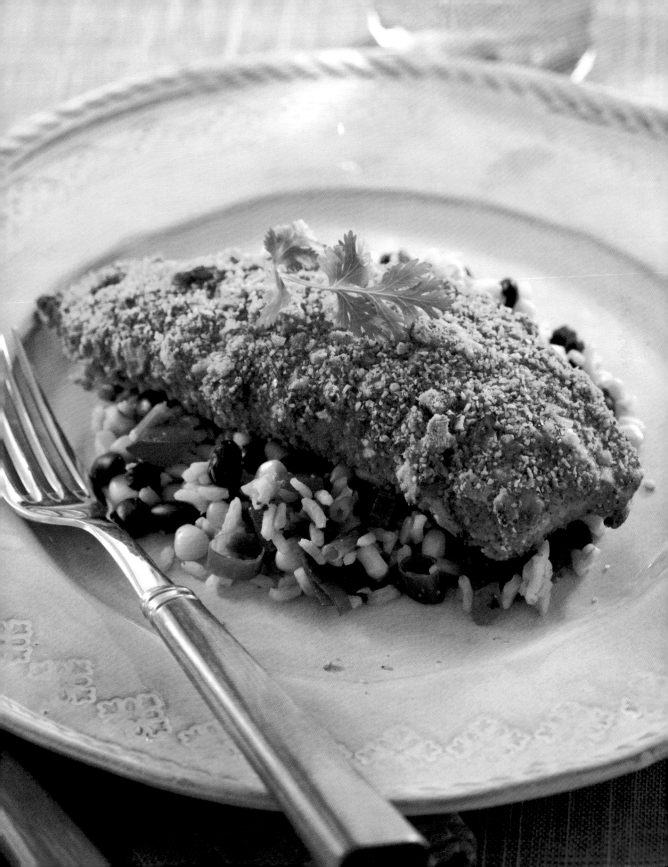

Nut-Crusted Fish Fillets

GO NUTS! And enjoy these fish fillets coated with a delectable nutty crust. This recipe strikes the perfect balance of almonds versus breadcrumbs—resulting in fabulous flavor and crunch—while keeping the carbs and fat in check. Prepare this with any mild white fish and feel free to use your favorite nuts.

MAKES **4** SERVINGS

1 pound fresh or thawed tilapia filets or other mild white fish

4 teaspoons Dijonnaise

1 teaspoon honey

¼ cup almonds, finely chopped

¼ cup panko breadcrumbs

¼ teaspoon garlic powder

½ teaspoon salt

¼ teaspoon black pepper

½ teaspoon dried dill

1. Preheat the oven to 425°F. Spray a baking sheet with cooking spray. Pat the fish filets dry with a paper towel. Combine the Dijonnaise and honey and spread one side of each filet with 1 teaspoon of the mixture.

2. In a small bowl, combine the almonds, breadcrumbs, garlic powder, salt, pepper, and dill. Sprinkle the almond mixture evenly over the coated side of each filet, pressing the crumbs lightly to help them stick. Transfer the filets, coating side up, to the prepared baking sheet, and coat lightly with non-stick cooking spray.

3. Bake the filets for 10 minutes or until the fish is golden brown and flakes easily when tested with a fork.

Marlene Says: *With a bag (or two) of fish filets in the freezer it's easy to meet the dietary recommendation of eating delicious fish twice a week. Individually sealed packets of frozen fish can be thawed in about 15 minutes by placing a packet in warm water.*

NUTRITION INFORMATION PER SERVING (1 Filet): Calories 200 | Carbohydrate 7g (Sugars 2g) | Total Fat 8g (Sat Fat 1.5g) | Protein 26g | Fiber 1g | Cholesterol 25mg | Sodium 470mg | Food Exchanges: 4 Lean Meat, ½ Starch | Carbohydrate Choices: ½ | Weight Watcher Plus Point Comparison: 5

Honey Walnut Shrimp

IF YOU LOVE HONEY WALNUT SHRIMP, you can thank my kitchen assistant Judy, as she suggested we tackle this highly addictive dish. The combination of the sweet crunchy nuts, crispy shrimp, and creamy honey dressing is a definite winner—and now it is also completely guilt-free. If you have never tasted Honey Walnut Shrimp, now is a good time.

1 large egg

½ cup walnut halves

3 tablespoons granulated no-calorie sweetener, divided (or 4 packets)

3 teaspoons honey, divided

2 tablespoons light mayonnaise

2 tablespoons light sour cream

½ teaspoon lemon juice

1 pound extra-large shrimp, peeled and deveined

¼ cup all-purpose flour

1 tablespoon canola oil, divided

3 cups green or Napa cabbage, finely shredded

1. Preheat the oven to 350°F. In a medium bowl, whisk the egg until light and frothy. Place 1 teaspoon of the egg and ½ teaspoon of honey in a small bowl, add the walnuts and toss to coat. Add 2 tablespoons of the sweetener and toss well. Place nuts on a baking sheet and cook for 8 to 10 minutes or until golden. Set aside.

2. For the sauce, in a large bowl, combine the mayonnaise, sour cream, lemon juice, 1 tablespoon sweetener, and 2½ teaspoons honey. Set aside.

3. Dip each shrimp in the egg and then roll in the flour to coat. Heat ½ tablespoon of the oil in a large non-stick skillet over medium heat. Add half of the shrimp and cook for 2 to 3 minutes per side, turning when the underside is well browned. Transfer the shrimp to a plate and keep warm. Heat the remaining oil and cook the remaining shrimp.

4. Transfer the shrimp to the bowl, add honey sauce, and toss to coat. Spread the cabbage on a serving platter, pile the sauced shrimp on top and scatter half the walnuts over (reserve the remaining nuts for another use).

DARE TO COMPARE: A restaurant order of Honey Walnut Shrimp can have over 1,000 calories, 50 grams of fat and more than an entire day's worth of added sugar!

NUTRITION INFORMATION PER SERVING: Calories 290 | Carbohydrate 16g (Sugars 7g) | Total Fat 12g (Sat Fat 2.5g) | Protein 27g | Fiber 2g | Cholesterol 230mg | Sodium 600mg | Food Exchanges: 3 Lean Meat, 1 Starch, 1 Fat | Carbohydrate Choices: 1 | Weight Watcher Plus Point Comparison: 7

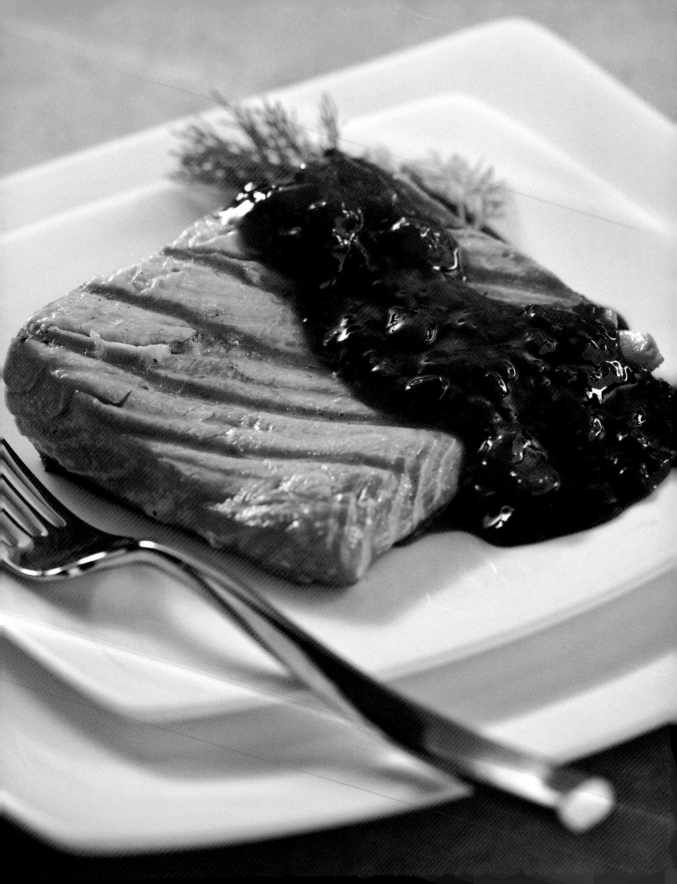

Grilled Salmon with Raspberry Chipotle Sauce

ELEGANT, YET BOLD, this salmon recipe is worthy of any dinner party. The "sweet with a kick" raspberry chipotle sauce is a true show-stopper both in flavor and presentation. No need for fresh raspberries, as frozen berries work best. Canned chipotle peppers can be found in the Mexican foods section. Be prepared for recipe requests from delighted guests after they taste this one!

MAKES **4** SERVINGS

¾ cup frozen unsweetened raspberries

¼ cup sugar-free raspberry jam

1 tablespoon rice vinegar

1 tablespoon brown sugar

4 teaspoons soy sauce

1 teaspoon canned chipotle pepper in adobo sauce, chopped, or more to taste*

4 (5-ounce) salmon filets, rinsed and dried

1. Combine first 6 ingredients (raspberries through chipotle pepper) in a small saucepan and bring to a boil. Reduce the heat and simmer on low for 3 minutes. Remove from heat and set aside.

2. Grill salmon over high heat, cooking each side approximately 5 minutes (for 1-inch filets) or until fish flakes apart easily.

3. Place the salmon on plates and spoon the sauce over the filets.

Marlene Says: *Canned chipotle peppers are smoked jalapeño peppers and a little goes a long way. They freeze very well and add a nice spicy, smoky piquancy to many foods. Try adding a bit to mayonnaise.*

* As an alternative, you can use 1 teaspoon of Tabasco Chipotle sauce.

NUTRITION INFORMATION PER SERVING: Calories 250 | Carbohydrate 8g (Sugars 2g) | Total Fat 11g (Sat Fat 2.5g) | Protein 31g | Fiber 2g | Cholesterol 70mg | Sodium 410mg | Food Exchanges: 4 Medium Fat Meat, ½ Fruit | Carbohydrate Choices: ½ | Weight Watcher Plus Point Comparison: 6

Easy 20-Minute Fish Stew

*RESTAURANT-QUALITY AT THE READY—that's what I think about this stew. Chop up some onion and celery and while it sautés, prepare the rest of the ingredients. Once you start adding them to the pan you will have a lovely fish stew finished before you know it. My husband often makes this stew by himself. His favorite fish mix is one pound of tilapia filets with ½ pound of shrimp. With a bottle of clam juice and fish in the freezer it's a dinner he can throw together any time. Did I say how much I **really** like this stew?*

MAKES **4** SERVINGS

1 tablespoon olive oil

1 cup onion, chopped

1 stalk celery, finely chopped

3 large garlic cloves, minced

½ cup fresh parsley, chopped

1 cup fresh chopped tomato or petite diced (without juice)

1 (8-ounce) bottle clam juice

¾ cup dry white wine

2 tablespoons tomato paste

½ teaspoon oregano

¼ teaspoon thyme

1½ pounds white fish filets, cut into 2-inch pieces

Salt and pepper to taste

1. Heat the oil in a large saucepan over medium heat. Add chopped onion and celery and cook for 5 minutes or until softened. Add the garlic and sauté for 1 minute. Add ¼ cup parsley and sauté with the garlic for 1 minute. Add second ¼ cup parsley and tomatoes. Cook for one minute.

2. Stir in the clam juice, dry white wine, tomato paste and seasonings (crushing the thyme and oregano with your fingers). Tuck the fish into the pan. Cover and cook 5 minutes. Uncover, stir, and simmer for 5 more minutes or until fish is cooked through. Add remaining parsley and adjust salt and pepper to taste. Ladle into bowls and serve.

Marlene Says: *Sourdough bread is my bread of choice to sop up all the pan juices. Did you know that the "sour" in sourdough lowers the glycemic index, making sourdough bread easier on blood sugar than other white breads?*

NUTRITION INFORMATION PER SERVING: Calories 290 | Carbohydrate 16g (Sugars 7g) | Total Fat 12g (Sat Fat 2.5g) | Protein 27g | Fiber 2g | Cholesterol 230mg | Sodium 600mg | Food Exchanges: 3 Lean Meat, 2 Vegetable, 1 Fat | Carbohydrate Choices: 1½ | Weight Watcher Plus Point Comparison: 7

pies, puddings, and specialty desserts

Fast Fix Fruit Pies

Free Form Apple Pie

Amazing Pecan Pie Cups

Chocolate Pavlova Pie

Impossible Cheesecake Pie

Cheesecake-Stuffed Strawberries

Pumpkin Pie Cheesecake Squares

Quick and Creamy Cinnamon Rice Pudding

Crème Caramel Pudding Squares

Fresh Peach and Blueberry Cobbler

Easy Lemon Ice Cream with Raspberry Sauce

5-Ingredient Dark Chocolate Souffles

Like a delectable dessert buffet, this chapter offers an *amazing array of happy endings*. From the simple to the sublime—with an extra helping or two of fun tossed in—the only thing missing from these nutty, *crunchy*, creamy, fruity, *chocolatey* desserts is the customary sugar, fat and calories. Some of the recipes in this chapter use only real sugar, such as the Chocolate Pavlova Pie, while others use a mixture of sweeteners. In most of the recipes in this section, the only job of the sweeteners is to *sweeten* (instead of, say, helping baked goods to rise or to brown), so you can more easily substitute one for another. See page 54 for all your sweetening options.

One of my *favorite creations* is the Fast Fix Fruit Pies. These "hand" pies take advantage of ready-to-use pie dough to create individual *fresh fruit* pies that can be eaten out of hand. The smiles they'll inspire are priceless. The most *amazing* creation is my Amazing Pecan Pie Cups. If you love pecan pie, you will love these. They have all the sweetness and *buttery nutty* flavor of pecan pie, with 90% less sugar and one-third the fat. They're a pecan pie *delight* that actually loves you back!

Moving from crunchy to *creamy*, the Creme Caramel Pudding Squares are a wonderful example of how ordinary ingredients, perfectly combined, can be *transformed* into something *extraordinary*. Garnering two big thumbs up from everyone who has tried them, these beautiful *tote–able* squares are perfect for church get-togethers or family gatherings. "Fruity" makes its mark in desserts like *homey* Fresh Peach and Blueberry Cobbler, and easy, *elegant* Cheesecake Stuffed Strawberries, but the grand finale of course belongs to chocolate. Deep, dark, and *utterly delicious*, the 15-Minute 5-Ingredient Dark Chocolate Soufflés are simple to make and impressive to serve.

Fast Fix Fruit Pies

PIES ARE BACK IN FASHION in a big way and these easy-to-make "hand" pies deliver big pie satisfaction in a perfectly portioned package. Fill with apples, peaches, or berries and freeze extra pies for a steady supply of seasonal desserts year round. These beauties are also kid-friendly and a great way to get little bakers into the kitchen. (Note: It's usually the case that a bit of fruit juice escapes the pie during baking, so line the baking sheet with foil or parchment for easy clean-up.)

Apple Hand Pies

½ package refrigerated pie crust

¼ teaspoon cornstarch

¾ teaspoon cinnamon

3 tablespoons granulated no-calorie sweetener (or 4 packets)

1 teaspoon granulated sugar

2 medium apples, peeled and diced, about 3 cups

1. Preheat the oven to 400°F. Place the pie crust on a cutting board or flat surface. Using a 3½-inch round cutter, cut out seven rounds (it's easiest to cut three rounds across the center, two above and two below). Roll out scraps and cut out one more round. Lightly roll each round to 5-inch diameter. Transfer the crusts to a baking sheet.

2. In a small bowl, whisk together ⅓ cup water, cornstarch, cinnamon, and sweetener. Heat a medium-size non-stick sauté pan over medium heat. Add the apples and sauté for 3 minutes. Stir in cornstarch mixture and cook for 5 minutes or until sauce is thickened and apples softened. Remove from heat and cool slightly.

3. Spoon scant 2 tablespoons apple filling onto half of each crust. Fold the empty crust over the filling (to form a half moon) and crimp the edges closed with a fork. With a sharp knife, cut two small vents on the top. Repeat with the remaining crusts and pie filling.

4. Sprinkle sugar over pies and bake for 18 to 20 minutes or until the crusts are golden brown and the filling is bubbly. Let cool slightly before serving.

Peach Hand Pies: For peach filling, in a small bowl, combine 1 cup diced peaches, peeled fresh or drained water-packed canned (drained), and 2 tablespoons low-sugar apricot jam. (Subtract 10 calories and 3 grams of carbohydrate per pie.)

Mixed Berry Hand Pies: For berry filling, in a small bowl, combine 2 tablespoons sweetener, 1 tablespoon cornstarch, and 1 tablespoon granulated sugar. Measure out ½ cup each halved blackberries and raspberries. Place 4 blackberry and 4 raspberry halves on each crust round. Sprinkle berries with scant teaspoon of the cornstarch mixture, fold, and bake as directed. (Subtract 10 calories and 3 grams of carbohydrate per pie.)

Marlene Says: *These perfectly sized pies can also be frozen and baked when needed. Bake the frozen pies right out of the freezer at 425°F for the first 10 minutes, then reduce the oven temperature to 400°F and bake an additional 20 minutes.*

NUTRITION INFORMATION PER SERVING (1 apple pie): Calories 135 | Carbohydrate 19g (Sugars 7g) | Total Fat 6g (Sat Fat 2.5g) | Protein 1g | Fiber 2g | Cholesterol 5mg | Sodium 120mg | Food Exchanges: 1 Carbohydrate, 1 Fat, ¼ Fruit | Carbohydrate Choices: 1 | Weight Watcher Plus Point Comparison: 4

Free Form Apple Pie

A SPEEDIER VERSION OF A PIE, this rustic yet elegant apple galette is effortless to make—lay down the crust, top it, and go! It's definitely a dessert worthy of company and on first look **and** first bite, I guarantee your guests will ooh and aah. It's up to you whether or not to tell them how little time you spent putting it together.

1 tablespoon dark brown sugar

¼ cup granulated no-calorie sweetener (or 6 packets)

1 tablespoon plus 2 teaspoons all-purpose flour, divided

1 teaspoon cinnamon

1½ teaspoons vanilla

4 to 5 medium Golden Delicious or other baking apples (about 1¾ pounds)

½ package refrigerated pie crust

1 tablespoon butter, melted

1 tablespoon granulated sugar

1. Preheat oven to 400°F. Line a baking sheet with parchment paper or silicone sheet.

2. In a medium bowl, combine the brown sugar, sweetener, 1 tablespoon flour, cinnamon, and vanilla. Peel, core and slice apples into ½-inch slices, add to the sugar mixture, and toss well to coat.

3. Sprinkle 2 teaspoons of flour on a flat surface, place the pie crust on it, roll it out lightly to a 12-inch diameter, and place on baking sheet. Gently pile the apples on the crust, leaving a 1-inch border of plain dough. Gently fold the edges of the dough over the apples, crimping as necessary.

4. Brush the apples with the melted butter and sprinkle evenly with the granulated sugar. Bake for 30 to 35 minutes until the crust is golden brown and apples are cooked. Let cool at least 10 minutes before serving.

Marlene Says: *For a beautiful summer galette, substitute fresh peaches and berries, omit the cinnamon, and bake for 25 to 35 minutes. No top crust required!*

NUTRITION INFORMATION PER SERVING (1 slice): Calories 180 | Carbohydrate 27g (Sugars 13g) | Total Fat 8g (Sat Fat 3.5g) | Protein 1g | Fiber 2g | Cholesterol 10mg | Sodium 120mg | Food Exchanges: 1 Starch | Carbohydrate Choices: 2 | Weight Watcher Plus Point Comparison: 5

Amazing Pecan Pie Cups

OH MY, PECAN PIE. A traditional pecan pie is made with at least one cup each of corn syrup and sugar. Toss in the pecans and butter, and the richest of all pies is born. It took at least a dozen attempts and an entire week to create a great-tasting pecan pie that everyone could enjoy guilt-free—but I did it! Each delectable pecan pie cup has a mere teaspoon (that's right, one teaspoon) of added sugar. I still find the numbers amazing and I'm sure once you taste one, you will too.

MAKES **12** SERVINGS

1 package refrigerated pie crust

¾ cup pecan halves

¼ cup brown sugar

1 teaspoon cornstarch

½ cup granulated no-calorie sweetener (like Splenda)

2 eggs, beaten

1 cup sugar-free maple syrup

1½ teaspoons vanilla

3 tablespoons melted butter

1. Preheat the oven to 350°F. Place one pie crust on a cutting board or flat surface and roll out lightly to an 11-inch diameter. Using a 4-inch round cutter, cut out six rounds. Set scraps aside. Repeat with the second pie crust.

2. Lightly press the pastry rounds into 12 muffin cups, pressing into the bottom and up the sides. Set aside. Reserving 12 pecan halves, chop the remaining pecan halves and set aside.

3. In a medium bowl, whisk together the brown sugar, sweetener and cornstarch. Add the eggs, syrup, vanilla and melted butter and mix well. Stir in the chopped pecans. Divide the filling evenly among the 12 cups. Top each with a pecan half.

4. Bake for 30 to 35 minutes or until the tops and crust are nicely browned. Let cool slightly before serving.

DARE TO COMPARE: Winning the dubious honor of Thanksgiving's most fattening (and sugary) food, a regular piece of pecan pie has 600 calories, 40 grams of fat, and 12 teaspoons of sugar (or 4 carb servings) per *piece*!

NUTRITION INFORMATION PER SERVING (1 pie cup): Calories 200 | Carbohydrate 17g (Sugars 3g) | Total Fat 13g (Sat Fat 4g) | Protein 3g | Fiber 1g | Cholesterol 45mg | Sodium 200mg | Food Exchanges: 1 Carbohydrate, 2 Fat | Carbohydrate Choices: 1 | Weight Watcher Plus Point Comparison: 5

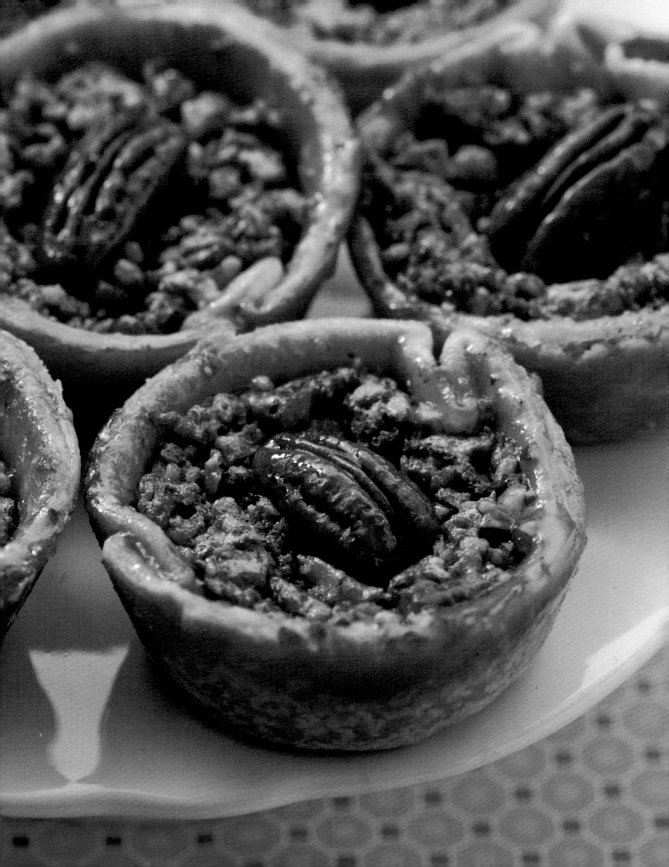

Chocolate Pavlova Pie

HAILING FROM AUSTRIA, a Pavlova is a dessert consisting of a free form meringue shell filled with whipped cream and topped with fresh fruit. Crispy, chewy, and a bit messy, a Pavlova is a marvelous treat, but creating a shell that holds together can be tricky. I solve the problem with the use of a pie plate—hence the "pie" in the title of this dessert. Cocoa powder is added to the meringue for a delicious chocolatey twist and beautiful fresh red strawberries crown the top. If you've never tried Pavlova, this one makes it easy. (A serrated knife eases cutting the sticky meringue.)

MAKES **6** SERVINGS

3 large egg whites

¼ teaspoon cream of tartar

⅔ cup granulated sugar

1½ tablespoons cocoa powder, Dutch-process preferred

1½ teaspoons cornstarch

1 teaspoon vanilla extract

1½ cups light whipped topping, thawed

1 pound of fresh strawberries, stemmed and halved

1. Preheat the oven to 300°F. Spray a 9-inch glass pie plate well with non-stick cooking spray.

2. Whisk together the egg whites, cream of tartar, and sugar in a medium bowl and place over simmering water. Heat for 2 to 3 minutes or until the sugar dissolves.

3. Remove the bowl from the heat and beat with an electric mixer on high for 5 minutes or until stiff peaks form. Using a sifter, sift in cocoa powder and cornstarch, and then fold it in using a large spatula. Stir in vanilla, taking care to not deflate the egg whites.

4. Spoon the meringue into the pie pan, pushing it halfway up the sides to create a wide shallow well in the center. Bake for 50 to 60 minutes or until the outside is dry and crisp (some cracking is normal). Turn off the oven, open the oven door slightly, and leave the Pavlova in the oven to dry for one hour.

5. When cooled, spread the whipped topping evenly over the Pavlova and top with strawberries. (The shell can be made up to one day in advance. Wrap tightly or store in an airtight container.)

Marlene Says: *Because they require no flour, meringue-based desserts are naturally lower in carbohydrates. Sugar provides not only the sweetness, but all of the structure.*

NUTRITION INFORMATION PER SERVING (1 piece): Calories 140 | Carbohydrate 26g (Sugars 22g) | Total Fat 2g (Sat Fat 6g) | Protein 3g | Fiber 2g | Cholesterol 35mg | Sodium 30mg | Food Exchanges: 1 Carbohydrate, ½ Fruit | Carbohydrate Choices: 1½ | Weight Watcher Plus Point Comparison: 3

Impossible Cheesecake Pie

THIS THROWBACK COMES FROM THE EARLY 1980's when plenty of pies were "impossible." Deceptively named, this delectable dessert is neither a pie nor is it impossible to make—the adjective in the title refers to the uncanny way the pie forms its own style of crust as it bakes. My new twist includes the addition of a bit of brown sugar to the cheesecake and a luscious topping of peaches and cream. I promise that once you dig in you'll forget all about its name.

MAKES **8** SERVINGS

8 ounces light cream cheese

8 ounces nonfat cream cheese, room temperature

1¾ teaspoons vanilla extract, divided

⅜ teaspoon almond extract, divided

⅔ cup, plus 2 tablespoons granulated no-calorie sweetener (like Splenda), divided

2 tablespoons brown sugar

¼ cup reduced-fat baking mix

2 large eggs, room temperature

1 cup light sour cream, divided

1 teaspoon granulated sugar

1 large peach, peeled, pitted and sliced

1. Preheat the oven to 300°F. Spray a 9-inch glass pie plate with non-stick cooking spray.

2. Place the cream cheeses, 1½ teaspoons vanilla, ¼ teaspoon almond extract, ⅔ cup sweetener, brown sugar, and baking mix in a large bowl and beat with an electric mixer at medium speed until smooth. Decrease the speed to low and beat in eggs one at a time, beating just until blended. Stir in ¼ cup sour cream and pour into the prepared pie plate.

3. Bake for 30 to 35 minutes or until the cheesecake no longer jiggles and is set. While the cheesecake bakes, combine ¾ cup sour cream, ¼ teaspoon vanilla, ⅛ teaspoon almond extract, 2 tablespoons sweetener, and granulated sugar. Stir until well blended.

4. Pour the topping over the warm cheesecake and spread evenly with a small spatula. Cool to room temperature. Chill in the refrigerator until firm, at least 4 hours. Before serving, arrange the peach slices in a circle in the center of the cheesecake.

Marlene Says: *Impossible pies are reputed to form a magic "crust" during baking. This cheesecake does not have an appreciable crust, but the baking mix does create a thin layer that settles between pie pan and cheesecake, making it easy to cut and serve.*

NUTRITION INFORMATION PER SERVING (1 slice): Calories 140 | Carbohydrate 12g (Sugars 7g) | Total Fat 6g (Sat Fat 3.5g) | Protein 9g | Fiber 0g | Cholesterol 60mg | Sodium 270mg | Food Exchanges: 1 Lean Meat, 1 Carbohydrate, ½ Fat | Carbohydrate Choices: 1 | Weight Watcher Plus Point Comparison: 4

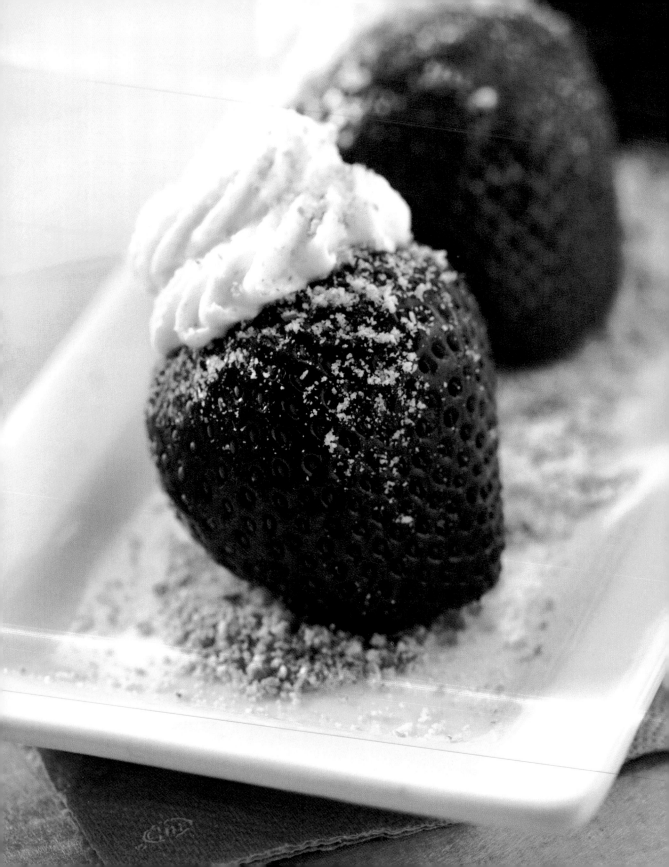

Cheesecake-Stuffed Strawberries

LUSCIOUS, CREAMY, JUICY, DREAMY—here's a dessert that turns decadent strawberry cheese-cake inside out. With only 50 calories per stuffed berry, life doesn't get much sweeter. Mini-desserts are "in" and these no-bake sweet bites are meant for sharing.

½ cup light tub-style cream cheese

⅓ cup nonfat cream cheese

3 tablespoons granulated no-calorie sweetener (or 4 packets)

⅛ teaspoon lemon zest

2 drops almond extract

½ cup light whipped topping, thawed

12 large whole strawberries, about one pound

2 graham cracker squares, finely crushed

1. In a small mixing bowl, by hand or with an electric mixer, beat cream cheeses with the sweetener, lemon zest, and almond extract until smooth. Stir in the light whipped topping. Transfer the mixture to a pastry bag with a ½-inch fluted tip; alternately, you can use a zip-top bag with a small hole cut in the bottom.

2. With a sharp knife or apple corer, remove the stem and hull from the strawberries, creating a small cavity. Slice a ¼-inch strip from the side of each strawberry (so it can sit on its side without rolling).

3. Place the graham cracker crumbs on a small plate. Pipe 1 table-spoon of the cream cheese filling into and on top of each straw-berry. Sprinkle ½ teaspoon of crumbs over the filling. Place strawberries in the refrigerator until time to serve. Arrange the strawberries on a platter and serve.

Marlene Says: *These little gems are great for entertaining. You can stuff the strawberries up to 6 hours ahead and sprinkle with the gra-ham cracker crumbs (or crushed vanilla or chocolate wafer crumbs) just before serving.*

NUTRITION INFORMATION PER SERVING (**1 stuffed strawberry**): Calories 50 | Carbohydrate 5g (Sugars 3g) | Total Fat 2g (Sat Fat 1g) | Protein 2g | Fiber 1g | Cholesterol 35mg | Sodium 70mg | Food Exchanges: ½ Fruit, ½ Fat | Carbohydrate Choices: ½ | Weight Watcher Plus Point Comparison: 1

Pumpkin Pie Cheesecake Squares

THE LUXURY OF PUMPKIN PIE AND CHEESECAKE rolled into one—all for only 90 calories per serving. What's not to love? Ideal for fall and fun for the holidays, these layered beauties are sure-fire crowd-pleasers. Make and serve them straight out of a pretty dish or after cutting, place each square into a cupcake liner for a festive presentation and neat, convenient nibbling.

MAKES **16** SERVINGS

Crust

3 tablespoons butter or margarine, melted

1 cup graham cracker crumbs

3 tablespoons no-calorie granulated sweetener (like Splenda)

Filling

8 ounces light tub-style cream cheese

2 large eggs, divided

⅓ cup plus ½ cup no-calorie granulated sweetener (like Splenda), divided

1 teaspoon vanilla

1 (15 ounce) can 100% packed pumpkin

1 teaspoon cinnamon

½ teaspoon ginger

⅛ teaspoon cloves

1. Preheat the oven to 325°F. Spray an 8 x 8-inch baking dish with non-stick baking spray.

2. Mix together crust ingredients in a small bowl. Pat crumbs firmly into the bottom of the baking dish. Bake for 8 minutes. Let cool and set aside.

3. While the crust is baking, in a medium bowl, using an electric mixer, beat the cream cheese, 1 egg, ⅓ cup sweetener, and vanilla. When crust has cooled, gently spoon the mixture over the crust and smooth. Set aside.

4. In the same bowl, beat the pumpkin, 1 egg, ½ cup sweetener, and spices until smooth. Gently spoon dollops of the filling onto the cream cheese mixture and smooth the layer.

5. Bake for 30 minutes. Allow to cool 25 minutes at room temperature. Refrigerate for 4 hours or overnight. Cut cheesecake into 16 2 x 2-inch squares.

Marlene Says: *Just like pumpkin pie, these squares are perfect when served with a little dollop of light whipped topping and a sprinkle of cinnamon or pumpkin pie spice.*

NUTRITION INFORMATION PER SERVING (1 square): Calories 90 | Carbohydrate 9g (Sugars 5g) | Total Fat 4.5g (Sat Fat 1.5g) | Protein 3g | Fiber 1g | Cholesterol 30mg | Sodium 125mg | Food Exchanges: ½ Carbohydrate, ½ Vegetable, 1 Fat | Carbohydrate Choices: ½ | Weight Watcher Plus Point Comparison: 2

Quick and Creamy Cinnamon Rice Pudding

THE CHOICE IS YOURS—you can make this pudding the old-fashioned way (see "Marlene Says") or with one of today's most popular milk alternatives— almond milk. Made from pressed almonds, nutritious almond milk is a creamy, easy to find, and low-cal alternative to cow's milk (only 40 calories and 2 grams of carb per cup compared to 110 calories and 12 grams of carb). The slightly nutty flavor also pairs great with better-for-you brown rice and cinnamon. Nonfat half-and-half brings a rich and creamy texture.

MAKES **6** SERVINGS

¾ cup cold water

½ cup quick-cooking brown rice (like Uncle Ben's Fast and Natural)

2¼ cups unsweetened or Vanilla almond milk

½ cup granulated no-calorie sweetener (or 12 packets)

1 teaspoon cinnamon

⅛ teaspoon salt

¾ cup nonfat half-and-half

2 teaspoons cornstarch

1 teaspoon vanilla

1. In a medium saucepan, bring the water to a boil and stir in the rice. Reduce to a simmer, cover, and cook for 10 minutes or until the water is absorbed.

2. Stir in the milk, sweetener, cinnamon and salt, and cook over medium heat, uncovered, for 20 minutes, stirring occasionally.

3. In a small bowl, whisk together the cornstarch and half-and-half and add to the rice. Stir in the vanilla and cook until bubbling. Cook on low for another minute and remove from heat (pudding will continue to thicken as it cools). Pour into a serving bowl or dessert dishes and let cool. Serve immediately, or cover and refrigerate until served.

Marlene Says: *To make **Old-Fashioned Cinnamon Rice Pudding**, substitute white rice for quick-cooking brown rice (add 10 minutes cooking time in Step 1, for a total of 20 minutes) and 1% milk for almond milk. (Adds 25 calories and 6 grams of carbohydrate per serving.)*

NUTRITION INFORMATION PER SERVING (½ cup): Calories 105 | Carbohydrate 19g (Sugars 0) | Total Fat 2g (Sat Fat 0g) | Protein 3g | Fiber 1g Cholesterol 0mg | Sodium 80mg | Food Exchanges: 1 Carbohydrate | Carbohydrate Choices: 1 | Weight Watcher Plus Point Comparison: 2

Crème Caramel Pudding Squares

LOOKING FOR AN EASY, IMPRESSIVE DESSERT? Look no further. Out of all of the desserts I tested for this book, this was one of the biggest crowd-pleasers. I have to admit that when I first looked at the ingredient list for the full fat, full sugar version, I was not overly impressed, but the combination of ingredients creates something far richer tasting and more beautiful than I ever expected. The 9 x 13-inch pan makes it a perfect tote 'n go dessert.

MAKES **20** SERVINGS

3 tablespoons margarine or butter, melted

1½ cups graham cracker crumbs

¼ cup plus 2 tablespoons granulated no-calorie sweetener, divided

4 ounces light tub-style cream cheese

4 ounces nonfat cream cheese, room temperature

3¼ cups low-fat milk, divided

1 tub (8-ounces) light whipped topping, thawed

1 (4-serving size) package sugar-free instant vanilla pudding mix

1 (4-serving size) package sugar-free instant butterscotch pudding mix

¼ cup sugar-free caramel ice cream topping

1. Place the melted margarine in a 9 x 13-inch dish. Add the graham cracker crumbs and 2 tablespoons of the sweetener. Mix well and pat crumbs onto bottom of pan. Refrigerate while preparing fillings.

2. In a medium bowl, beat the cream cheeses, ¼ cup of milk and ¼ cup of sweetener with an electric mixer until smooth. Gently fold in 1 cup of the whipped topping and spread evenly over the crust.

3. Whisk vanilla pudding mix with 1½ cups of milk for 2 minutes or until smooth. Spoon dollops of vanilla pudding on top of cream cheese layer and smooth the entire layer. Place in refrigerator while you whisk the butterscotch pudding mix with 1½ cups of milk. Carefully spoon the butterscotch pudding on top of vanilla pudding and smooth.

4. Top with the remaining whipped topping. Refrigerate for at least 4 hours. Just before serving, drizzle on the caramel topping. Cut into 20 squares.

NUTRITION INFORMATION PER SERVING (1 Square): Calories 130 | Carbohydrate 17g (Sugars 10g) | Total Fat 5g (Sat Fat 3g) | Protein 3g | Fiber 0g | Cholesterol 5mg Sodium 220mg | Food Exchanges: 1 Carbohydrate, 1 Fat | Carbohydrate Choices: 1 | Weight Watcher Plus Point Comparison: 3

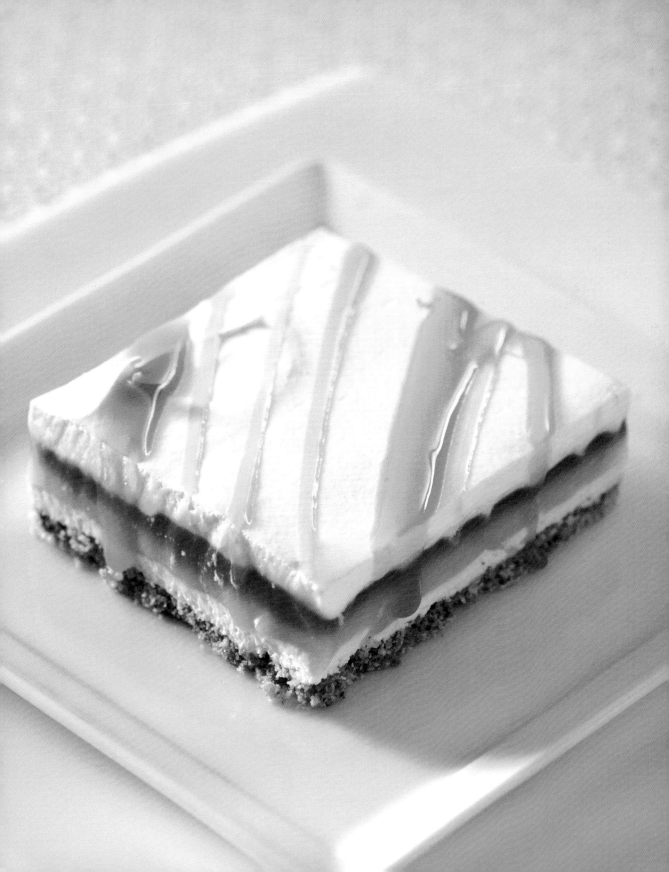

Fresh Peach and Blueberry Cobbler

THERE IS NOTHING BETTER on a lazy, hazy summer's day than kicking back and enjoying a time-honored dessert showcasing the season's finest fruits. One of the most popular requests I've ever received was for a healthier cobbler recipe and with just a few tweaks to the original recipe, I was able to deliver. While peaches ranked as the most popular summer fruit among my readers, this recipe works great with any summer fruit.

MAKES 6 SERVINGS

Filling

3 cups sliced fresh peaches

1 cup blueberries

1 cup blackberries or raspberries

¼ cup granulated no-calorie sweetener (or 6 packets)

1 tablespoon all-purpose flour

Topping

½ cup low-fat milk

2 tablespoons butter or margarine, melted

1 cup all-purpose flour

3 tablespoons granulated no-calorie sweetener (or 4 packets)

1 teaspoon baking powder

¼ teaspoon baking soda

1 teaspoon granulated sugar

1. Preheat the oven to 375°F. Lightly spray an 8 x 8-inch glass baking dish or a 9-inch glass pie plate with non-stick cooking spray.

2. For the filling, in a large bowl, toss the peaches and berries lightly with the sweetener and flour, and place in the baking dish.

3. To make the topping, in a small bowl, whisk together the milk and melted butter and set aside. In a medium bowl, whisk together the flour, sweetener, baking powder, and baking soda.

4. Add the milk mixture to the flour mixture and stir just until the dough comes together. Using a spoon or with floured hands, drop the dough in dollops over the fruit, lightly spreading to cover most of the fruit. Sprinkle the dough with sugar.

5. Bake for 35 to 40 minutes or until berries are bubbly and crust is light brown. Let cool 15 minutes before serving.

NUTRITION INFORMATION PER SERVING (about ¾ cup): Calories 180 | Carbohydrate 32g (Sugars 14g) | Total Fat 4g (Sat Fat 1g) | Protein 4g | Fiber 4g | Cholesterol 0mg | Sodium 135mg | Food Exchanges: 1 Carbohydrate, 1 Fruit, ½ Fat | Carbohydrate Choices: 2 | Weight Watcher Plus Point Comparison: 4

Easy Lemon Ice Cream with Quick Raspberry Sauce

PREPARE "HOMEMADE" ICE CREAM in just 10 minutes! In the world of easy desserts, this one ranks near the top of the list. Adding the juice and zest of a fresh lemon to store-bought vanilla ice cream is my trick for creating rich-tasting, yet low-fat lemon ice cream in a flash. Finish with a quick drizzle of raspberry sauce and a few fresh berries and you'll get maximum kudos with minimal effort.

MAKES **4** SERVINGS

2½ cups light no-sugar-added ice cream

1 medium lemon, washed and dried

4 tablespoons low-sugar raspberry jam

2 tablespoons water

2 tablespoons granulated no-calorie sweetener (or 3 packets)

Fresh raspberries, optional

1. Scoop ice cream into a medium bowl and set out at room temperature for 10 minutes, or until slightly softened.

2. Zest the lemon directly into the ice cream. Cut lemon in half and squeeze juice into the bowl. Using a spoon or fork (a fork helps to mash the zest into the ice cream if it is still a bit hard), mix the lemon into the ice cream until it is smooth. Place back into the freezer for at least 30 minutes to firm up.

3. Just before serving, place jam, water, and sweetener in a small microwave-safe bowl. Place in microwave and cook on high for 30 to 45 seconds or until warm. Stir. Scoop ½ cup lemon ice cream into small bowl or glass and drizzle with 1½ tablespoons raspberry sauce. Garnish with fresh raspberries, if desired.

Marlene Says: *Active time for this recipe is only 10 minutes! Do plan ahead, however, so that your "homemade" ice cream has time to re-freeze to the consistency you desire.*

NUTRITION INFORMATION PER SERVING (½ cup ice cream plus sauce): Calories 140 | Carbohydrate 23g (Sugars 10g) | Total Fat 4g (Sat Fat 2.5g) | Protein 4g | Fiber 4g | Cholesterol 0mg | Sodium 100 mg | Food Exchanges: 1 Carbohydrate, ½ Low-Fat Milk | Carbohydrate Choices: 1½ | Weight Watcher Plus Point Comparison: 3

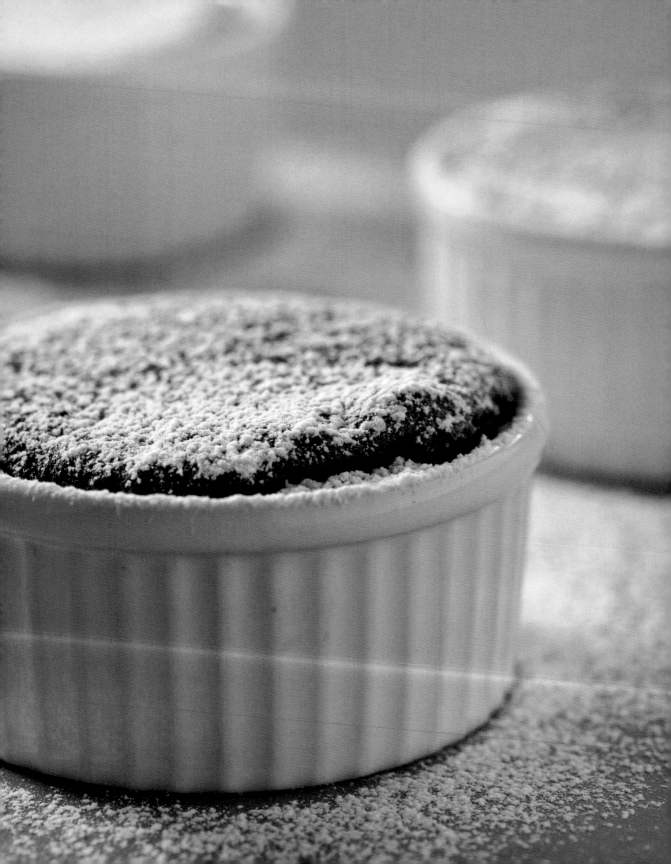

5-Ingredient Dark Chocolate Soufflés

FIVE INGREDIENTS, 15 MINUTES, AND JUST 160 CALORIES—wow! The first time through may take a few extra minutes, but after making these once you will be amazed at how fast these impressive soufflés come together. To serve, dust with cocoa or powdered sugar, adorn with fresh raspberries or add a dollop of light whipped topping.

MAKES **5** SERVINGS

4 large eggs

½ cup semisweet chocolate chips

¼ teaspoon instant coffee

1 tablespoon cocoa powder, preferably Dutch-processed

2 tablespoons granulated sugar

Additional cocoa powder or powdered sugar (optional)

1. Preheat oven to 400°F. Lightly spray five 6-ounce ramekins with baking spray and place on a sheet pan.

2. Separate the eggs, placing all the egg whites in one large bowl and two yolks in a small bowl (reserve remaining two yolks for another use).

3. Place the chocolate chips in a small microwave-safe bowl and heat for 1 to 1½ minutes or until chips are partially melted and appear shiny. Remove and stir. Set aside. In a medium bowl, whisk together 3 tablespoons warm water, instant coffee and cocoa powder. Whisk in the two egg yolks. Add the melted chocolate and whisk until smooth.

4. With an electric mixer on high speed, beat the egg whites until foamy. Gradually add the sugar and beat to stiff, but not dry, peaks. Gently fold half the chocolate mixture into the egg whites, taking care to not deflate the egg whites. Repeat with the remaining chocolate mixture.

5. Fill ramekins and place the pan in oven on center rack. Bake for 9 to 11 minutes or just until firm to the touch. Dust with cocoa powder or powdered sugar, if desired. Serve immediately

Marlene Says: *You can substitute 3 tablespoons brewed coffee for the ¼ teaspoon of instant coffee and water. You can also add ½ teaspoon of almond, vanilla, or orange extract, if desired. For a more intense chocolate flavor, use bittersweet chocolate.*

NUTRITION INFORMATION PER SERVING (1 souffle): Calories 160 | Carbohydrate 17g (Sugars 15g) | Total Fat 9g (Sat Fat 4.5g) | Protein 6g | Fiber 1g | Cholesterol 170mg | Sodium 55mg | Food Exchanges: 1½ Fat, 1 Carbohydrate, ½ Lean Meat | Carbohydrate Choices: 1 | Weight Watcher Plus Point Comparison: 5

homestyle cookies and cakes

Snickerdoodle Softies

Krispy Meringues

One Bowl Three-Bite Brownies

Raspberry Oat Bars

No-Bake Chocolate Sandwich Cookies

Sugar-Free Lemon Shortbread

Unbelievable Whoopie Pies

Old-Fashioned Chocolate Mayo Cake

Fresh Orange and Almond Cake

Double Pineapple Upside Down Cake

Heavenly Pumpkin Spice Cake

Unbelievable Chocolate Cake

There's nothing like coming home to the smell of *fresh-baked cookies* or the sight of a *homemade cake*. I like to cook, but I *love* to bake. Give me a bad day, and I'll bake the stress away with *warm* cookies and *comforting* cupcakes. Food, especially baked goods, often means more to us than simply what we put on our plate. I know how hard it is to try to modify your diet or resist the *foods you love*, for the sake of your health. That's why I'm delighted to tell you that no matter what your diet, with my recipes, you *can* have your cake (and *cookies*), and eat it too.

This chapter starts with cookies, among them three *stellar* recipes to add to your healthy cookie collection: cinnamon Snickerdoodle Softies, *fudgy* One Bowl Three-Bite Brownies, and *Unbelievable* Whoopie Pies. If you have ever tried to reduce the sugar (not to mention the fat) in cookies, you know how challenging it can be. Don't worry, though, I've already done the hard work (all three of these recipes have *less* than half the usual *sugar*, but the same great *classic taste*). All you have to do is get out your mixing bowl and stir up some fun!

Next up are more classic cake recipes. The Double Pineapple Upside Down Cake is a sure-fire *crowd pleaser*, and of course there are plenty of *chocolate* recipes in this chapter, starting with an Old-Fashioned Chocolate Mayo Cake. If you have never had a cake made with mayonnaise, you are going to love how *moist* this one is. Speaking of chocolate *cake*, over the years my signature Unbelievable Chocolate Cake has been enjoyed by countless readers. I am excited to share it once again—this time with a *new taste twist* I have dubbed the Unbelievable Almond Joy.

For the Love of
CHOCOLATE

Every chocoholic knows that chocolate has a unique ability to deliver comfort and blissful satisfaction in a way that few other foods can. It probably won't surprise you to learn that surveys rank chocolate as the most-craved food in America. What may surprise you (and delight you) is that irresistibly scrumptious chocolate can be as good for you as it is delicious!

- **Chocolate not only tastes great, it makes you feel great.** Chocolate stimulates endorphin production, creating feelings of pleasure, raises serotonin levels, improving mood, and affects hormones that can help reduce stress. Chocolate is a feel-good food!

- **Heart-healthy dark chocolate, when eaten regularly in moderation,** has been shown to reduce blood pressure and cholesterol, as well as lower the risk of a heart attack by as much as 50%!

- **Over a dozen vitamins and minerals are found in cocoa,** including Vitamins A, B1, C and E, along with calcium, iron and potassium. Cocoa offers the highest natural source of magnesium, which can help keep blood sugar in check and lower blood pressure.

- **Cocoa powder is low in fat and high in chocolatey goodness.** Two tablespoons of natural cocoa powder delivers more antioxidants than 3½ cups of green tea or 1½ glasses of red wine. Oleic acid, the healthy monounsaturated fat found in olive oil, is also found in dark chocolate.

- **Low in sugar and carbohydrates, unsweetened cocoa powder packs a fiber punch and has little effect on blood sugar.** Great for beverages and baking, it's chocolate heaven for those watching their weight or with diabetes.

- **Alkalizing natural cocoa powder reduces bitterness and darkens the color.** Alkalized cocoa powder (also known as Dutch-processed) works exceptionally well in reduced-sugar recipes.

- **Tempt your tastebuds with delectable dark chocolate.** Chocolates with 60% or more cocoa offer the most health benefits and deliver a richer chocolate flavor than milk chocolate.

- **Eat More of What You Love, including chocolate!** In this book you will find dozens of delicious recipes guaranteed to (healthfully) satisfy every chocolate craving.

Snickerdoodle Softies

I LOVE THE OLD-FASHIONED TASTE of cinnamon and vanilla sweetly rolled together—and that's what you get when you bite into one of these soft cookie jar cookies. No one is really sure how the whimsical Snickerdoodle got its name, but what I do know is that once my son James smells "doodles" in the kitchen he's all smiles. (P.S. You don't have to wait until the holidays to enjoy my Holiday Doodles—the homey taste of nutmeg is always in season.)

MAKES **26** COOKIES

2 cups all-purpose flour

1½ teaspoons cream of tartar

½ teaspoon baking soda

½ cup margarine or butter, room temperature

5 tablespoons granulated sugar, divided

2 tablespoons corn syrup

1½ teaspoons vanilla

1 large egg

¾ cup granulated no-calorie sweetener (like Splenda)

⅓ cup light sour cream

2 teaspoons cinnamon

1. Preheat oven to 375°F. Lightly spray baking sheet with non-stick cooking spray.

2. In a large bowl, combine flour, cream of tartar, and baking soda. Whisk to combine. Set aside.

3. In a medium bowl, with an electric mixer, beat the margarine or butter, 2 tablespoons of sugar, and corn syrup until light and fluffy. Beat in the vanilla, egg and sweetener until creamy. Turn the mixer to low and beat in the sour cream and flour until just combined.

4. With moist hands, roll dough into 1-inch balls. Mix together last 2 tablespoons sugar with cinnamon. Roll the balls in the sugar-spice mix and place on a cookie sheet that has been sprayed with cooking spray. Flatten cookies with the bottom of a drinking glass.

5. Bake for 7 to 8 minutes. Cookies should be soft on top. Remove to a wire rack to cool.

Marlene Says: *To create Holiday Doodles add 1 teaspoon nutmeg to the flour mix. To make Eggnog Snickerdoodles, add 1 teaspoon nutmeg and ¾ teaspoon rum extract to the egg mixture.*

NUTRITION INFORMATION PER SERVING (one cookie): Calories 80 | Carbohydrate 11g (Sugars 3g) | Total Fat 3g (Sat Fat 2g) | Protein 1g | Fiber 2g | Cholesterol 25mg | Sodium 20mg | Food Exchanges: 1 Carbohydrate | Carbohydrate Choices: 1 | Weight Watcher Plus Point Comparison: 1

Krispy Meringues

THE HALLMARK OF A PICTURE-PERFECT PLAIN MERINGUE COOKIE is its snowy white color. When baked as directed these meringues stay white and have a crisp exterior with a slightly soft chewy inside. If you bake them at a slightly higher temperature, they turn light brown as the sugar caramelizes and you get a crunchier cookie with a taste reminiscent of toasted marshmallows. If you like the idea of the "toasted" effect, bake the cookies at 275°F for 45 minutes, turn off the oven and let cool in the oven for one hour.

MAKES **24** COOKIES

4 large egg whites

¼ teaspoon cream of tartar

⅔ cup granulated sugar

¾ teaspoon vanilla

¼ teaspoon almond extract

1¼ cups crispy rice cereal (like Rice Krispies)

1. Preheat oven to 225°F. Line cookie sheets with silicone liners or parchment. Set aside.

2. Place egg whites, cream of tartar, and sugar in a metal mixing bowl and place over simmering water (make sure the bowl does not touch the water). Heat for 2 to 3 minutes or until sugar dissolves and egg whites are slightly warm. Remove the bowl from the heat and beat the egg whites with an electric mixer on high for 4 to 5 minutes or until stiff peaks form. With a spatula, fold in extracts and then rice cereal, being careful not to deflate meringue mixture.

3. Using a tablespoon, immediately spoon batter onto cookie sheets. Bake for 45 to 50 minutes or until you can lift a cookie cleanly off the cookie sheet. Turn off oven and leave cookies in for 15 more minutes. Remove and let cool. Store cookies in an airtight container.

Marlene Says: *I find the easiest way to separate eggs is to use my hands. Simply crack an egg on a work surface or the edge of a bowl and drop the egg into your cupped hand. Carefully let the white slip through your fingers into the bowl while the yolk remains in your hand. Be sure to wash your hands thoroughly (to rid them of grease) before you begin and again when you finish.*

NUTRITION INFORMATION PER SERVING (2 cookies): Calories 60 | Carbohydrate 12g (Sugars 6g) | Total Fat 0g (Sat Fat 0g) | Protein 2g | Fiber 0g | Cholesterol 0mg | Sodium 50mg | Food Exchanges: 1 Carbohydrate | Carbohydrate Choices: 1 | Weight Watcher Plus Point Comparison: 1

One Bowl Three-Bite Brownies

DEEP, DARK, AND OH-SO-CHOCOLATEY, who can resist fudgy brownies? I refused to give up until I made a brownie deserving of the name—and these deliver. They are easy to make, requiring only one bowl, and have ⅓ fewer calories and half the fat and sugar of regular brownies! The extra "bite" is a bonus when you compare these to the popular two-bite brownie brands. (P.S. Be sure to bake these in a regular-size muffin pan, not a mini.)

MAKES **12** BROWNIES

½ cup bittersweet or semisweet chocolate chips

1½ tablespoons butter

¼ cup (or 3.5 ounce container) prune puree

¼ teaspoon instant coffee crystals

1½ teaspoons vanilla extract

¼ cup dark brown sugar

½ cup granulated no-calorie sweetener

1 egg, beaten*

¼ cup cocoa powder

½ teaspoon baking powder

¼ cup all-purpose flour

1. Preheat the oven to 325°F. Lightly spray a 12-cup muffin tin with non-stick baking spray.

2. Place chocolate chips and butter in medium bowl and microwave on high for 45 to 60 seconds or until chocolate looks shiny and partially melted. Remove bowl from the microwave and whisk until completely melted. Whisk in prune puree, instant coffee, vanilla, and brown sugar (it should be lump free), blending until smooth.

3. Stir in beaten egg. Add cocoa powder, baking powder, and flour, mixing after each addition.

4. Spoon batter evenly into prepared muffin tins, using about 2 tablespoons each. Bake for 10 to 12 minutes or until the center springs back when lightly touched. Cool pan on wire rack for 5 to 10 minutes (if you can wait) before removing brownies.

Marlene Says: *Prune puree is the secret to cutting the fat in half while keeping these brownies moist and delicious. I use Gerber brand baby food prunes and apples. It's easy to find, has a long shelf life, and is sold in a two-pack. Each container is ¼ cup.*

* *For cakier brownies, add one additional egg.*

NUTRITION INFORMATION PER SERVING (1 brownie): Calories 100 | Carbohydrate 15g (Sugars 7g) | Total Fat 4g (Sat Fat 2g) | Protein 3g | Fiber 2g | Cholesterol 25mg | Sodium 20mg | Food Exchanges: 1 Carbohydrate, ½ Fat | Carbohydrate Choices: 1 | Weight Watcher Plus Point Comparison: 2

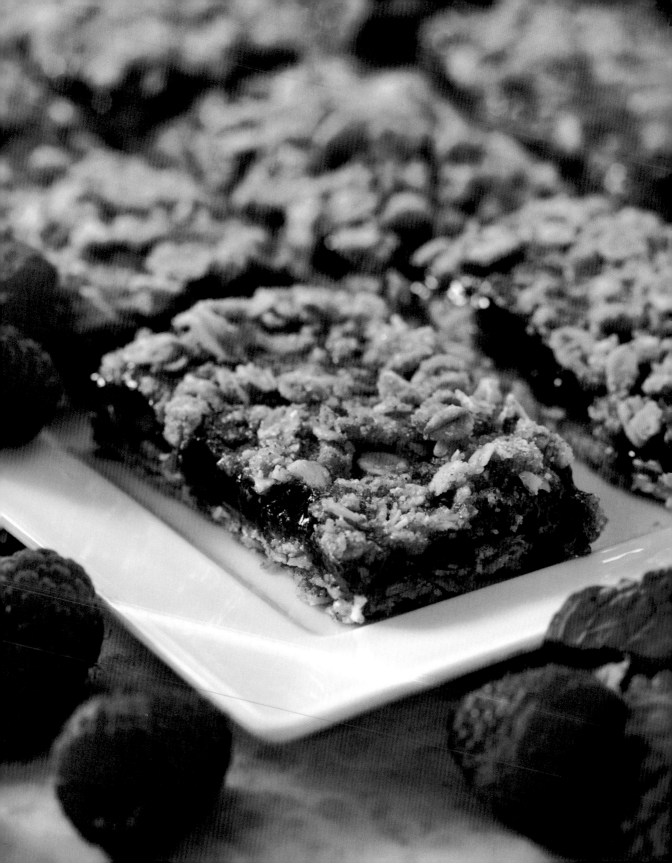

Raspberry Oat Bars

THIS SIMPLE RECIPE COMBINES THE GOODNESS of hearty oats, the sweetness of raspberry, and the scent of cinnamon to tie it all together. One batch can serve a crowd or be parceled out through the week as an after-school snack or a better-for-you dessert. If you prefer, you can substitute another fruit jam flavor.

MAKES **15** SERVINGS

1 cup rolled oats

½ cup all-purpose flour

1 teaspoon cinnamon

⅛ teaspoon salt

3 tablespoons brown sugar

¼ cup granulated no-calorie sweetener (or 6 packets)

⅓ cup margarine or butter, softened

1 cup sugar-free raspberry jam

1. Preheat the oven to 325°F. Lightly spray an 8-inch square baking pan with non-stick baking spray.

2. In a medium bowl, with an electric mixer on low speed, combine the first 7 ingredients (oats through margarine), until the mixture starts to come together. Increase to medium speed and continue mixing until margarine is fully incorporated and the mixture forms a coarse crumb.

3. Press two-thirds of the crumb mixture into the prepared pan. Spread the jam onto the crust. Sprinkle the rest of oat mixture on top of jam.

4. Bake for 25 to 30 minutes or until the edges are golden brown. Cool in the pan on a wire rack. Cut 5 times across and 3 lengthwise for 15 squares.

Marlene Says: *Did you know that oats in all forms are equally nutritious? Steel cut, old-fashioned (rolled), quick-cooking, and instant oats are all whole-grain oats. Their appearance differs—i.e., how they are cut or rolled—and that affects texture and cooking time, but not nutritional value.*

NUTRITION INFORMATION PER SERVING (1 bar): Calories 90 | Carbohydrate 14g (Sugars 3g) | Total Fat 4g (Sat Fat 2.5g) | Protein 1g | Fiber 1g | Cholesterol 10mg | Sodium 20mg | Food Exchanges: 1 Carbohydrate, 1 Fat | Carbohydrate Choices: 1 | Weight Watcher Plus Point Comparison: 2

No-Bake Chocolate Sandwich Cookies

THESE ARE THE EASIEST TO MAKE cream-filled cookies *ever*. Luscious cream filling is sandwiched between two deliciously thin store-bought chocolate wafers and then refrigerated to set and soften. Just as when you make an icebox cake, the fridge does most of the work. The hardest part of this recipe is the waiting!* Ideal chill time is 4 to 6 hours, then store the cookies in the freezer and thaw for 20 minutes before eating.

MAKES **19** COOKIES

1 box Nabisco Famous Wafer cookies

½ cup light cream cheese

½ cup light sour cream

3 tablespoons granulated no-calorie sweetener (or 5 packets)

½ teaspoon vanilla extract

1½ cups light whipped topping, thawed

1. Carefully lay 19 chocolate cookies on a baking sheet and set aside 19 more.

2. In a small bowl, using an electric mixer, beat the cream cheese on low speed until smooth. Add the sour cream, sweetener, and vanilla and beat until smooth.

3. With a rubber spatula, gently fold in half of the whipped topping, and then add the other half, folding until just combined.

4. Spoon 1½ tablespoons of filling onto each cookie. Top with additional chocolate cookie.

5. Cover the pan and refrigerate for 4 to 6 hours before serving. To hold longer, wrap and freeze cookies.

Marlene Says: *The filling options for these sandwich cookies are endless: For a Double Chocolate Sandwich Cookie, add 3 tablespoons cocoa powder in Step 2; for a lovely orange-tinged filling, add 1 teaspoon orange zest. You can also fill the cookies with Strawberry Cream Frosting (page 333), Whipped Cream Cheese Frosting (page 332), or even Peanut Butter Mousse (page 423 of Eat What You Love), which adds 5 calories per sandwich cookie.*

* *The cookies need to soften for the filling to stay intact. Biting into them when still crunchy will cause the filling to spurt out.*

NUTRITION INFORMATION PER SERVING (1 cookie): Calories 85 | Carbohydrate 11g (Sugars 5g) | Total Fat 3g (Sat Fat 3g) | Protein 2g | Fiber 0g | Cholesterol 5mg | Sodium 115mg | Food Exchanges: 1 Carbohydrate, ½ Fat | Carbohydrate Choices: 1 | Weight Watcher Plus Point Comparison: 2

Sugar-Free Lemon Shortbread

A FEW YEARS BACK, a desperate reader contacted me asking for a sugar-free version of her father's favorite lemon shortbread cookie. After several rounds of testing, I was delighted to tell her that I had succeeded. In true shortbread fashion, these cookies are buttery rich, so save them for special occasions (and special people).

MAKES **30** COOKIES

1¾ cups all-purpose flour

½ cup whole almonds, finely ground

¼ teaspoon baking powder

1 cup butter

⅔ cup granulated no-calorie sweetener (like Splenda)

2 tablespoons lemon zest (from 2 large lemons)

1 egg yolk

1. In a small bowl, combine the flour, ground almonds, and baking powder. Set aside.

2. In a large bowl, with an electric mixer, cream the butter, sweetener, and lemon zest until light and creamy, around 2 to 3 minutes. Add the egg yolk and beat until combined.

3. Add the dry ingredients to the butter mixture, and beat on low until the dough barely comes together. Roll the dough into 2 logs, each about 1¾-inch diameter and 6 inches long. Wrap in plastic wrap or waxed paper and chill until completely firm, around 1 to 2 hours.

4. Preheat the oven to 350°F. Line a baking sheet with parchment. Slice the dough into 3/8-inch slices and place onto prepared baking sheet.

5. Bake for 15 minutes or until lightly golden. Remove and cool on rack. Store in an airtight container.

Marlene Says: *While these cookies have no added sugar, like all good shortbread cookies, they are not low in fat. They are deliciously decadent, make a lovely gift, and freeze perfectly.*

NUTRITION INFORMATION PER SERVING (1 cookie): Calories 100 | Carbohydrate 6g (Sugars 0g) | Total Fat 8g (Sat Fat 4g) | Protein 1g | Fiber 0g | Cholesterol 25mg | Sodium 65 mg | Food Exchanges: 1½ Fat, ½ Starch | Carbohydrate Choices: ½ | Weight Watcher Plus Point Comparison: 3

Unbelievable Whoopie Pies

OH MY, WHOOPIE PIES! I must give credit where credit is due. Betsey, a kind reader who bakes for Meals on Wheels, shared with me how she converted my Unbelievable Chocolate Cake into whoopie pies for her clients. She was thrilled with her results and so was I —and now you will be, too.

MAKES **12** COOKIES

¼ cup canola oil

1 large egg

1 teaspoon vanilla

¼ cup packed brown sugar

1 cup granulated
no-calorie sweetener
(like Splenda)

½ cup low-fat buttermilk

1¼ cups cake flour

1 teaspoon baking soda

1 teaspoon baking powder

¼ cup Dutch-process
cocoa powder (like
Hershey's European)

1 Recipe Whipped
Cream Cheese Frosting
(page 332) or Chocolate
Whipped Cream Frosting
(page 334)

1. Preheat oven to 325°F. Spray a baking sheet, parchment or silicone liner with cooking spray.

2. In a large bowl, whisk together the oil and egg for 1 minute until the mixture is frothy. Add the vanilla, brown sugar, and sweetener. Beat with a whisk for 2 more minutes until the mixture is thick and smooth. Whisk in buttermilk. Sift the remaining dry ingredients into the batter and stir until smooth.

3. Spoon 1 tablespoon of batter onto the cookie sheet for each cookie, rounding off edges, if necessary. Bake for 7 to 8 minutes, rotating halfway through. Cookies should be soft.

4. Store cookies in an airtight container. To fill whoopie pies, make frosting according to directions. Spread 1 ½ tablespoons of frosting on one half and top with another. Cookies are best eaten the day you bake them. To store when filled, wrap tightly and place in the fridge.

Marlene Says: *A one tablespoon scoop makes it easy to scoop the batter and creates uniform whoopies (no special pan required!). Look for one at your local kitchen supply store.*

NUTRITION INFORMATION PER SERVING (1 whoopie pie): Calories 130 | Carbohydrate 17g (Sugars 5g) | Total Fat 4g (Sat Fat 3g) | Protein 4g | Fiber 1g | Cholesterol 20mg | Sodium 220mg | Food Exchanges: 1 Starch, 1 Fat | Carbohydrate Choices: 1 | Weight Watcher Plus Point Comparison: 3

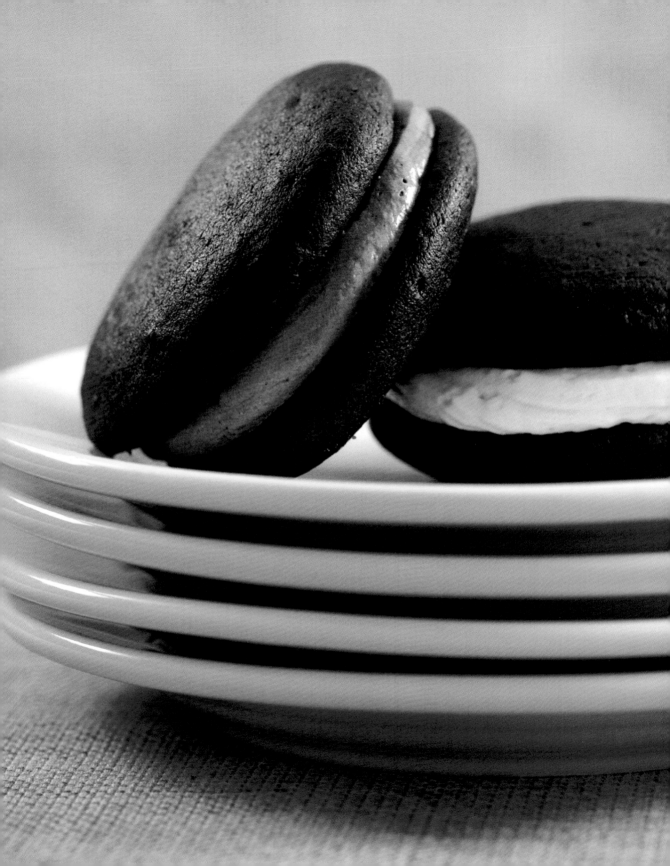

Old-Fashioned Chocolate Mayo Cake

MAYONNAISE IN CAKE—YOU BET! The idea of adding mayonnaise to cake became popular during World War II when food staples like eggs and butter were rationed. This modern take on the famous chocolate mayonnaise cake pays homage to resourceful bakers everywhere (mayonnaise is made from eggs and oil, after all). There's good reason this recipe has survived over the years—mayo makes a super moist fudgy cake. My version cuts down on the sugar, but is just as easy, chocolatey, and moist.

MAKES 8 SERVINGS

¼ cup and 2 tablespoons cocoa powder

½ cup hot water

¾ cup granulated no-calorie sweetener (like Splenda)

2 tablespoons brown sugar

⅓ cup low-fat milk

1½ teaspoon vanilla extract

1 large egg

½ cup light mayonnaise

1 cup all-purpose flour

1 teaspoon baking powder

1 teaspoon baking soda

1. Preheat the oven to 350°F. Spray a 9-inch round baking pan with non-stick baking spray.

2. Place the cocoa powder in a large bowl. Add the hot water and whisk until smooth.

3. Whisk in the sweetener until smooth, then add the brown sugar, milk, vanilla extract, egg, and mayonnaise and continue whisking until smooth.

4. Gradually sift the in flour, baking soda, and baking powder and stir until well mixed.

5. Pour the batter into the prepared pan and smooth the top. Bake for 13 to 15 minutes or until the center of the cake springs back when touched or a toothpick inserted into the center comes out clean.

Marlene Says: *An extra thank-you for this cake goes out to Megan Waldrop, who helped test this cake (over and over and over again). We tested it with various sweeteners but found sucralose-based ones (like Splenda) worked best, as did regular or light mayonaise.*

NUTRITION INFORMATION PER SERVING: Calories 130 | Carbohydrate 19g (Sugars 2g) | Total Fat 5g (Sat Fat 0.5g) | Protein 2g | Fiber 1g | Cholesterol 20mg | Sodium 320mg | Food Exchanges: 1 Starch, 1 Fat | Carbohydrate Choices: 1 | Weight Watcher Plus Point Comparison: 2

Fresh Orange and Almond Cake

AN ENTIRE ORANGE (rind and all) provides a fresh burst of citrus flavor that perfectly complements the nuttiness of ground almonds in this simple yet elegant cake. The nuts keep the carb count down, while the fresh orange puree keeps the cake wonderfully moist. A dollop of light whipped topping is a perfect garnish.

MAKES **8** SERVINGS

1 medium orange

¾ cup almonds

¾ cup all-purpose flour

2 teaspoons baking powder

½ teaspoon salt

3 large eggs

2 tablespoon canola oil

1 teaspoon vanilla extract

1 cup granulated no-calorie sweetener (like Splenda)

2 teaspoons powdered sugar

1. Place the whole orange in a medium pot, fill two-thirds full with water, and bring to boil. Reduce heat to medium, cover, and simmer orange for one hour. Remove orange from pot, quarter, and remove seeds. Place orange pieces (rind and all) in a food processor and purée (you should have about 1 cup orange pulp).

2. Preheat the oven to 350°F. Spray a 9-inch springform pan with non-stick baking spray.

3. Place the almonds in a food processor and grind until fine. Place in a medium bowl and combine with the flour, baking powder, and salt. Set aside.

4. In a large bowl, using an electric mixer, whip the eggs, oil, vanilla, and sweetener on high speed until it becomes light in color and triples in volume, about 5 minutes. Using a spatula or wooden spoon, lightly fold the almond mixture into the egg mixture. Fold in the orange purée until just combined.

5. Pour the batter into the prepared pan and bake for 35 minutes or until a toothpick inserted into the center comes out clean. Cool cake on wire rack. Remove from pan and dust the cake with powdered sugar before serving.

Marlene Says: *For **Gluten-Free Fresh Orange and Almond Cake**, replace the all-purpose flour with ¾ cup Bob's Red Mill or King Arthur Gluten-Free Flour and ¼ teaspoon xanthan gum. (Xanthan gum is available online and at most natural food stores.)*

NUTRITION INFORMATION PER SERVING (one piece): Calories 200 | Carbohydrate 16g (Sugars 3g) | Total Fat 12g (Sat Fat 1.5g) | Protein 7g | Fiber 2g | Cholesterol 80mg | Sodium 230mg | Food Exchanges: 1 Starch, 1 High-Fat Meat, 1 Fat | Carbohydrate Choices: 1 | Weight Watcher Plus Point Comparison: 7

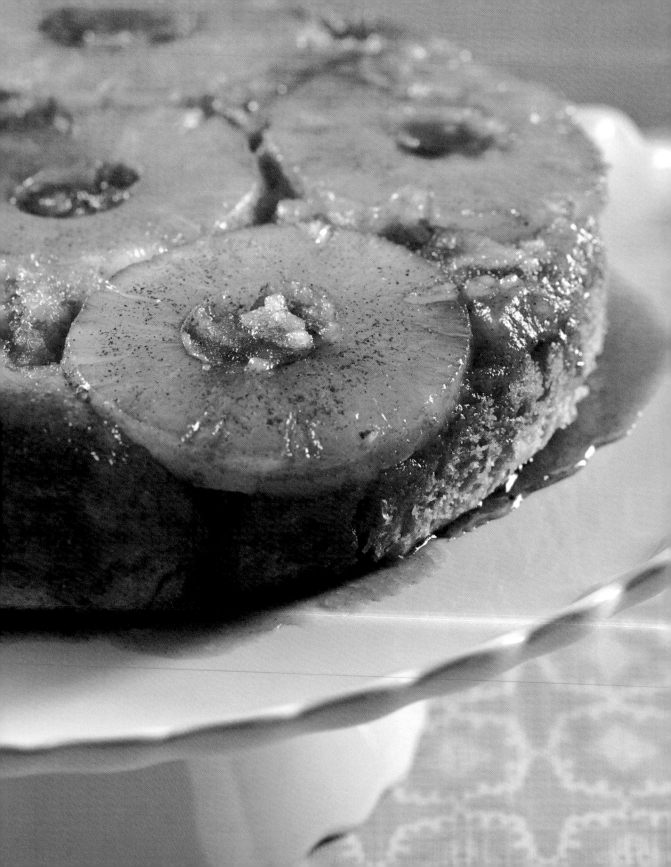

Double Pineapple Upside Down Cake

DECKED OUT WITH A RICH BUTTERY BROWN SUGAR TOPPING and a double dose of pineapple, this cake truly takes the cake. If I had to describe it in a single word, it would be: YUMMY! The fact that I have slashed an entire cup of sugar and a full stick of butter from the traditional recipe is, well, downright upright. (Warning: this cake has been known to inspire fights over who gets the last piece— serve at your own risk.)

MAKES **8** SERVINGS

2 tablespoons butter

3 tablespoons brown sugar, divided

1 cup granulated no-calorie sweetener (like Splenda), divided

1 teaspoon cinnamon, divided

6 pineapple rings, packed in juice (drain and reserve juice)

¼ cup margarine or butter, softened

1 large egg

1 teaspoon vanilla

1⅓ cups all-purpose flour

1½ teaspoons baking powder

½ teaspoon baking soda

½ cup reserved pineapple juice

¼ cup low-fat milk

1. Preheat the oven to 350°F. Set oven rack to lower third of oven. Spray an 8-inch round cake pan with non-stick baking spray.

2. Melt the butter in the prepared pan in the oven. After the butter is melted, evenly sprinkle with 2 tablespoons brown sugar, ¼ cup sweetener, and ¾ teaspoon cinnamon. Arrange the pineapple slices in the pan and set aside.

3. In a medium bowl, using an electric mixer, cream butter, 1 tablespoon brown sugar, and ¾ cup sweetener. Add egg and vanilla and beat until smooth.

4. In a small bowl, sift together the flour, baking powder, baking soda, and ¼ teaspoon cinnamon. In another small bowl or liquid measure, combine the pineapple juice and milk. Alternate mixing the dry ingredients and pineapple juice into the egg mixture.

5. Pour the batter over the pineapple rings and bake for 30 to 35 minutes or until a toothpick inserted into the middle comes out clean. Cool the cake 10 minutes in the pan. Using a knife, loosen around the edges of the pan and invert the cake onto a plate.

NUTRITION INFORMATION PER SERVING (one piece): Calories 195 | Carbohydrate 26g (Sugars 11g) | Total Fat 8g (Sat Fat 2.5g) | Protein 5g | Fiber 1g | Cholesterol 60mg | Sodium 250mg | Food Exchanges: 1 Carbohydrate, ½ Fruit | Carbohydrate Choices: 1½ | Weight Watcher Plus Point Comparison: 5

Heavenly Pumpkin Spice Cake

THIS ULTRA-EASY, REDUCED-FAT PUMPKIN CAKE is lightly textured like a chiffon cake and perfectly scented with pie spices. Baked as a sheet cake, it's perfect for a potluck or last-minute dinner guests. Finish it off with light whipped topping and a sprinkle of cinnamon to keep it extra light or top with whipped cream cheese frosting for a little bite of heaven.

MAKES **15** SERVINGS

1 box angel food cake mix

¾ cup canned pumpkin

1¼ teaspoons cinnamon

½ teaspoon nutmeg

¼ teaspoon ginger

⅛ teaspoon cloves (optional)

1. In a large bowl, with an electric mixer, make angel food cake according to package directions. In a small bowl, mix spices into pumpkin and then carefully fold pumpkin by spoonfuls into angel food cake batter, taking care not to deflate batter.

2. Spoon batter into an ungreased 9 x 13-inch pan and smooth. Bake for 35 minutes or until cake looks dry and springs back when touched. Remove from oven and cool cake upside down. When cool, frost, or serve the cake with whipped topping, if desired.

Marlene Says: *Frosting the cake with 1 (8-ounce) tub light whipped topping adds 30 calories and 3 grams of carbohydrate per piece. Be sure your bowl and beaters are clean and free of any grease or oil before making this cake.*

NUTRITION INFORMATION PER SERVING (1 piece): Calories 115 | Carbohydrate 26g (Sugars 23g) | Total Fat 0g (Sat Fat 0g) | Protein 3g | Fiber 0g | Cholesterol 0mg | Sodium 30mg | Food Exchanges: 2 Carbohydrate | Carbohydrate Choices: 1½ | Weight Watcher Plus Point Comparison: 2

Unbelievable Chocolate Cake

MY SIGNATURE UNBELIEVABLE CHOCOLATE CAKE has appeared in every one of my cookbooks and here it is again. Why? Because it takes just a whisk and a bowl and 10 short minutes to whip up, and it has allowed thousands to enjoy good health and chocolate cake! Be sure to check out my new Almond Joy variation below.

¼ cup canola oil

1 large egg

1 teaspoon vanilla

¼ cup packed brown sugar

1 cup granulated no-calorie sweetener (like Splenda)

1 cup low-fat buttermilk

1¼ cups cake flour

1 teaspoon baking soda

1 teaspoon baking powder

¼ cup Dutch-process cocoa powder (like Hershey's European)

2 teaspoons powdered sugar

1. Preheat oven to 350°F. Spray an 8 x 8-inch baking pan with non-stick baking spray.

2. In a large bowl, whisk together the oil and the egg for 1 minute until the mixture is frothy and thick. Add the vanilla, brown sugar, and sweetener. Beat for 2 more minutes until the mixture is smooth and the sugars have been thoroughly incorporated into the mixture. Add the buttermilk and continue to mix.

3. Sift the flour, baking powder, baking soda, and cocoa powder. Whisk vigorously for 1 to 2 minutes until the batter is smooth. Add ¼ cup hot water to the batter and whisk again until the batter is smooth. Pour the batter into the prepared cake pan and tap the pan on the counter to level the surface and remove any air bubbles.

4. Bake for 18 to 20 minutes or just until the center springs back when touched and a cake tester or toothpick comes out clean. Do not overbake. Place on a rack to cool. Dust with powdered sugar just before serving.

Marlene Says: *For **Almond Joy Cake** variation, replace flour with ⅓ cup finely ground almonds plus 1 cup all-purpose flour. Add 1 teaspoon almond extract in Step 2. Bake 22 to 24 minutes. Top with Coconut Whipped Cream Cheese Frosting (page 332) and garnish each piece with 2 teaspoons toasted coconut (adds 65 calories and 5 grams fat).*

NUTRITION INFORMATION PER SERVING (one piece): Calories 160 | Carbohydrate 22g (Sugars 8g) Total Fat 7g (Sat Fat 1g) | Protein 3g | Fiber 1g | Cholesterol 25mg | Sodium 180mg | Food Exchanges: 1½ Carbohydrate, 1 Fat | Carbohydrate Choices: 1½ | Weight Watcher Plus Point Comparison: 5

cupcakes, cupcakes, cupcakes!

Red Velvet Cupcakes

Best-Ever Banana Cupcakes

90-Calorie Chocolate Cupcakes

Triple Strawberry Stuffed Cupcakes

Ooey-Gooey Peanut Butter Stuffed Chocolate Cupcakes

Heavenly Angel Cupcakes with Luscious Lemon Frosting

Tuxedo Cheesecake Cupcakes

No-Bake Red, White and Blue Cheesecake Cupcakes

Basic Whipped Cream Cheese Frosting

Strawberry Sour Cream Frosting

Chocolate Whipped Cream Frosting

Chocolate Fudge Glaze

Friendly, *sweet*, portable, *and oh-so-easy* to make, there is SO much to love about cupcakes. The term "cupcake" is said to have originated in 1828 when bakers first broke with the *tradition* of weighing ingredients and instead started to measure them in "cups." The batter was baked in teacups, to *expedite* baking, so these small cakes also got their name from the cup. Today the little cakes known as cupcakes are a big deal! *Cupcakes* have taken the nation by storm: they're *just the right size* when you're looking for a few bites *of indulgence*. After all, how bad could a single cupcake be? Holy cupcake!—the average gourmet cupcake from a bakery is reported to have as much as 750 calories and up to 2 days' worth of added sugar!

In this chapter you will find a *wonderful assortment* of better-for-you cupcakes that look and taste fantastic—all with 175 calories or less! I have to admit that it was challenging to find just the right ingredient mix, but the results are so worth it! In this section you'll find several types—*classic, stuffed, and cheesecake* cupcakes. First up is one of the most beloved cupcakes of all times—Red Velvet. Moist, light, and *royally* red, these whipped-cream-frosted cakes are a sight to behold. Looking for something really *decadent?* The Ooey-Gooey Peanut Butter Stuffed Chocolate Cupcakes offer rich chocolate cake stuffed with peanut butter mousse and topped with chocolate glaze. *So yummy*. For entertaining, the No-Bake Red, White, and Blue Cheesecake Cupcakes take just minutes, but the *oohs and aahs* from your family or guests will last hours.

TIP: *For perfect cupcakes every time, make sure to use and prepare the cupcake liners as suggested. These moist cupcakes have a tendency to stick to the liner.*

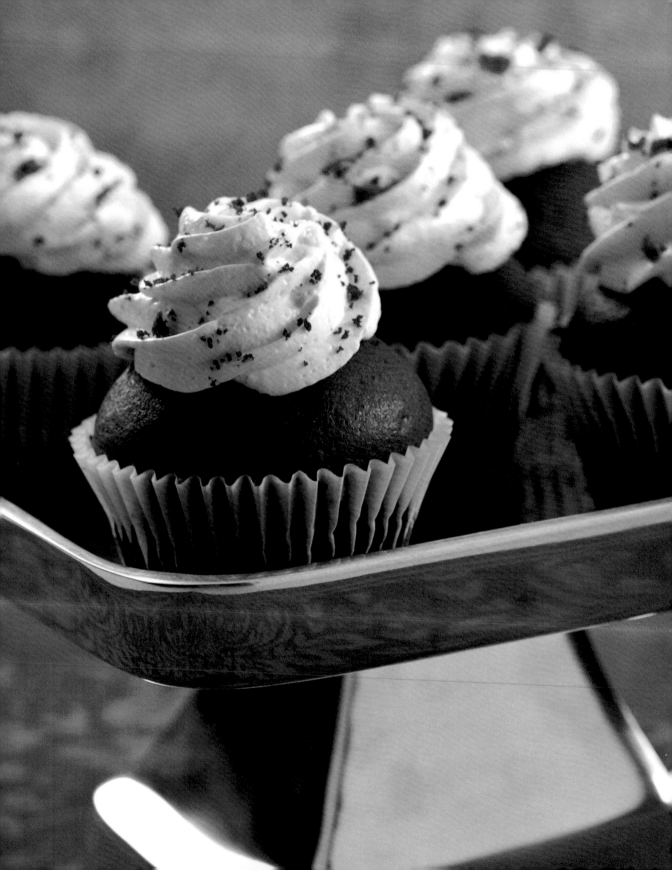

Red Velvet Cupcakes

FOR A GLORIOUS HANDHELD TREAT one need look no further than a Red Velvet cupcake. These cupcakes took more tries to get right than I care to count, but it was worth it. With a tender cake, a rich red color, and luscious whipped cream frosting they are everything you'd expect from a Red Velvet cupcake— for a whole lot less (see my shocking "Dare to Compare" below). And just like my Unbelievable Chocolate Cake (page 317), a whisk, one bowl, and a few minutes is all you need to make them.

MAKES **12** SERVINGS

1 large egg

⅓ cup oil

¼ cup sugar

1 teaspoon vanilla extract

¾ cup buttermilk

¾ cup granulated
no-calorie sweetener
(like Splenda)

2 tablespoons red
food coloring

1½ cups plus 2
tablespoons cake flour

2 tablespoons cocoa
powder

1 teaspoon baking powder

¾ teaspoon baking soda

1 recipe Basic Whipped
Cream Cheese Frosting
(page 332)

1. Preheat the oven to 350°F. Line a non-stick 12-cup muffin tin with cupcake liners or spray with non-stick baking spray.

2. In a medium bowl, whisk the egg until at least double in volume. Mix in the oil, sugar, vanilla extract, buttermilk, sweetener, and red food coloring.

3. Sift the flour, cocoa powder, baking powder, and baking soda into the wet mixture (the batter will be thin). Scoop the batter evenly into prepared muffin tins.

4. Bake for 15 to 17 minutes, until the center springs back when touched or a toothpick comes out clean. Cool completely and frost with Basic Whipped Cream Frosting.

DARE TO COMPARE: A Red Velvet cupcake at the famous Sprinkles cupcake shop serves up 497 calories, 27 grams of fat (including close to a day's worth of saturated fat), and 45 grams of sugar (for my Weight Watchers friends that equals 14 + points!).

NUTRITION INFORMATION PER SERVING (1 cupcake): Calories 170 | Carbohydrate 20g (Sugars 6g) | Total Fat 8g (Sat Fat 2g) | Protein 3g | Fiber 1g | Cholesterol 20mg | Sodium 225mg | Food exchanges: 1 | Carbohydrate, 1½ Fat | Carbohydrate Choices: 1 | Weight Watcher Plus Point Comparison: 4

Best-Ever Banana Cupcakes

MY GOAL WAS TO CREATE A VERY LIGHT, tender banana cupcake, but I had no idea how difficult that would be. After much research, Martha Stewart's "Best" recipe for Banana Cupcakes with Honey-Cinnamon Frosting finally got me on the right track. I cannot tell you how delighted I am with this recipe. These cupcakes are light and tender and the hint of honey in them is incredibly delicious. These really are my best-ever banana cupcakes.

MAKES **12** SERVINGS

1⅔ cups cake flour

1½ teaspoons baking powder

½ teaspoon baking soda

¼ cup shortening

1 tablespoon honey

¾ cup granulated no-calorie sweetener (like Splenda)

2 large eggs

2 medium bananas, broken into pieces

½ teaspoon vanilla

½ cup buttermilk

Touch of Honey Whipped Cream Cheese Frosting (page 332)

1. Preheat the oven to 325°F. Place cupcake liners in 12-cup muffin tin and spray them with non-stick baking spray (cupcakes will stick to liner otherwise).

2. In a medium bowl, sift together the flour, baking powder, and baking soda. Set aside.

3. In a large bowl, with an electric mixer, cream the shortening on medium speed for 2 minutes. Add the honey and sweetener and beat 2 more minutes. Beat in eggs, one at a time, and then beat batter for 2 minutes on high speed, scraping the bowl as needed. Set aside.

4. Add the bananas to a medium bowl and beat them with the mixer on low until pureed. Beat in the vanilla and buttermilk. Using a spatula, gently mix one-half of the flour mixture into the shortening mixture. Mix in one-half of the banana mixture. Repeat. *Do not overmix.* Scoop the batter into the prepared muffin cups.

5. Bake for 20 to 22 minutes or until the center springs back when touched or a toothpick comes out clean. Set cupcakes on a wire rack to cool. Frost with Touch of Honey Whipped Cream Cheese Frosting.

Marlene Says: *These cupcakes have 60% fewer carbs and calories, 66% less fat, and 80% less sugar than Martha Stewart's "Best" Banana Cupcakes!*

NUTRITION INFORMATION PER SERVING (1 cupcake): Calories 175 | Carbohydrate 22g (Sugars 8g) | Total Fat 7g (Sat Fat 3g) | Protein 5g | Fiber 1g | Cholesterol 5 mg | Sodium 220mg | Food Exchanges: 1½ Carbohydrate, 1 Fat | Carbohydrate Choices: 1½ | Weight Watcher Plus Point Comparison: 5

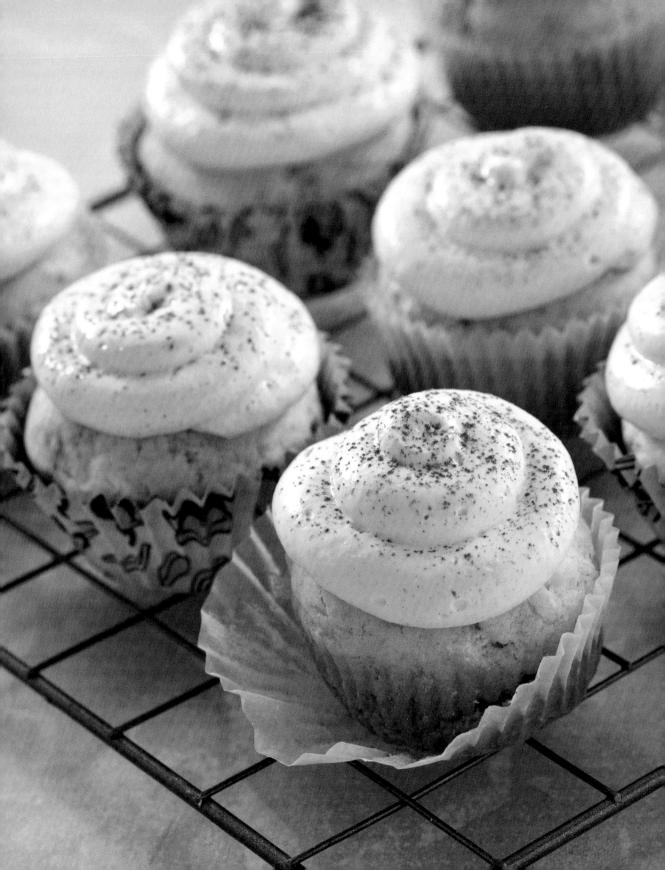

90-Calorie Chocolate Cupcakes

I AM DOUBLE DIPPING WITH THIS RECIPE, but some recipes deserve to be shared twice. Made with my Old-Fashioned Chocolate Mayo Cake (page 312), these moist little beauties are my slimmest, moistest, most chocolatey cupcakes yet. Tip: If you don't spray the cupcake liners with cooking spray, these exceptionally moist cupcakes will stick to the liners.

MAKES 12 SERVINGS

¼ cup and 2 tablespoons cocoa powder

½ cup hot water

¾ cup granulated no-calorie sweetener (like Splenda)

2 tablespoons brown sugar

⅓ cup low-fat milk

1½ teaspoons vanilla extract

1 large egg

½ cup light mayonnaise

1 cup all-purpose flour

1 teaspoon baking powder

1 teaspoon baking soda

1. Preheat the oven to 325°F. Line 12 muffin cups with liners and spray with non-stick cooking spray (alternately, foil liners can be used and do not require spraying).

2. Place cocoa powder in a large bowl. Add hot water and whisk until smooth.

3. Whisk in sweetener until smooth, then add brown sugar, milk, vanilla extract, egg, and mayonnaise and continue to whisk until smooth.

4. Gradually sift in flour, baking soda, and baking powder and stir until well mixed.

5. Scoop ¼ cup of batter into each muffin cup. Bake for 13 minutes or until the center springs back when touched or a toothpick comes out clean.

Marlene Says: *Made with granulated no-calorie sweetener these sweet treats have just 2 grams of sugar and fewer carbs than your average slice of bread. Enjoy!*

NUTRITION INFORMATION PER SERVING (1 cupcake): Calories 90 | Carbohydrate 13g (Sugars 2g) | Total Fat 3.5g (Sat Fat 1g) | Protein 2g | Fiber 1g | Cholesterol 5mg | Sodium 220mg | Food Exchanges: 1 | Carbohydrate Choices: 1 | Weight Watcher Plus Point Comparison: 2

Triple Strawberry Stuffed Cupcakes

STRAWBERRY LOVERS, HERE IS YOUR ULTIMATE CUPCAKE. You get a triple whammy of strawberry taste—a soft, cakey batter flavored with sweet strawberry jam, a burst of more jam in the middle, and to top it off, luscious strawberry sour cream frosting. For an extra hit of flavor and flourish, garnish each cupcake with a slice of fresh strawberry.

MAKES **12** SERVINGS

1¼ cups all-purpose flour

1 teaspoon baking powder

½ teaspoon baking soda

¼ cup shortening

⅔ cup granulated
no-calorie sweetener
(like Splenda)

1 large egg

½ cup reduced-sugar
strawberry jam, divided

1 teaspoon vanilla extract

⅔ cup low-fat milk

1 recipe Strawberry Sour
Cream Frosting (page 333)

Sliced or halved fresh
strawberries, optional

1. Preheat the oven to 350°F. Place cupcake liners in a 12-cup muffin tin and spray liners with non-stick baking spray. Set aside.

2. In a medium bowl, sift together flour, baking powder, and baking soda. Set aside.

3. In a large bowl, with an electric mixer on medium speed, cream the shortening for 2 minutes. Add the sweetener and cream for 2 more minutes. Add the egg, ¼ cup jam, and vanilla extract, and continue mixing until all ingredients are incorporated.

4. Using a spatula, gently mix one-third of the flour mixture into the wet mixture by hand. Mix in one-third of the milk. Repeat until all the ingredients are combined. *Do not overmix.*

5. Scoop about ¼ cup batter into each of the muffin cups. Bake for 13 to 15 minutes or until the center springs back when touched or a toothpick comes out clean. Cool on a rack.

6. Once cupcakes have cooled completely, using an apple corer, remove a cake plug from the center of each cupcake. Fill each cupcake with 1 teaspoon strawberry jam. Gently spoon or pipe 2 tablespoons of frosting onto each cupcake. Garnish each cupcake with an optional strawberry slice.

NUTRITION INFORMATION PER SERVING: Calories 160 | Carbohydrate 18g (Sugars 5g) | Total Fat 7g (Sat Fat 3g) | Protein 3g | Fiber 0g | Cholesterol 25mg | Sodium 140mg | Food Exchanges: 1 Carbohydrate, 1 Fat | Carbohydrate Choices: 1 | Weight Watcher Plus Point Comparison: 4

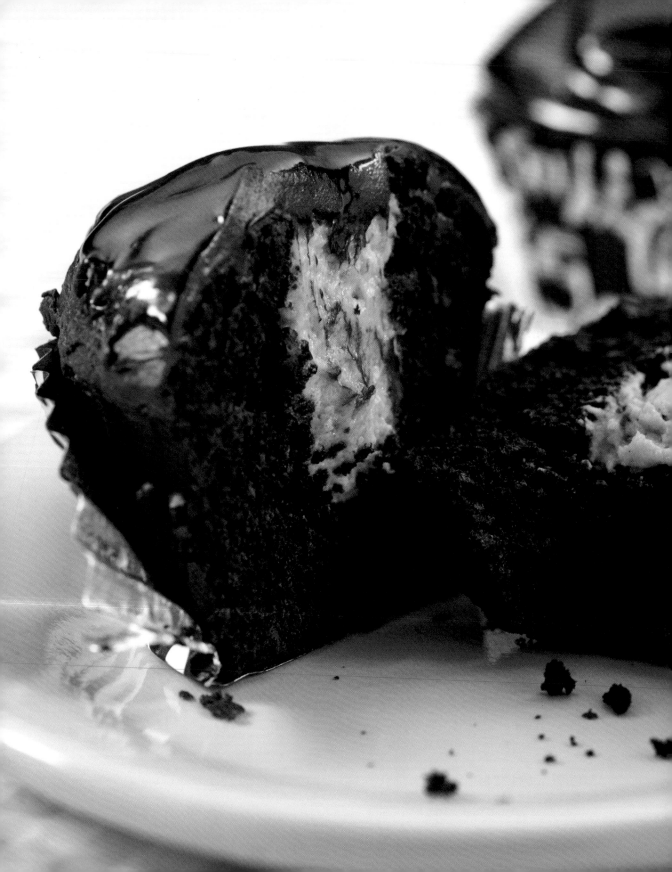

Ooey Gooey Peanut Butter Stuffed Chocolate Cupcakes

IMAGINE RICH, CHOCOLATEY CAKE, creamy peanut butter mousse, and sticky fudgy frosting in every delicious bite. You won't believe (and I can hardly believe it myself) that each sinfully rich-tasting cupcake is only 160 calories!! My advice is to make these for someone special, even if it's just yourself.

MAKES **12** CUPCAKES

1 recipe 90-Calorie Chocolate Cupcakes (page 324)

1 recipe Chocolate Fudge Glaze (page 335)

2 tablespoons creamy peanut butter

2 tablespoons light cream cheese, room temperature

2 tablespoons granulated no-calorie sweetener (or 3 packets)

⅓ cup light whipped topping, thawed

1. Bake the cupcakes according to recipe directions. Let cool.

2. Prepare the Chocolate Fudge Glaze according to the recipe and set aside.

3. In a small bowl, stir together the peanut butter, cream cheese, and sweetener. Gently fold in the whipped topping.

4. To assemble the cupcakes, use an apple corer to remove a plug from the center of each cupcake. Fill each cupcake with 1½ teaspoons of the peanut butter mixture. Frost each cupcake with 2 teaspoons of the chocolate glaze.

DARE TO COMPARE: Whoa, cupcake! It's estimated there are over 500 calories in a Peanut Butter Cup Chocolate Cupcake from Crumbs, a premier cupcake bakery in New York City. Just think how much money and calories you can save by eating one (or even two or three) of these at home!

NUTRITION INFORMATION PER SERVING (1 cupcake): Calories 160 | Carbohydrate 23g (Sugars 9g) | Total Fat 6g (Sat Fat 2g) | Protein 4g | Fiber 2g | Cholesterol 20mg | Sodium 270mg | Food Exchanges: 1½ Carbohydrate, 1 Fat | Carbohydrate Choices: 1½ | Weight Watcher Plus Point Comparison: 4

Heavenly Angel Cupcakes with Luscious Lemon Frosting

IT'S SIMPLY HEAVENLY MAKING CUPCAKES with an angel food cake mix, especially when you are busy and looking for airy, low-calorie, fat-free perfection. Here I've taken these ethereal cakes and adorned them with a topping that will have lemon lovers cheering. Note: Using one-half of a box of Angel Food cake mix yields 15 cupcakes, leaving you enough for another batch. Feel free to double!

MAKES **15** SERVINGS

1 cup, plus 2 tablespoons dry angel food cake mix (one-half 16-ounce box)

½ tablespoons cornstarch

⅔ cup granulated no-calorie sweetener (like Splenda)

2 tablespoons granulated sugar

¼ cup fresh lemon juice

1 large egg yolk

1⅓ cups light whipped topping, thawed

4 teaspoons lemon zest, optional

1. Preheat the oven to 350°F. Place foil cupcake liners in 15 muffin cups and set aside. Prepare angel food batter according to the package directions, using half the recommended water. Scoop batter into muffin cups (about ¼ cup each). Bake for 12 to 15 minutes or until lightly browned. Set muffin tin on a baking rack to cool.

2. While the cupcakes are cooling, whisk together the cornstarch, sweetener and sugar in a small non-aluminum saucepan. Thoroughly whisk in ¼ cup water, lemon juice and egg yolk. Place the pan over medium heat and cook, whisking constantly, until mixture comes to a boil. Cook for 1 additional minute or until clear. Transfer lemon mixture to a medium bowl and let cool completely.

3. Fold half of the whipped topping into the lemon mixture. Repeat with the remaining whipped topping, folding lightly.

4. Frost each cupcake with 1 ½ tablespoons of the lemon frosting and top with a light sprinkle of lemon zest, if desired.

Marlene Says: *These cupcakes release best from foil liners. Most foil liners come with a paper liner inside. Remove paper liner and save them for other cupcakes. For best results, bake cupcakes shortly after mixing the batter. If baking in batches, bake the second batch shortly after the first.*

NUTRITION INFORMATION PER SERVING (1 cupcake): Calories 105 | Carbohydrate 17g (Sugars 13g) | Total Fat 4g (Sat Fat 0g) | Protein 2g | Fiber 0g | Cholesterol 25mg Sodium 115mg | Food Exchanges: 1 Carbohydrate, 1 Fat | Carbohydrate Choices: 1 | Weight Watcher Plus Point Comparison: 2

Tuxedo Cheesecake Cupcakes

WITH A DARK CHOCOLATE CRUST, a creamy cheesecake middle, and a sweet topper of luscious sour cream, these cupcakes are sugar-free perfection (with only 8 grams of carb). Perfect for entertaining, they are already individually portioned and hold well for up to three days in the refrigerator (if no one eats them first!).

MAKES **12** SERVINGS

½ cup crushed chocolate graham crackers (about 8 crackers)

2 tablespoons margarine or butter, melted

¾ cup granulated no-calorie sweetener (like Splenda), divided

1 tablespoon unsweetened cocoa powder, preferably Dutch-process

8 ounces light tub-style cream cheese

8 ounces nonfat cream cheese, room temperature

1 large egg

2 large egg whites

2 teaspoons lemon juice

2 teaspoons vanilla extract, divided

¾ cup light sour cream, divided

1. Preheat the oven to 325°F. Place cupcake liners in 12-cup muffin tin and spray with non-stick cooking spray.

2. In a small bowl, stir together the crushed graham crackers, margarine, 2 tablespoons sweetener, and cocoa powder. Sprinkle a heaping tablespoon of crust mixture into each cup. Press gently to form a compact crust. Set aside.

3. In a large bowl, using an electric mixer, beat the cream cheeses and ½ cup sweetener until combined. Add the egg, egg white, lemon juice and 1 teaspoon vanilla. Continue beating until all ingredients are incorporated. Stir in ½ cup sour cream.

4. Spoon 2 tablespoons of cheesecake mixture into each cup and gently spread until level. Bake for 13 to 15 minutes or until cheesecakes are just set. Remove from oven. Let cool slightly before topping.

5. In a small bowl, mix the sour cream, 2 tablespoons sweetener, and 1 teaspoon vanilla until combined. Spread 2 teaspoons of mixture on each cheesecake. Cool to room temperature and chill at least 2 hours before serving.

NUTRITION INFORMATION PER SERVING (one cupcake): Calories 130 | Carbohydrate 9g (Sugars 4g) | Total Fat 7g (Sat Fat 4g) | Protein 7g | Fiber 0g | Cholesterol 35mg | Sodium 190mg | Food Exchanges: ½ Carbohydrate, 1 Fat | Carbohydrate Choices: ½ | Weight Watcher Plus Point Comparison: 3

No-Bake Red, White and Blue Cheesecake Cupcakes

WITH THEIR FESTIVE SHADES OF RED, WHITE AND BLUE, and featuring a bounty of summer berries, these are perfect for picnics and holiday barbecues. No need to turn on the oven in the hot weather, or fuss with whether the cheesecake is done. Just mix, pour and stick in the fridge. Two hours later, dessert is ready to party.

MAKES **12** SERVINGS

⅔ cup crushed graham crackers

2 tablespoons granulated no-calorie sweetener (or 3 packets)

3 tablespooons butter, melted

8 ounces tub-style reduced-fat cream cheese

8 ounces nonfat cream cheese, room temperature

⅓ cup granulated no-calorie sweetener (or 8 packets)

½ cup light sour cream

1 cup light whipped topping, thawed

¼ teaspoon almond extract

1 cup blueberries

6 medium strawberries, stemmed and halved

1. Line 12 muffin cups with cupcake liners. Lightly spray the liners with cooking spray.

2. In a medium bowl, mix together the graham cracker crumbs, 2 tablespoons sweetener, and butter. Press 1 rounded tablespoon into the bottom of each muffin cup. Place in the refrigerator to chill.

3. In a medium bowl, with an electric mixer on low speed, beat the cream cheeses, ⅓ cup sweetener, and sour cream until smooth. Beat in ½ cup of whipped topping and the almond extract. Fold in the remaining topping.

4. Spoon the cheesecake filling into the crusts and smooth the tops. Place a strawberry half in the center of each cheesecake and arrange the blueberries around the strawberry. Place cheesecakes in the refrigerator and chill until set, at least 2 hours.

Marlene Says: *The cheesecake base is as versatile as it is easy. Top with light cherry pie topping for Christmas or Valentine's Day, double the strawberries for Easter, or crown with fresh-picked blackberries in August.*

NUTRITION INFORMATION PER SERVING (1 cupcake): Calories 150 | Carbohydrate 13g (Sugars 6g) | Total Fat 7g (Sat Fat 5g) | Protein 6g | Fiber 1g | Cholesterol 20mg | Sodium 250 mg | Food Exchanges: 1 Starch, ½ Lean Meat, 1 Fat | Carbohydrate Choices: 1 | Weight Watcher Plus Point Comparison: 4

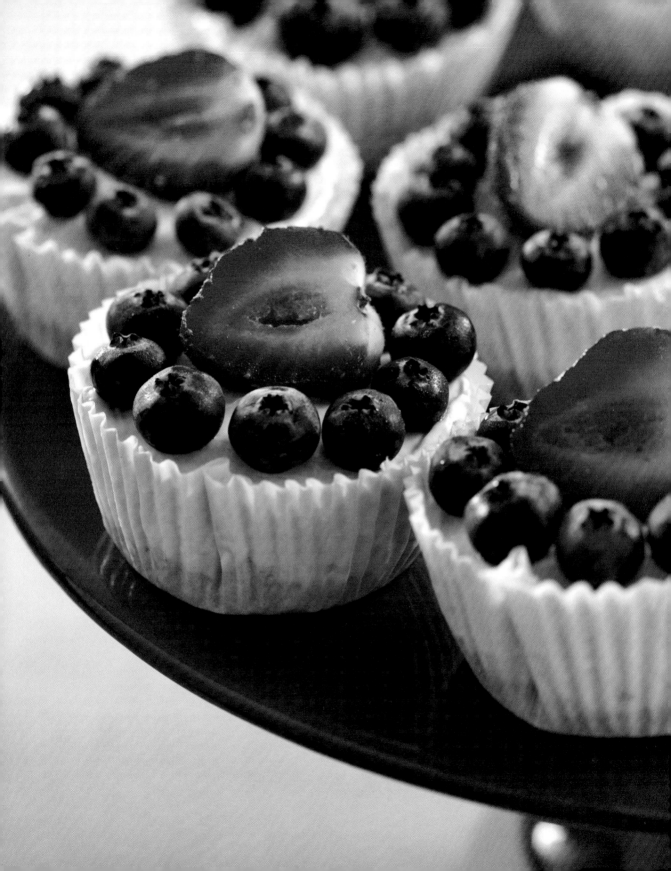

Basic Whipped Cream Cheese Frosting

LIKE A PERFECT WHITE SHIRT, this frosting goes well with everything! When I was searching for a frosting base that was not too high in fat or sugar, I lucked out when I thought of using cream cheese. The result is a light, fluffy frosting graced with the great taste of cheesecake. This frosting stands tall all by itself and elevates everything it touches.

MAKES **1½** CUPS

½ cup tub-style reduced* fat cream cheese, softened

⅓ cup nonfat cream cheese, softened

4 tablespoons granulated no-calorie sweetener (or 6 packets)

¾ cup light whipped topping, thawed

1. In a small bowl, beat the cream cheeses with an electric mixer until smooth. Add the sweetener and beat for 1 minute longer.

2. On slow speed, beat in half of the whipped topping until fluffy and just combined. Using a rubber spatula, carefully fold in the remaining whipped topping.

Marlene Says: *To make a delicious **Touch of Honey Whipped Cream Cheese Frosting**, replace 1 tablespoon of sweetener with 2 teaspoons of honey and beat in ⅛ teaspoon cinnamon. For **Coconut Whipped Cream Frosting**, add ½ teaspoon coconut extract to cream cheese mixture.*

NUTRITION INFORMATION PER SERVING (2 tablespoons): Calories 40 | Carbohydrate 2g (Sugars 1g) | Total Fat 2g (Sat Fat 1g) | Protein 2g | Fiber 0g | Cholesterol 0mg | Sodium 40mg | Food Exchanges: ½ Fat | Carbohydrate Choices: 0 | Weight Watcher Plus Point Comparison: 1

Strawberry Sour Cream Frosting

THIS FROSTING WAS MEANT TO ADORN my Triple Strawberry Stuffed Cupcakes, but it wound up being a star on its own. The sour cream adds a soft tang to the subtle flavor of strawberry jam. It can also be used as a filling for my No-Bake Chocolate Sandwich Cookies (page 308) and makes a great topper for the Old-Fashioned Chocolate Mayo Cake (page 312) or Heavenly Angel Cupcakes (page 328).

MAKES **1½** CUPS

⅓ cup light cream cheese

⅓ cup light sour cream

3 tablespoons granulated no-calorie sweetener (or 4 packets)

3 tablespoons reduced sugar strawberry jam

½ teaspoon vanilla extract

1 cup light whipped topping, thawed

1. In a small mixing bowl, beat the cream cheese on low speed with an electric mixer until smooth. Add the sour cream, sweetener, jam and vanilla extract. Continue beating until smooth.

2. Gently mix in one-half of the whipped topping with a spatula. Fold in the remaining whipped topping until just combined.

3. Cover the bowl and refrigerate until ready to use.

NUTRITION INFORMATION PER SERVING (1½ tablespoons)**:** Calories 30 | Carbohydrate 2g (Sugars 1g) | Total Fat 1.5g (Sat Fat .5g) | Protein 1.5g | Fiber 0g | Cholesterol 0mg | Sodium 40mg | Food Exchanges: ½ Fat | Carbohydrate Choices: 0 | Weight Watcher Plus Point Comparison: 1

Chocolate Whipped Cream Frosting

BECAUSE I AM A CHOCOLATE LOVER, this recipe is an absolute staple for me. It's light, deca-dent-tasting, and making it is as easy as can be. It is the finishing touch on my Unbelievable Chocolate Cake (page 317) and has more recently found its way onto my Old-Fashioned Chocolate Mayo Cake (page 312) and 90-Calorie Chocolate Cupcakes (page 324). After tasting this frosting once, I guarantee you'll find multiple uses for it.

MAKES **2** CUPS

4 ounces tub-style light cream cheese

¼ cup cocoa powder

⅓ cup granulated no-calorie sweetener (or 8 packets)

½ teaspoon vanilla extract

2 cups light whipped topping, divided

1. In a small mixing bowl, beat the cream cheese, cocoa powder, sweetener, and vanilla with an electric mixer until well blended.

2. On slow speed, beat in 1 cup of the whipped topping to incorporate. Add the remaining 1 cup and beat on low very briefly until fluffy and combined.

NUTRITION INFORMATION PER SERVING (2 tablespoons): Calories 40 | Carbohydrate 3g (Sugar 1g) | Total Fat 2g (Sat Fat 1.5g) | Protein 2g | Fiber 0g | Cholesterol 0mg | Sodium 80mg | Food Exchange: ½ Fat | Carbohydrate Choice: 0 | Weight Watcher Plus Point Comparison: 1 point

Chocolate Fudge Glaze

WITH A DOUBLE DOSE OF CHOCOLATE, this decadent, sticky, shiny, chocolatey glaze was originally created for my Ooey-Gooey Peanut Butter Stuffed Chocolate Cupcakes (page 327), but it's equally good when smeared onto a Best-Ever Banana Cupcake (page 323) or a 90-Calorie Chocolate Cupcake (page 324). It can also be warmed in the microwave and drizzled over ice cream or fresh strawberries.

MAKES ½ CUP

3 tablespoons semi-sweet chocolate chips

¼ cup non-fat half-and-half

¾ cup granulated no-calorie sweetener (like Splenda)

½ teaspoon vanilla extract

½ cup powdered sugar, sifted

⅓ cup cocoa powder, preferably Dutch-process

1. Place the chocolate chips in a medium microwave-safe bowl. Add the nonfat half-and-half and the sweetener. Place in the microwave and heat for one minute. Remove, add the vanilla, and stir until the chocolate chips are melted and the mixture is smooth.

3. With an electric mixer on low speed, or whisk, beat in the powdered sugar until smooth. Sift in the cocoa powder and beat again until smooth. (Glaze will thicken as it cools. To thin, re-warm for 15 to 20 seconds.)

DARE TO COMPARE: A tablespoon of chocolate glaze made with cream and chocolate (also known as chocolate ganache) has 8 grams of fat—half of them saturated—in each tablespoon.

NUTRITION INFORMATION PER SERVING (2 teaspoons): Calories 35 | Carbohydrate 7g (Sugars 3g) | Total Fat 1g (Sat Fat 0g) | Protein 0g | Fiber 0g | Cholesterol 0mg | Sodium 0mg | Food Exchanges: ½ Carbohydrate | Carbohydrate Choices: ½ | Weight Watcher Plus Point Comparison: 1

MENUS

sunday brunch

Fresh Fruit with Creamy Fruit Dip *(page 96)*
Triple Lemon Blueberry Muffins *(page 55)*
Canadian Bacon
Quick 'n Easy Quiche *(page 85)*
Fresh Brewed Coffee

Marlene Says: *Make the dip, cut your fruit, and mix your quiche filling the night before for an easy Sunday morning. Pour the refrigerated filling into the crust just before baking.*

sunday dinner southern-style

Ranch Slaw *(page 152)*
Chicken Chicken Fried Steak with Cream Gravy *(page 240)*
Sour Cream and Onion Smashed Potatoes *(page 227)*
Smoky Garlicy Greens *(page 218)*
Pecan Pie Cups *(page 286)*

Marlene Says: *Prepare the pie cups up to a day ahead but dress your salad within 2 hours of serving.*

DARE TO COMPARE: Ready to splurge Southern-style? The Southern-Style menu on this page has just ⅓ of the usual calories (and a fraction of the sugar and fat!). A traditional Chicken Fried Steak dinner with all the fixings clocks in at 2100 calories including over 100 grams of fat and close to a days' worth of carbs! Enjoy this one y'all!

easy everyday italian family supper

Everyday Mixed Greens with Balsamic Vinaigrette *(page 148)*
Pizza Pasta Pie *(page 204)*
Easy Lemon Ice Cream with Quick Raspberry Sauce *(page 297)*

Marlene Says: *Cook your spaghetti ahead of time or use leftovers to make this even quicker. Six ounces dry spaghetti is about 3 cups cooked.*

a celebration dinner for everyone*!

Green Leafy Salad with Green Goddess Dressing *(page 147)*
Steak Diane *(page 263)*
Classic Creamed Spinach *(page 213)*
Sour Cream and Smashed Potatoes *(page 227)* or
Creamy Golden Mashed Potatoes *(page 226)*
5-Ingredient Dark Chocolate Soufflés *(page 299)*

Marlene Says: *The dressing can be made ahead of time. Having all the soufflé ingredients measured out before you sit down to eat, makes assembling and popping them into the oven after dinner quick and easy.*

This menu is also gluten-free.

slim 'n speedy weeknight special

Good 'ol Iceberg with Classic French Dressing *(page 145)*
Good 'n Easy Garlic Chicken *(page 238)*
Lemony Buttery Green Beans *(page 214)*
Small Wheat Roll

Marlene Says: *The dressing can be doubled and leftovers kept in the fridge all week long.*

game day for 8 to 10 of your favorite people

Ooey Gooey Pizza Dip *(page 97)*
Susan's "Zero" Point Wonder Dip *(page 100)*
Fresh Veggies (for dipping and munching)
Store bought or More Baked Pita Chips *(page 101)*
Wendy's Style Chili *(page 177)*
Chili Toppings (grated cheese, etc...optional)
Crème Caramel Squares *(page 294)*

Marlene Says: *Susan's "Zero" Point Wonder Dip will keep for several days in the fridge. The Crème Caramel Squares can be refrigerated for up to 1 day or frozen for up to 3 days. Serve the pizza dip piping hot and the chili right from the crock!*

An entire week's worth of calorie/carb controlled menus (with calculations) can be also be found at www.marlenekoch.com

Extra Tasty Menus

These tasty menus use recipes from the original
Eat What You Love: More than 300 Incredible Recipes Low in Sugar, Fat and Calories.
Mix and match the recipes and menus for even more incredible meals!

easy fast food fix

Easy Sonic-Style Cherry Lemonade *(page 36)*
Crispy Spicy Chicken Sandwich *(page 216)*
Sweet Potato Wedges *(page 276)*
Amazing Peanut Butter Cookie *(page 383)*

DARE TO COMPARE: This entire menu clocks in with 100 fewer calories
and 45% less fat than just the chicken sandwich alone from your typical fast
food restaurant. Total fast food fix menu = 500 calories. You save 700 calories!

meatless monday—soups on!

5-Minute Skinny Slaw *(page 180)*
Speedy Black Bean Soup with Jalapeño Cream *(page 154)*
Country Cornbread Muffins *(page 290)*

Marlene Says: *The cool crunchy salad and slightly sweet corny muffins
are perfect partners to the creamy, spicy black bean soup.
Bonus: This inexpensive meatless menu is packed with a whopping
15 grams of fat fighting fiber!*

weeknight wonder—dinner for four in a flash

Bagged Salad Mix with Reduced Fat Dressing*
Marlene's Favorite Go-To Italian Chicken *(page 310)*
Stewed Italian Zucchini Parmesan *(page 261)*
Penne Pasta (whole grain blend or fiber fortified suggested)

Marlene Says: *Start the water boiling for the pasta while you prep
the Stewed Italian Zucchini Parmesan. While the pasta and zucchini are cooking,
season and cook the chicken.*

** Use your favorite bottled dressing or try one of my favorites,
the Balsamic Dressing on page 176.*

asian inspiration

5-Minute Egg Drop Soup *(page 153)*
Stephen's Stir-Fried Rice *(page 284)*
Quicker-Than-Take-Out-Orange Chicken *(page 304)*

Marlene Says: *This one of my son Stephen's favorite "take-out" menus.*
The orange chicken is always a hit, but when served with his favorite fried rice and a bowl
of steaming soup there's no place better to "order" take-out than at home.

everyday's a holiday

Pork Tenderloin with Cranberry Pan Sauce *(page 340)*
Sweet Potato Puff *(page 279)* OR
Parmesan Garlic Smashed Potatoes *(page 277)*
Seared, Steamed Glazed Green Beans *(page 252)*
Creamy Instant Pumpkin Mousse *(page 100)* OR
All-Purpose No-Bake Vanilla Cheesecake *(page 413)*

Marlene Says: *Who say's you need a holiday when food tastes this good!*
Countless guests have been treated to this menu in my home. In fall and winter
I often opt for sweet potatoes or pumpkin mousse, the rest of the year I
switch it up with smashed potatoes and cheesecake.

better-than-take-out mexican fiesta

Spicy Jalapeno Carrots *(page 127)*
Shredded Spinach, Lettuce, and Fresh Orange Salad *(page 178)*
Baja Fish Tacos *(page 222)*
Simple Southwest Black Beans *(page 288)*
Fresh Pineapple or
Key Lime Cheesecake Cupcakes *(page 416)*

Marlene Says: *Make the cheesecake cupcakes and carrots ahead of time and*
the rest of this flavorful meal will come together in a snap. Use a colorful table
runner and serve it family style. By having one taco instead of two, even the
lightest eaters can enjoy the entire menu!

acknowledgments

FIRST AND FOREMOST I WOULD LIKE TO THANK ALL THE INCREDIBLE READERS who have bought my books over the years, especially the predecessor to this book, *Eat What You Love*, as without your support this book would never have come to fruition. Hearing that my recipes make your life better is truly priceless and there is no better compliment than knowing you have shared my work with your own family and friends.

While incredibly delicious at times, the enormity of creating a brand-new cookbook never ceases to amaze me. Hours of research and daily trips to the supermarket multiply into even more hours in the kitchen leading to never-ending nights on the computer. Fortunately, in the effort to get everything done just right (including oft times testing and tweaking a single recipe a dozen times or more), I have not been alone.

With sincere gratitude many thanks go to:

- Roberta Cuneo and chef Judy LaCara, my tireless kitchen assistants who never waivered at the fact we had to make it "just one more time." From shopping to cooking to clean-up and beyond, your work ethic and support was beyond measure.

- Chefs Michele Musel, Michele Dudash, Anne-Marie Ramo, and Sophia Ortiz along with Charisse Petruno, Miriam Rubin and especially Ms. Megan Waldrop for your extraordinary enthusiasm and tasty contributions.

- Colleagues Patricia O'Keefe Girbal, Paulette Thompson and Diane Welland for your delicious assistance.

- Interns Krista Douglass and Noelle Stephens. You both will go far!

- Deanna Segrave-Daly, August Terrier and longtime friend PJ Dempsey for your love of the written word.

- My styling and photography team extraordinaire, photographer Steve Legato, stylists Carole Haffey, John Haffey and Bonne DiTomo, and prop stylist Mary Ellen . . .

- Chris Navratil and editor Jennifer Kasius at Running Press for their unwavering support and art directors Frances Soo Ping Chow and Susan Van Horn for creating a beautiful book.

- The wonderful folks at QVC; Jessica Hart, Christina Pennypacker, Lauren Baker, and all the stellar hosts including the ultimate foodie, Mr. David Venable.

- Family and friends far-and-wide (like Ms. Nancie Crosby), and last but never least, Chuck, Stephen and James for your patience, love and constant support.

index

MORE FROM MARLENE

Visit Marlene online at **www.marlenekoch.com** *today for:*

- A weeks worth of sample weight loss/carb controlled
menus featuring delicious *Eat More of What You Love* recipes

- Marlene's Free Monthly Newsletter and Sensational New Recipes

- Healthy Eating Tips

- "Plus" Point comparisons for all recipes in *Eat What You Love:
More than 300 Incredible Recipes Low in Sugar, Fat, and Calories.*

You will also find personalized nutrition tools to help you feel your best!

- Personal Calorie Calculator

- Carbohydrate Budget Calculator

- Body Mass (BMI) Calculator

- Activity Fitness Calculator

- Blood Sugar and Weight Tracking Logs

Have a Question? Comment? Just click on:
"Ask Marlene" at **www.marlenekoch.com** *where*
Good Health is always delivered with Great Taste!